# *M*ENTAL HEALTH
# &
# NURSING PRACTICE

D1809954

# MENTAL HEALTH
# &
# NURSING PRACTICE

Edited by
## Michael Clinton & Sioban Nelson

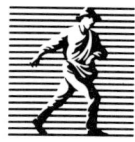

## PRENTICE HALL

Sydney  New York  Toronto  Mexico  New Delhi
London  Tokyo  Singapore  Rio de Janeiro

Aquisitions Editor: Joy Whitton
Production Editor: Andrew Brock
Text design: Kim Webber
Cover design: The Modern Art Production Group, Prahran, Victoria
Typeset by Southern Star Design, South Tacoma, NSW
Printed in Australia by Star Printery, Erskineville, NSW

1 2 3 4 5 00 99 98 97 96

ISBN 0 7248 0824 8.

---

**National Library Of Australia**
**Cataloguing-in-Publication Data**

---

Clinton, Michael
    Mental health and nursing practice.


    Includes index.
    ISBN 0 7248 0824 8.


    1. Psychiatric nursing. I. Nelson, Sioban. II. Title.


610.7368

---

Prentice-Hall of Australia Pty Ltd, *Sydney*
Prentice Hall, Inc., *Englewood Cliffs, New Jersey*
Prentice Hall Canada, Inc., *Toronto*
Prentice Hall Hispanoamericana, *SA, Mexico*
Prentice Hall of India Private Ltd, *New Delhi*
Prentice Hall International, Inc., *London*
Prentice Hall of Japan, Inc., *Tokyo*
Prentice Hall of South East Asia Pty Ltd, *Singapore*
Editora Prentice Hall do Brasil Ltda, *Rio de Janeiro*

 PRENTICE HALL

A division of Simon & Schuster

# **F**OREWORD

As a nurse whose experience has been largely in general health care settings I am aware of the strong relationship between health, thinking, feeling and behaving. It is heartening to find, in this comprehensive book, a perspective on the person and health which is inclusive of these elements. Mental health and physical health are inseparable, yet modern health care systems frequently encourage their separation.

Historically mental health and mental health care have been a low priority on the national health care agenda, not only in Australia but globally. Often changes to mental health care practices and delivery have been in the form of knee jerk reactions to political imperatives. We have seen a move from custodial care in large institutions to community-based care, but often without the requisite infrastructure to support such a move or adequate followup and evaluation of the effects that such changes have had on those the changes were designed to help. Often these measures appear to be thinly disguised cost cutting exercises.

Recently mental health has again been on the political agenda. The rural recession has focused attention on the plight of rural communities and the soaring suicide rate in 'the bush'. Likewise the tragedy of youth suicide, both rural and urban, has been reported in the media with youth suicide now overtaking road accidents as the leading cause of death in under 25-year olds. Coupled with this was the publication of the Australian Human Rights and Equal Opportunities Commission of Inquiry into the Rights of People with Mental Illness (The Burdekin Report) in 1993. This report was critical of the treatment of and existing services for people with mental illness, as well as the education and training of mental health professionals. And as Commissioner Burdekin noted, the political will to implement the recommendations of his report seems to be lacking.

The National Mental Health Strategy outlines the policy directions for mental health into the next century. However, while some policy directions such as mainstreaming appear to be on track, (again, a policy which is likely to save governments money with questionable benefits to the mentally ill) primary preventative measures which would be of real benefit to the community do not appear to be receiving the attention they deserve.

Mental health care delivery is complex, demanding and expensive and mental health problems cost the community and individuals of our communities dearly. Problems in the cost-effective delivery of an equitable and efficient service which takes into account the rights and human dignity of those who access this care are many. The solutions to these problems are unlikely to come from one source. Solutions will require a willingness on the part of the community to see mental health as an issue for all. This will require professional and public education of a type we have not previously seen, and the setting up of primary preventive measures which are seen as being just as essential as immunisation is to our physical health. Governments also will need to see the long-term benefits to the community (including economic benefits) inherent in the provision of high quality primary, secondary and tertiary mental health care and services in all settings.

This book will, I believe, make a major contribution to the promotion of mental health in all sectors of society. It is largely written, with consumer involvement, by members of a research centre who are committed to quality research in mental health nursing and who clearly demonstrate credible understandings of current issues. The text concisely examines mental health and its promotion throughout the lifespan, across cultures and in the many settings in which health care is delivered. I commend this book to nursing students and nursing practitioners at all levels, in all specialties. The editors and authors are to be congratulated on the development of a timely, comprehensive text and on the contribution they are making to the promotion of mental health and the care of those with a mental illness through both the production of this book and their ongoing research endeavours.

ALAN PEARSON
The University of Adelaide
September 1995

# CONTENTS

# PREFACE

This book was initiated and written largely by the staff of the Centre for Mental Health Nursing Research at Queensland University of Technology, which was funded under the Vice-Chancellor's Research Initiatives Program with a grant of $750 000 for the three-year period 1993–95. The Centre is located in the School of Nursing and is a collaborative project with the Faculty of Arts. We are grateful to staff of the Centre and the School of Nursing, who have contributed to the writing of this book. We are also grateful to the other authors, from Tasmania to Townsville, who have broadened and enriched the project. The style and content of the book evolved as the diverse work of the authors began to take shape. The editorial challenge has been to keep the aim and focus of the book and to tailor the diversity of the contributions into a well-rounded and coherent text. We hope we have succeeded. In our view it is appropriate that this is a heterogeneous work, embracing consumer perspectives, diagnostic criteria, Aboriginal health, Primary Health Care and ethical issues, to name a few important themes. Mental health nursing itself is an eclectic and heterogeneous pursuit and the practitioner has many areas of practice and requires many skills.

The view of mental health nursing presented here encompasses models of mental disorder, the social context of mental health and illness, and the significance of the nurse–patient relationship. The contributions and limitations of the medical model are discussed, together with the importance of meeting the mental health needs of families, groups and communities, as well as those of individuals. The dangers of cultural bias are highlighted and a research-based approach has been adopted throughout. The 19 chapters are presented in seven sections: Consumers, Stress, Needs, Clinical Focus, Clients, Practice Settings and Professionalisation. General themes are illustrated with examples, case studies and 'voice boxes' to assist the application of theory to practice. Each chapter concludes with exercises and discussion questions. Key terms appear in bold in the text and—for ease of reference—are defined in a glossary at the end of the book. Care has been taken to emphasise variability in the manifestation of mental disorder and in the reactions and needs of clients, including those with physical illnesses.

Our aim has been to provide undergraduate students with the means to embrace mental health nursing as part of their everyday practice on graduation. We hope that this text will help them understand that one does not stop being a mental health nurse when a client has a physical condition, any more than one should ignore the mental health needs that attend physical conditions. But unless the beginning practitioner possesses the skills and knowledge of mental health nursing, the claims of the classroom to a holistic approach to nursing are merely rhetorical. It is hoped that this book will in some modest way build a bridge to mental health nursing for practitioners of the future, so that all nurses will eventually possess mental health nursing skills that they can and will apply in their everyday practice. Furthermore, we hope that an introduction to these skills will instil in nurses a high regard for their colleagues who are specialist mental health nurses and, perhaps, inspire more nurses to take that path.

We would like to voice our appreciation to our editors, Joy Whitton and Chris Lowe of Prentice Hall, who shared the task of overseeing this book, for their enthusiasm and boundless encouragement. Tim Owen's kind assistance in compiling the photographs, as well as his own fine photography, is much appreciated, as is Sarah Feek and Lila Pratap's skill with the figures and tables. Professor Max Abbott, Dean of Health, Auckland Institute of Technology, Pauline Climo of the Nursing Council of New Zealand, Dr Sue Hallwright of the Northern Regional Health Authority, Auckland, and Dr Janice Wilson, Director of Mental Health, Wellington, New Zealand, have all been more than generous with published and unpublished documents and data and, of course, helpful advice.

We also wish to acknowledge the generous efforts of those who have contributed to the lengthy process of review that occurs in preparing a text such as this. We wish to thank: Professor Sandra Speedy, University of the Southern Cross; Pro Vice Chancellor Janice Reed, QUT; Merinda Epstein, Independant Member of the National Mental Health Community Advisory Committee (NCAG); Associate Professor Jan Horsfall, University of Sydney; Professor Christine Duffield, University of Technology, Sydney; Dr Peter Isaacs, QUT; John Fanshawe, QUT; Rhonda Holland, Rozelle Hospital, Sydney; Pat Swan, Aboriginal Medical Service, Redfern, Sydney; Patsy Yates, QUT; Eric Smith, Northern Metropolitan Mental Health Services, Melbourne; and Neil McCloud, NT Health, East Arnhem Region.

MICHAEL CLINTON
SIOBAN NELSON

## NOTE

Keyterms have been highlighted in bold within the chapters. The definitions for keyterms can be found in the consolidated glossary beginning on page 397.

# CONTRIBUTORS

Jennie Barr
Research Fellow, Centre for Mental Health Nursing Research, QUT

Professor Michael Clinton
Director, Centre for Mental Health Nursing Research, QUT

Debra Creedy
Senior Lecturer, School of Nursing, Griffith University, Brisbane

Anne Dewar,
Lecturer, School of Nursing, QUT

Helen Edwards
Senior Lecturer, Centre for Mental Health Nursing Research, QUT

Professor Gary Easthope
Chair of Sociology, University of Tasmania

Marilyn Harris
Lecturer, School of Nursing, QUT

Professor Gail Hart
Centre for Mental Health Nursing Research, QUT

Kim Jewell is a primary consumer of mental health services. He is a former member of the Queensland Mental Health Consumer Advisory Group, past vice-president of Friends of the Mentally Ill. Kim is currently studying visual arts.

Jill Mannion
Lecturer, School of Nursing, QUT

Robyn Nash
Senior Lecturer, School of Nursing, QUT

Sioban Nelson
Senior Research Assistant, Centre for Mental Health Nursing Research, QUT

Associate Professor Tian Oei
Reader in Clinical Psychology, University of Queensland

Dr Wendy Patton
Senior Lecturer, School of Learning and Development, QUT

Dr Natasha Posner
Senior Research Fellow, Centre for Mental Health Nursing Research, QUT

John Quinn
Special Service Leader, Assessment and Acute Care Service, West Moreton
Integrated Mental Health, Ipswich, Queensland

Dr Roberta Julian
Lecturer, Department of Sociology, University of Tasmania

Fran Sanders
Senior Lecturer, Centre for Mental Health Nursing Research, QUT

Gracelyn Smallwood
Director, Kumbari Ngurpai Lag Higher Education Centre, University of
Southern Queensland

Dr Barbara Tooth
Senior Lecturer, Centre for Mental Health Nursing Research, QUT

Dr Gail Tulloch
Lecturer, Faculty of Humanities, Griffith University, Brisbane

Derek Weir
Senior Lecturer, Centre for Mental Health Nursing Research, QUT

Tania Yegdich
Nurse Therapist, Alcohol and Drug Program, Northern Regional Health
Authority, Queensland Health, Brisbane

# ■S OURCES

Copyright material used in this book, pertaining to photographs, figures, tables and boxes has been reproduced courtesy of the following organisations. The publisher has made every effort to trace the source of the copyright material used. All material referenced below is also included in the general references at the end of the relevant chapter.

## Chapter 1

**Page 1**   Photograph, *A thinking approach*, artist Lionel Cooper, photographer David Sanderson. Poster produced by ARTRIGHT Brisbane as part of a community arts project at the St Vincent de Paul Homeless Person Hostel in South Brisbane. Reproduced with permission.

## Chapter 2

**Page 22**   Photograph, *Lunch hour*, photographer Tim Owen. Reproduced with permission.

## Chapter 3

**Page 40**   Photograph, *Covering up*, photographer Tim Owen. Reproduced with permission.

**Page 45**   Table 3.1, 'Injuries sustained as a result of abuse' Queensland Domestic Violence Task Force (1988), *Beyond these walls*, Brisbane: QLD Government Printing Service, p. 18. Reproduced with permission.

**Page 45**   Voice box 3.1 'Breaking point' Human Rights and Equal Opportunities Commission (1993) *Human Rights and Mental Illness: Report of the National Inquiry into the Human Rights of People with Mental Illness*, vols 1 & 2, Canberra: AGPS, p. 593. Commonwealth of Australia copyright, reproduced with permission.

**Page 47**   Voice box 3.2 'Father's honour' Legge, K. (1994) 'Living two lives', *The Australian Magazine*, Sept. 3-4, p. 20. Reproduced with permission.

**Page 48**    Voice box 3.3 'Why didn't you seek help' Excerpt from *Battered Wives*, copyright 1976/81 by Del Martin. All rights reserved. Cited in Derouard, M., Marz, C. & Cava, M. (1993) *The Road Beyond Violence against Women: A Public Education Manual for Nurses*, North York, Ontario: North York Public Health Department, pp. 141-2. Reproduced with permission.

**Page 51**    Table 3.2 'Questions to use to uncover violence', King, C. & Ryan, J. (1989) 'Abused women: Dispelling myths and encouraging intervention', *Nurse Practitioner* 14(5), pp. 47-58. Reproduced with permission.

## Chapter 4

**Page 58**    Photograph, *The headache*, photographer George Cruickshank (1835). Reproduced with permission of the Wellcome Institute Library, London.

## Chapter 5

**Page 80**    Photograph, *Bromham Place*. Reproduced with permission of Bromham Place, Richmond, Melbourne.

**Page 87**    Table 5.1 'Why people consult GPs (reasons for encounters across body systems) Bridges-Webb, C., et al. (1992) 'Morbidity in general practice', *Medical Journal of Australia*, 157 (Supp.) Oct.19, S1 - S55.

**Page 88**    Table 5.2 'Estimates of one-year prevalence of mental disorders in Australia: people aged 20 years and over'. Henderson cited in National Health Strategy (1993) *Help where Help is Needed*, National Health Strategy, Issues Paper No. 5, Melbourne.

**Page 89**    New Zealand Ministry of Health (1993), 'Major causes of first psychiatric admission', *Mental Health Data 1992*. Wellington: Ministry of Health.

**Page 90**    Table 5.3: Involuntary and law enforcement admissions in New Zealand Abbott, M.W. & Kemp, D.R. (1993) 'New Zealand' in D. Kemp (ed.) *International Handbook on Mental Health Policy*, New Zealand: Greenwood Press, p.221.

## Chapter 6

**Page 102**    Photograph (untitled), photographer David Houlder. Reproduced with permission.

**Page 105**    Box 6.1 'Devastated lives' Adapted from Swan, P. (1991) '200 years of unfinished business', *The Lamp* 48 (11), pp. 40-3. Reproduced with permission.

**Page 114**    Box 6.3 'Working with the community' Adapted from McCloud, N. (1993) 'Early Intervention in East Arnhemland rural mental health', *Mental Health in Australia* 5(2), pp. 76 - 81. Reproduced with permission.

## Chapter 7

**Page 120**   Photograph, *Dance*, photographer Roberta Julian. Reproduced with permission of the Migrant Resource Centre, Hobart Tasmania.

## Chapter 8

**Page 139**   Photograph, *Structure*, photographer Tim Owen. Reproduced with permission.

**Page 141**   Department of Health, Housing, Local Government and Local Government (Aus) (1993) *Annual Report*, Canberra: AGPS.

**Page 143**   New Zealand Ministry of Health (1994) *Ministry of Health Corporate Plan 1994/95*, p.5. Reproduced with permission.

## Chapter 9

**Page 160**   Photograph, *Classification*, photographer Tim Owen. Reproduced with permission.

## Chapter 10

**Page 180**   Photograph, *Fear*, photographer, Graham Burstow. Reproduced with permission.

## Chapter 11

**Page 200**   Photograph, *Listening*, photographer Tim Owen. Reproduced with permission.

## Chapter 12

**Page 228**   Photograph, *Bonds*, photographer Bronwyn Jewell. Reproduced with permission.

**Page 233**   Voice box 12.1 'Isolated mothering' Donnelly, C. et al. (1986) *The Parents Book Collective. Feeling our Way*, Maryborough, Penguin, p.225. Reproduced with permission.

**Page 235**   ibid., p.81. Reproduced with permission.

## Chapter 13

**Page 250**   Photograph, *Youth*, photographer Tim Owen. Reproduced with permission.

**Page 254**   Buckmaster, C. (1989) 'To the mind undeveloped', *Collected Poems*, ed. D. McDonald, St Lucia: Queensland University Press. Reproduced with permission.

**Page 262** Box 13.2 'Questions raised during assessment' West, P. & Evans, C.L. (1992) *Psychiatric and Mental Health Nursing with Children and Adolescents*, Maryland: Aspen Publishers, p.44.

## Chapter 14

**Page 274** Photograph, *Health*, photographer Tim Owen. Reproduced with permission.

## Chapter 15

**Page 294** Photograph, *Typhoid fever ward at the Royal Brisbane Hospital circa 1898*, John Oxley Library, Queensland. Reproduced with permission.

**Page 299** American Psychiatric Association (1994) *Diagnostic and Statistics Manual of Mental Disorders* (4th edn.), Washington D.C. Reproduced with permission.

## Chapter 16

**Page 312** Photograph, *Birdsville*, John Oxley Library, Queensland. Reproduced with permission.

## Chapter 17

**Page 334** Photograph, *Thoughts*, photographer, Phillip Keefe-Jackson. Reproduced with permission.

## Chapter 18

**Page 356** Photograph, *Action*, photographer, *Nursing New Zealand*. Reproduced with permission.

**Page 365** Figure 18.1 'Mental health standards in Queensland — minimum service standards' Mental Health Branch Queensland Health (1993) *Minimum Standards for Mental Health Services in Queensland. The Standards Implementation Kit.* Internal document, Queensland Health, pp. 5-6.

**Page 366** Figure 18.2 'Standards for mental health nursing practice' Australian and New Zealand College of Mental Health Nurses (1995) *Standards for Mental Health Nursing Practice (revised).* Greenacres, SA: ANZCMHN, p.4.

# PART I

# CONSUMERS

THE FIRST CHAPTER of this book is written by a 'primary consumer', or user of mental health services, and a social scientist. This chapter does not, however, represent two perspectives. For consumers can be analysts, and social scientists may well be consumers, if not in the past, then in the future. This focus in Chapter 1 on 'the consumer' sets the tone for the book as a whole by drawing attention to the human and social consequences of mental illness. As you read through the other chapters try to keep this focus in mind, because it is easy to forget that the primary role of mental health nurses is to meet the needs of the consumer, and that to do this effectively involves taking an empathic and critical stance on mental health policy and mental health care.

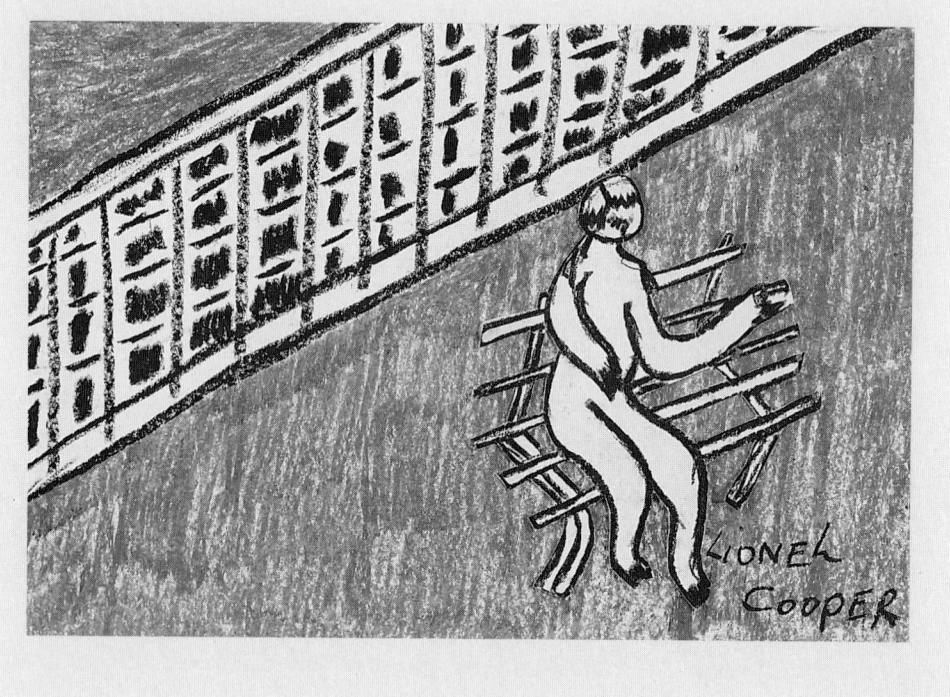

Artist Lionel Cooper, design Lawrence Mullins, photograph David Sanderson. Lionel Cooper was a homeless person with a chronic mental illness who participated in an ARTRIGHT community arts project at the St Vincent de Paul Homeless Person Shelter in South Brisbane. Lionel is now in permanent accommodation and an active artist.

ARTRIGHT is a voluntary group of artworkers dedicated to raising public awareness of human rights abuses and other problems in the community.

CHAPTER 1

# A CONSUMER FOCUS

Kim Jewell and Natasha Posner

# CONTENTS

- recognise that deinstitutionalisation does not guarantee adequate community care;
- appreciate the enabling and empowering role of self-help, support and advocacy groups;
- understand the role and broader possibilities of non-government organisations (NGOs).

# INTRODUCTION

In this chapter a 'consumer' and a social scientist discuss some contemporary issues facing consumers of mental health services in Australia and New Zealand today, and provide an analytical treatment, informed by lived experience. The implications of moving people with mental illness out of institutional care into the community, the role of self-help, support and advocacy groups, and the growing participation of consumers in the public arena are reviewed.

The word 'consumer' (meaning consumer of mental health services) has gained wide currency primarily because it has been chosen and accepted by the people usually affected. In this chapter we will adopt the current terminology which divides consumers of mental health services into two groups: primary and secondary consumers. **A primary consumer** is defined as a person who has, or has had, a diagnosed mental illness, while a **secondary consumer** is someone other than a health professional, who cares for such a person.

# THE EXPERIENCE OF MENTAL ILLNESS

'Mental illness', as a generic term, can be applied to a continuum of difficulties, varying from temporary problems to intractable and disabling conditions (see Chapters 9 and 10). A temporary inability to cope following excessive stress, or the vaguely defined 'nervous breakdown', are generally seen as isolated and non-recurring events and are, perhaps, familiar enough. More disabling conditions such as **schizophrenia** or manic-depressive illness may be less familiar. It is important to appreciate, however, that such conditions are often episodic, so that the person enjoys a relatively normal life for much or most of the time. In other cases, illness may be constant and unrelenting, presenting the person with difficult challenges.

The subjective or personal experience of mental illness will of course vary with the nature and severity of the condition, but many of the emotional, psychological and social consequences will be similar. Even temporary incapacity following a major life event, such as divorce, will be disconcerting and disorienting. Feelings of powerlessness, loss of control of one's affairs and reduced self-confidence will tend to produce anxiety. As emotional reserves are called on to accommodate these extraordinary needs, the capacity to cope with new stresses will be impaired (see Chapter 2). Since feelings of self-worth are often linked to competence, performance and an ability to cope, even temporary failure may lower self-esteem and engender **depression**.

Where temporary absence from employment becomes necessary, the person may be isolated from a helpful source of social support from fellow workers. Unemployment, even temporary unemployment, is associated in our society with failure. Family and friends tend to be less supportive of emotional incapacity than physical incapacity. Mental health difficulties are often perceived to be under the control of individuals, so that blame attaches to those who fail to adjust. Should the incapacity persist, the person may become more and more isolated, insecure and depressed. Any kind of illness that becomes a continuing disability will tend to attract a degree of prejudice and even repugnance. Disabled people, for whatever reasons, are often perceived as a source of fear, as a burden and as somehow responsible for their own condition.

Due to prejudicial community attitudes and poor levels of education in this area, the experience of seeking help for a mental health problem or disorder can be frightening, humiliating and **stigmatising**. Traditionally, training in the mental health field has not given strong emphasis to an understanding of the patient's perspective or the social context of illness. Since the causes of mental illness are often uncertain, and treatment options limited, the traditional role of the clinician has been largely restricted to 'managing' the illness. The legacy of this paternalistic and pessimistic approach for those affected has been a deep sense of frustration and powerlessness (see Chapter 19 for further discussion of paternalism).

In this way the person becomes an identified 'psychiatric patient', the descendant of the feared and reviled 'mental patient' of old. As friends, family and others become aware of this development, prejudice and discrimination may exacerbate the isolation already experienced. The clinical response to the condition will commonly be sedative, antidepressant or psychotropic drugs, often with little or no explanatory information or indication of prognosis. Many of these medications, particularly the family of drugs known as the 'major tranquillisers', will profoundly affect the brain and have severe and often bizarre side effects, such as parkinson-like involuntary limb movements (see Chapter 11). These side effects, combined with disturbing feelings of loss of the integrity of one's mind, and a drug-induced flattening of emotional life, can add a significant dimension to the personal experience of illness.

In the mind of many consumers the 'medication' becomes identified with the illness itself, and with loss of autonomy, free choice and self-determination. The humiliation of having to submit to such a drug regime may constitute the beginning of a life of resentment and frustration. Neither does the regime guarantee protection from relapse. A solution to this dilemma for consumers is to educate themselves about treatment alternatives, including drug therapy, and to participate as much as they are able in decisions concerning their therapy. Such participation is, however, rarely encouraged and will, as a principle, become a central focus of the growing demands of consumers for participation at all levels of decision making concerning their health.

The person with mental illness may thus be subject to isolation, insecurity, low self-esteem, depression, prejudice, repugnance, paternalism, powerlessness, mind-altering drugs, humiliation and frustration. As the perception and identification of mental illness and disability becomes more entrenched in loved ones and the community, the classical negative stereotype of the 'mental patient' will be more rigidly and indiscriminately applied.

The notion of **'labelling'** was popularised in the 1960s by Howard Becker in *Outsiders* (1963). The relevance of this work for the experience of mental illness is the identification of the distinction between a person's behaviour and society's application of a 'deviant' label (i.e. deviant from social norms). To labelling theory, Lemert contributed the notion of 'primary' and 'secondary' deviation. These ideas are well explained by Roach Anleu (1991, p.35):

> Primary deviation remains situational and is rationalised; it does not affect a person's self-conception or public identity as a conforming member of society. In contrast, secondary deviation involves an actor engaging in norm-breaking behaviour and assuming deviant roles and identities which are adaptations to the problems created by societal definitions and reactions to the initial deviance.

An important aspect of secondary deviation, for our purposes, is the concept of 'role engulfment' (Schur 1971, pp.69–73). The person may increasingly see themselves as 'nothing but' the label (in this case, as a psychiatric or 'mental' patient). Schur elaborates:

> A key element in role engulfment is the sudden or gradual collapse of the supports that uphold a person's conception of himself or herself as being socially acceptable ... One of the most insidious aspects of this self-altering process is the strong likelihood that deviators will begin to view themselves with contempt or even hatred. (Schur 1979, p.243)

Central to an understanding of labelling theory is the idea that society itself creates outsiders by applying 'deviant' labels to non-conforming members in an often arbitrary way. Societal perceptions of what is 'normal' differ across culture, geography and time. There is a difference between a person 'naming' a phenomenon for themselves and being labelled by, for example, the psychiatric profession. A phenomenon may be accepted by a person as, for example, 'my voices', but seen in diagnostic terms as 'auditory hallucinations'. Since little can be provided in terms of a causal explanation or cure for such a diagnosis, a person's own perceptions may be at least as useful as a formal diagnosis and far more empowering.

A further consequence of labelling, prejudice and stereotyping is a loss of credibility, perceived integrity and reputation of the person. The person with mental illness, irrespective of intelligence or ability, will tend to be seen as incompetent. Isolated criminal acts perpetrated by mentally ill people tend to be sensationalised by the media, contributing to negative stereotypes. The episodic nature of many psychiatric illnesses and the transient nature of situational mental health problems are poorly understood in the community. Often a primary preoccupation of carers, health service providers and government is the issue of control—control of the behaviour, environment and affairs of the person.

The tension between control and intensive therapeutic care is a critical feature of modern health service provision. Psychotropic drugs have been used for sedation and control of patients' behaviour as well as for medical treatment of their psychiatric illness. Confinement (including placing patients in cell-like seclusion rooms) has also been used in an attempt to modify patients' behaviour, sometimes in ways perceived to be arbitrary and punitive. Where patients are confined under detention orders and forced to submit to non-consensual treatment, it may be difficult for them to appeal against their treatment or protect their basic human rights. Concern about the use of confinement generally has led to the development of the principle of the 'least restrictive environment', which seeks to provide each person with the maximum degree of autonomy. Even where this principle is applied, the most modern mental health service facility may still present a frightening prospect to the consumer.

The full reality of mental illness and the fear of permanent impairment are brought home to the person on admission to a mental health service facility, an admission that, in many cases, will be involuntary. In the brisk, clinical and impersonal admission area, the gradual withdrawal of social support, what might be more appropriately described as a growing 'aloneness' than loneliness, and the hurtful effects of stigmatisation come to a climax. For many, the psychiatric unit or psychiatric hospital will be the ultimate defining metaphor of rejection and abandonment.

The grey half-life endured by inmates of a long-term asylum of a type still in existence has been powerfully and lyrically described in Janet Frame's *Faces in the Water* (1980). Her description of an inter-ward dance captures something of the pathos of the experience:

> Yes, we danced, the crazy people from Ward Two whom even the people from the observation ward and the convalescent ward looked upon as oddities and loonies. We dressed in our exotic party dresses, taffeta and rayons and silky jersey florals, and we lined up outside the clinic to have make-up put on our faces from the ward box with its stump of lipstick .... (Frame 1980, p.186)

Oddly, however, while there can be a strong sense of community, there is little companionship in a psychiatric ward or asylum, where individual patients may often be said to suffer from a confinement of the mind. The interior mental world of the individual can be a primal and fearful place, and one to which the term 'illness' fails to do justice. The experience of **psychosis**, for example, has been described as 'tearing, screaming through the corridors of my mind, searching for a place to hide'. A little appreciated element of psychosis, for those concerned, is that they may respond to the terrors of **paranoia** and other distortions of reality exactly as if they were real. Mental illness, then, can be an experience not only of great **stress** and trauma, but also one of enormous significance and meaning for the individual.

## At the Interface

Lying under
my bed contemplating
the universe
creation's hoary hearse.

Mattress button stars
swirl in flat space
sheet's night curtains
shut out the sun.

Blackness invades my soul
the howling vortex invites—

the unknowing
unconscious unleashes
searing agonies …

psychosis soaring
insane planing
high above
the pain.

Gunshot.
Warm blood washes
away the pain
sweet heaven's rain

In the healing days
a choice
to live or die
to fight or
fly

And at
the interface,
I

Kim Jewell

Attendant on interior mental experience may be the humiliation and embarrassment suffered on realising that one has acted abnormally or out of control with family, friends or others. Loss of control, distortions of reality (often recalled after the fact) and temporary incapacity as experienced, for example, in endogenous depression, will have a profound effect on one's sense of self following an episode of mental illness. The impact may be felt not just at the level of one's self-image, but in the 'core' of the self, one's essential being.

The stability of a person's personality depends partly on consistency of thought and behaviour. Mental health problems can present the individual with a perplexing inconsistency which threatens that stability. Coping strategies that seem to have worked over a lifetime now come into question. A person's ability to negotiate his or her way through life relies on accumulated knowledge about his or her physical and social environment—about 'reality'. When perceptions of reality are distorted or threatened, the experience can be disabling. Suddenly unsure of the validity of his or her perceptions of self, others and reality, the person may be vulnerable to an overwhelming anxiety. Such anxiety may have a cumulative and lasting effect on the capacity to cope and develop. Similarly, in as much as mental illness may be seen to be sensitive to stress, a fear of stress may be learned which contributes spirally to levels of incapacity.

People with mental illness can find themselves strangely isolated, even within their own family. With few exceptions, they will feel isolated in the community, stigmatised, labelled and reified, perceived as 'different'. Commonly, the personal response to stigmatisation will be disabling feelings of low self-esteem and self-worth, an aloneness that is beyond loneliness, deep insecurity and an overwhelming sense of rejection. Such isolation may in practice be associated with homelessness and an inability to access health services.

### Lost Soul

*A star falls from the sky today*
*Crying as it lands,*
*Burying itself to hide*
*In cold and distant sands.*

*No life, no breath to smile for us,*
*Nothing left inside,*
*Just desire to lose touch,*
*Nowhere to confide.*

*Once a bright and gleaming hope*
*For all to place their dreams*
*Now just full of empty space,*
*And terrifying screams.*

*A star fell from the sky today*
*Once so strong and bold*
*Sadness took its life away*
*And left it dull and cold.*

**Denise**

In an often literal as well as metaphorical sense, isolated people can be seen as displaced persons. The road back, for those with the ability and will to take it, can be a long and tortuous one. Others will see themselves as refugees from a society which has ridiculed and rejected them, and in which they have become part of a permanent underclass. At one end of the spectrum, a diagnosis of serious mental illness will mean a high level of disability and possibly a subsistence-level disability support pension. Stigmatisation, prejudice, poverty and poor community understanding will restrict access to meaningful work and recreational pursuits. Towards the other end of the spectrum, less disabling conditions may still marginalise the people affected, restricting their access to suitable accommodation, employment and leisure activities. While levels of disability vary, the effects of stigmatisation are largely constant.

For those with the tenacity and will to win for themselves an equal place in society, the most well-trodden path for stigmatised groups is through self-acceptance, adaptation and negotiation. It will be necessary to accept oneself as different but, equally worthwhile, to adapt to a situation which can be intermittently or even constantly disabling, and to negotiate for equality. **'Coming out'**, declaring oneself in public to be a person with a mental health problem or disorder, can empower a person to negotiate on a more equal footing. The social dynamics of the support group can be seen as a training ground for **self-advocacy** and a rehearsal for declaring oneself in the public arena. Coming out represents a refusal on the part of people with mental illness to accept society's negative perceptions of them, a refusal to be intimidated by prejudice, and a claim for an equal place in society.

## LIVING WITH MENTAL ILLNESS IN THE COMMUNITY

In this century, the mental hospital became an institution ostensibly embracing the notion of therapy as well as protection and confinement. However, it has increasingly been seen as degrading and dehumanising in character, unable to meet the human needs of patients or to provide an environment conducive to recovery, growth or development. There is evidence that many of today's psychiatric institutions continue not only to fail to meet the needs of patients, but violate their human rights through systemic neglect (see Chapters 8 and 18). Such neglect has been recently reported in detail for Australia in a major report for the Schizophrenia Australia Foundation by Dr John Hoult (Hoult 1993).

Recognition of the negative impact of institutionalisation across a range of disability areas provided, in part, the stimulus for a shift in public policy planning to community-based mental health services. Since the 1950s there has been a gradual trend towards deinstitutionalisation in the western world. Kathleen Jones (1993, p.254) attributes the trend to three primary factors—the discovery in the 1950s of psychotropic drugs, the libertarianism of the 1960s, and the philosophy of **'normalisation'** of the 1970s.

The term 'normalisation' has become a catch-phrase in the human services area. The concept has spawned various definitions, but representative is that proposed by Wolfensberger (1972, pp.27–9):

> Utilisation of means which are as culturally normative as possible, in order to establish and/or maintain personal behaviours and characteristics which are as culturally normative as possible.

The concept is allied to that of **'mainstreaming'**, or the provision of mental health services from within the mainstream of health services (see Chapter 8). To the degree that these principles are effective in practice, they will result in a decrease in the level of stigmatisation of individuals using the services. A possible disadvantage may be that such policies also tend to make the special needs of people affected by mental illness less visible.

Such concepts are based on an attempt to change societal perceptions of people affected by disability, by providing more culturally normal environments and encouraging less deviant behaviour. Mental illness, however, can involve behavioural consequences that are outside the control of the person. For someone affected by mental illness to a disabling degree, self-esteem rests crucially on self-acceptance, which may include a sense of essential difference. There will undeniably be superficial benefits for consumers in association with less stigmatising treatment modalities and environments. It can, however, be argued that to encourage people with a disabling and often unpredictable behavioural illness to deny their essential difference is to create a painful schism, and to injure their sense of identity, challenge and achievement.

A second factor suggested by Jones (1993) to influence the trend towards deinstitutionalisation was the discovery of psychotropic drugs. It is fair to say that these and associated drugs have revolutionised mental health care. Due to the hypnotic and tranquillising properties of many of these drugs, they are open to abuse in attempts to make consumers more easily manageable, but the beneficial effects, when they are used ethically, are undeniable. It is true that drug therapy has enabled the release of many patients from institutions into the community, and continues to provide one important weapon in the struggle of consumers for independence, self-reliance and dignity.

The necessary and essential concomitant of deinstitutionalisation is community-oriented health care. Predictably, while governments have been quick to seize on the cost savings from the scaling down of institutions, they have been slow to create the necessary infrastructure for community care (see Chapter 8). Australian Human Rights Commissioner, Brian Burdekin, in his definitive 1993 report, states:

> In general, the savings resulting from de-institutionalisation have not been redirected to mental health services in the community. Those remain seriously underfunded .... (Human Rights and Equal Opportunities Commission 1993, p.908)

Jones' third factor influencing the trend towards deinstitutionalisation is the libertarianism of the 1960s, or the advocation of liberty and self-determination. Scull (1977), however, contends that the growth of the welfare state has paradoxically contributed to deinstitutionalisation, as segregative forms of social control have become more and more expensive compared with the opportunity cost of caring for people in the community. Scull (1977, p.137) concludes that the appeal of deinstitutionalisation for fiscal conservatives and the support it receives (as suggested by Jones) from liberal adherents makes the policy politically irresistible.

As there has been a failure thus far to provide the necessary community care resources to accompany deinstitutionalisation, it is difficult to gauge the degree of success of the policy in returning people to the community and in providing alternative therapeutic programs. The Human Rights and Equal Opportunities Commission (HREOC) Report, *Human Rights and Mental Illness* (1993, p.40), reports that, in Australia, many deinstitutionalised patients are merely relocated in substandard boarding houses or other semi-institutional accommodation, or face homelessness. Such patients are arguably worse off than before.

Clearly, the emerging need in the area of mental health care is for an integrated institutional and community-based approach (see Chapter 8). The concept of asylum remains a valid and valued one to consumers. The challenge for policy makers is to provide, in meaningful consultation with consumers, integrated services which retain elements of asylum in a creative, developmental and dignified way.

## Community attitudes towards mental illness

Although the policy of deinstitutionalisation would tend to promote the reintegration of people with mental illness into the community, the attitudes of people in the community tend to discourage such integration. A recent study of community attitudes to mental illness (Reark Research 1993) for the Australian Health Ministers' Advisory Council, found that, while the principle of community integration was generally supported, there were very negative attitudes to the prospect of a group home for people who had been treated for mental illness in actual proximity. Their investigation of attitudes led the researchers to conclude that:

> ... the topic of mental illness arouses deep seated fears, and constant denial, through all levels of our society. There is almost a wall of silence about this issue. (Reark Research 1993, p.6)

They found that physical and mental illness generate a very different response from society, so that 'the traditions of "tender, loving care", flowers, sympathy and support that are showered on those who break a leg, are clearly denied to those with mental illness'. A consequence of this is that 'consumers and carers experience continual discrimination, injustice and rejection'.

This study included the views of mental health service consumers and their carers. Consumers spoke of support from within the family, as well as the pain resulting from lack of understanding and compassion from family members and, sometimes, exclusion from family activities. They also spoke of their awareness of the family stress and dislocation that could be caused by the illness. Carers spoke of how they too were subject to lack of support, understanding and acceptance by family and friends, reducing their quality of life. As parents they could feel themselves to be the object of speculative and hurtful notions of parental causation of psychiatric disorder.

Whereas a history of mental illness is unlikely to be hidden within the family, it may be hidden from a wider social network. The fact that a person has been mentally ill is likely to be a key piece of information in the development of a relationship, and its disclosure may alter the perceptions of others for the worse.

> The issue that consumers wrestle with constantly is whether to disclose some or all of the facts, and to whom ... Experience quickly teaches ... that disclosure brings rebuttal and rejection; the issue then becomes whether to live a lie or live with integrity. (Reark Research 1993, p.40)

The most common strategy reported was to conceal the truth. Some consumers, particularly those who were members of supportive groups encouraging the 'coming out' described above, felt able to take a more assertive stance in challenging prejudice and in being open about their history.

The issue of disclosure is also a highly significant one for people with other invisible and stigmatised disabilities. Any attempt to lead a normal life in spite of the condition may be made more difficult by lack of social acceptance and the discrimination that follows disclosure. On the other hand, to hide the condition is, in effect, to allow the prejudice to go unchallenged.

The research mentioned above found that consumers who had tried to get work all spoke of the discrimination that occurs when a history of mental illness is disclosed, and 'it seemed the occasions when a satisfactory work situation could be established were extremely rare' (Reark Research 1993, p.42). Where work was offered it tended to be of the most menial type. Both consumers and carers interviewed expressed a strong sense of injustice about this situation, which tends to deny the person with mental illness the means to avoid poverty and its concomitants—poor accommodation, and lack of money for hobbies, recreation and other opportunities. Without work there is a need to find some other meaningful activity to provide a sense of self-worth and purpose.

The cumulative effect of the attitudinal barriers described above, the researchers concluded, meant that the weight of societal rejection of people with mental illness could be 'just as damaging and painful as the torments of the condition itself' (Reark Research 1993, p.44). Without acceptance and integration within the community, 'normalisation' as a development in the care of people with mental illness means very little.

## The role of mutual aid: self-help, support and advocacy groups

One way to combat the effects of such prejudice and rejection on one's sense of self is to seek the understanding, companionship and support of other people living with the same condition. The role of mutual aid groups in supporting people living with problematic conditions and situations in life is well known. The numbers and influence of mutual aid groups have grown over the past two decades, alongside 'consumer' organisations. Such groups can be a forum for the exchange of practical information and experiential knowledge which those living with the condition can acquire, and which may contribute to a person's ability to manage the situation in day-to-day terms. The members can provide each other with the encouragement and help they are unlikely to find outside the group in the community at large, which can enable an individual to feel more confident and hopeful about living with the condition or situation.

Members of such groups are people living in the community who come together in a form of temporary or ongoing fellowship which has the potential to make a significant contribution to their psychological well-being. This can happen in a number of ways. The support and understanding of group members in similar situations may sustain an individual through a crisis period. The group meetings provide a venue for meeting people with something in common, and for the formation of friendships and the development of support networks that can exist outside the group meetings. Furthermore, the information exchanged is likely to encourage greater use of available services and resources in the community to help sustain people living in the community with varying degrees of disability. Above all, **support groups** help to counteract the isolation and despair which may accompany life with a problematic or disabling condition.

A fundamental feature of self-help groups is that the aid is mutual—the help given is reciprocal. It is this feature that enables members to receive the support when they need it, without feeling demeaned or inadequate. They themselves will have a chance to offer support to other members when they can. This has been termed serial reciprocity (Richardson & Goodman 1983). It is particularly important, with any condition that is stigmatised and in some degree disabling, that the group should be run by people who themselves have the condition, if the full benefits of mutual aid are to be realised. If well-meaning citizens, carers or professionals run the groups, the dynamics are altered, and there is a danger of reproducing the patriarchal attitudes of the wider society.

The solidarity of a mutual aid group is a powerful way of dealing with the impact of social stigma. As the stigmatised condition is shared by the members of the group, they can feel that within the social circle of the group they are 'normal' rather than 'deviant', they are entirely acceptable (in a way that people without the condition would not be) and they can thus enjoy the benefits of group membership. From within the group, they can draw strength from the fact that they are not alone with their stigmatised condition, need not feel any less valuable than any other citizen, and can learn ways to combat discrimination in the wider society.

Self-help, support and advocacy groups can provide a facilitative and nurturing environment for the development of self-acceptance, and for the learning process for adaptation and negotiation. For the primary consumer, joining a support or self-help group can be a first step towards **self-advocacy**. It is not uncommon for the person and the group to make this transition together, and move from self-help to group advocacy. Self-advocacy has the secondary benefits of increasing self-esteem and self-acceptance and lessening feelings of powerlessness. In this way, the group can play an important part in the process of adaptation for the consumer.

## CONSUMERS IN THE PUBLIC ARENA

In Australia and New Zealand, during recent decades, a growing consumer presence in the public arena has been seen in three distinct but overlapping areas—the development of mental health **non-government organisations** (NGOs), consumer participation, and the mental health 'consumer movement'. NGOs are usually formalised groups with specific aims and programs, generally directed towards the provision of support services for consumers, community education, advocacy, consultancy and the promotion of consumer participation. With the movement away from institutionalisation and towards community care, NGOs are increasingly expected to fill large gaps in service provision and to respond to increased demand for their services. Government funding to support NGO services however, has been patchy and limited, in the absence of any 'cogent national strategy' (Morgan 1994). The resultant pattern of NGO service provision ranges from isolated examples of outstanding programs to skeleton administrative functions or, more commonly, services provided on a completely voluntary basis.

In Australia, the National Mental Health Policy and Plan (1992), following a broad consultative process, provided for consumer participation in the policy making process (see Chapter 8). The Plan provided for the establishment of Federal and State peak consumer advisory groups to advise the respective ministers. Through a proposed national, State and regional network of officially constituted consumer advisory groups, consumers will have a forum for communication with senior levels of government. Such networks provide a mechanism with the potential for meaningful consumer participation in decisions which profoundly affect their lives. However, even when the mechanism is in place, this does not guarantee that the communication of consumers' views will receive a full hearing or be acted upon.

In New Zealand, consumer participation has had a more direct input into policy. In 1988 a nationwide group of consumers, the Aotearoa Network of Psychiatric Survivors, was formed. The organisation was constituted to facilitate input into the National Mental Health Consortium, a peak mental health policy making committee. Since the 1970s, in the United States and Holland, and latterly in Britain, 'survivors' organisations have developed and used activist strategies to promote user participation in mental health services. In the view of Pilgrim and Rogers (1993, p.173):

> User dissatisfaction has now reached such a point that in terms of numbers and organisations, it constitutes a nascent 'new social movement'.

The mental health consumer movement can be described as just such a social movement. The role of the movement is a political one, and represents a struggle for social change and power in the community. This is essentially different from that of NGOs or consumer advisory groups. While NGOs continue to have an important function in advocacy and service provision, to a great extent they have as yet achieved only low levels of participation by primary consumers. In the case of consumer advisory groups, while they will provide an essential avenue of communication between consumers and government, their members are appointed by government and are therefore not free to play a completely independent role in the political arena.

Whatever level of success is achieved by the consumer movement in terms of social change, and whatever the degree of participation in the movement by ordinary consumers, standing up for consumer rights in public as a group can only engender a sense of identity, pride and solidarity in people whose needs have been largely ignored.

As we move towards the 21st century, in a climate of increasing awareness of the human needs of consumers of mental health services and a declared commitment by government towards reform, the challenge for policy makers will be to place consumers themselves at the centre of education and training, research and policy development. The development of awareness is most imperative in relation to the need for consumer participation in decisions concerning individual therapy, treatment and accommodation, and the need for personal development, choice and, above all, dignity.

## SUMMARY

- The term 'mental illness' covers a continuum of difficulties.
- Experiencing a mental illness can be very isolating, disabling and undermining of a person's sense of self.
- Hospital treatment for mental illness can be frightening and traumatic.
- The stigma of mental illness has social consequences in terms of loss of relationships, employment and other opportunities. The person may be marginalised, disempowered and impoverished. The labelling of a person can in itself have serious consequences.
- The policy of deinstitutionalisation does not guarantee adequate community care. Integrated institutional and community-based services are required.
- Self-help, support and advocacy groups can be enabling and empowering.

- The growth of NGOs and consumer participation augur well for the communication of consumer needs to government. The consumer movement has broader possibilities, including social change and the development of a sense of identity, pride and communality.

## DISCUSSION QUESTIONS

*Note: It is strongly suggested that consumers be invited to participate in your discussions.*

1. You find yourself a patient legally detained in an acute psychiatric unit, following disturbed behaviour for which you have no explanation. Your family can no longer accept your behaviour and refuse communication. You have no money or close friends. What is your most pressing need? How would you expect the unit to meet that need?

2. You find yourself given to alternating bouts of crying and anger. These are emotions that you have not shown for a very long time. You overhear a senior nurse discussing your behaviour with a doctor, saying you are attention-seeking and manipulative. How would you feel? Would you challenge the nurse? If so, why? If not, why not?

3. You return home from shopping to find your neighbour asking condescendingly about your state of health. A community mental health nurse, finding you out, had apparently asked your neighbour if you appeared 'well'. Your neighbour had no previous knowledge of your psychiatric history. How do you feel? If you are unhappy with the situation, what can you do about it?

4. Discuss the reasons for and against disclosing a history of mental illness to the following people: an employer; a potential boyfriend/girlfriend; a work colleague.

5. 'The term "mental illness" covers a continuum of difficulties and only those who have experienced these difficulties at first hand can speak about what it feels like.' Discuss this statement from the perspective of (a) a person with a mental illness, (b) a close relative of a person with a serious mental illness, and (c) a member of a mental health profession (refer to other chapters as necessary).

## EXERCISES

1. Trace the incidence of mental illness in your own family tree. Note and explain the degree of readiness or otherwise with which your relatives discuss the issue.

2. Arrange a group visit to the nearest psychiatric facility. What is your first and most striking impression? What, if anything, is the observable difference between the clients and yourself? What are the principal differences between

this environment and your campus? Are these differences related to the needs of consumers? Are they, in fact, necessary at all?

3. Read the life story of a consumer, and present a brief impression to the group. Invite several consumers to participate in your group and repeat the exercise, using a different story.

4. Prepare headbands for each group member labelled: doctor, nurse, clinical nurse consultant (CNC), psychologist, psychiatrist, social worker, occupational therapist, patient, parent. The 'patient' has decided to leave hospital and immediately pursue a career as a rocket scientist. Role play the scenario and later remove the labels. Ask the 'patient' to comment on his or her experiences and feelings about the exercise. What has each member of the group learned about the dynamics of patient–staff relations?

# FURTHER READING

- Frame, J. (1980) *Faces in the Water*, London: The Women's Press. Frame, one of New Zealand's foremost writers, has an ability to convey the interior and exterior world of a person affected by mental illness that is to be found nowhere else in literature. Frame's autobiography has been made into the film, *An Angel at my Table*, directed by Jane Campion.

- Williams, D. (1992) *Nobody Nowhere*, Moorebank: Transworld Publishers. From childhood, Donna Williams felt herself to be different in ways she could not understand. Her book is about autism, disorganisation, challenge and achievement, and the pain and joy these things can bring.

- Trombley, S. (1981) *All that Summer she was Mad—Virginia Woolf and her Doctors*, London: Junction Books. Trombley examines the life and death by suicide of the famous feminist writer. The book details childhood sexual abuse, sexual failure in her marriage and the concept of 'moral madness' espoused by some of her doctors. Woolf's personal diaries reveal the social context of emotional disturbance in her life.

- Flach, F. (1990) *Rickie*, New York: Ballantine Books. A collaborative work by a young woman and her psychiatrist father. The book is a good description of the nightmare than can result from misdiagnosis and involuntary detention, and underscores the poverty of scientific knowledge in this area of health.

- Pierce, E. *Ordinary Insanity*, Dulwich Hill, NSW: P.E. Pierce. Well-titled, Emma Pierce's work weaves together the subjective experience of psychosis with the social pressures in her life. A very readable account.

- Sayer, P. (1988) *The Comforts of Madness*, London: Doubleday. Written by a staff nurse in a large psychiatric hospital, this prize-winning work expresses the fictional 'interior monologue' of a long-term 'catatonic' patient with a chilling and poignant sense of reality.

# REFERENCES

Becker, H.S. (1963) *Outsiders: Studies in the Sociology of Deviance*, New York: The Free Press.

Frame, J. (1980) *Faces in the Water*, London: The Women's Press, p.186.

Hoult, J. (1993) *Care of the Seriously Mentally Ill in Australia. A Rating of State and Regional Programs*, Schizophrenia Foundation.

Human Rights and Equal Opportunities Commission (1993) *Human Rights and Mental Illness. Report of the National Inquiry into the Human Rights of People with Mental Illness*, Canberra. AGPS.

Jones, K. (1993) *Asylums and After*, Cambridge: Cambridge University Press.

Morgan, E. (1994) 'Our rightful place: the participation of non-government sector agencies in the system of mental health services'. Paper delivered to the National Mental Health Conference on Realities, Resources and Research, Adelaide.

*National Mental Health Policy and Plan* (1992) Canberra: AGPS.

Pilgrim, D. & Rogers, A. (1993) *A Sociology of Mental Health and Illness*, Buckingham: Open University Press.

Reark Research Pty Ltd (1993) 'Community attitudes to mental illness: a report on qualitative research' (unpublished report), Sydney.

Richardson, A. & Goodman, M. (1983) *Self-help and Social Care: Mutual Aid Organisations in Practice*, London: Policy Studies Institute.

Roach Anleu, S.L. (1991): *Deviance, Conformity and Social Control*, Melbourne: Longman Cheshire.

Schur, E.M. (1971) *Labelling Deviant Behaviour*, New York: Harper & Row.

Schur, E.M. (1979) *Interpreting Deviance: A Sociological Introduction*, New York: Harper & Row.

Scull, A.T. (1977) *Decarceration: Community Treatment and the Deviant—A Radical View*, Englewood Cliffs, NJ:.Prentice Hall.

Wolfensberger, W. (1972) *The Principle of Normalization*, Toronto: National Institute of Mental Retardation.

# PART II

# STRESS

STRESS IS THE REACTION of a person to stressors. It is an inevitable aspect of life, and has both positive and negative effects. At its most positive, a reasonable level of stress can be exciting and empowering. At worst, stress can be an important contributor to mental illness in people who are personally susceptible, socially vulnerable or in other ways at risk.

Chapter 2 sets the scene for this section by defining stress and considering its physiological and psychological components. The stress management techniques discussed are a powerful resource for people who are personally susceptible to stress.

Chapter 3 picks up the stress theme by examining the prevalence and impact of violence against women. This theme has been chosen to highlight the vulnerability to mental health problems of women subjected to violence in the home. However, it would be untrue and misleading to attribute male violence against women to mental illness. Yet the stress management techniques described in Chapter 2 could help men to find more acceptable ways to cope with their anger, thus reducing a major source of social vulnerability.

Chapter 4 takes up another major risk factor for mental health problems—chronic illness—and examines the complex interaction between physical and mental health problems. Case studies demonstrate the need for holistic nursing care.

# Lunch hour

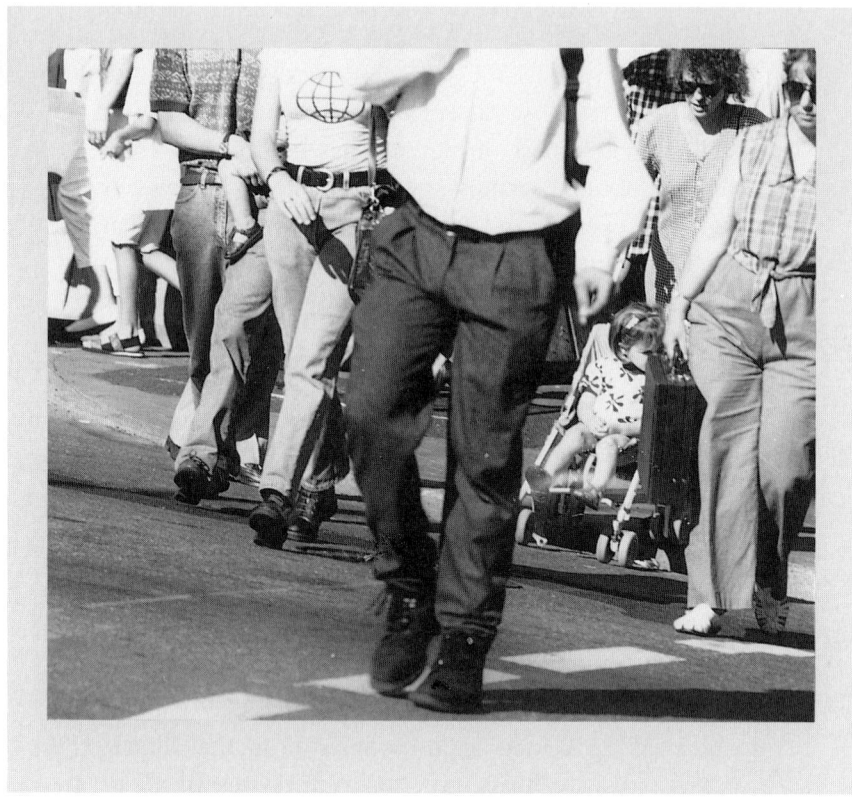

TIM OWEN

Everyone hurrying about their business: the stress of everyday life.

CHAPTER 2

# *L*IFE STRESSORS

Derek Weir and Tian Oei

# *C*ONTENTS

# LEARNING OBJECTIVES

This chapter will assist the reader to:
- understand the difference between mental health and mental disorder;
- discuss the parameters of mental health;
- understand typical responses to life stressors;
- differentiate between adaptive and maladaptive responses to stressors;
- consider the role of life stressors in mental well-being.

# INTRODUCTION

In order to understand health better, it is often necessary to distinguish the normal from the abnormal so that what is a healthy normal state can be differentiated from an abnormal state. This is particularly so when mental health and mental ill-health are considered. Much has been written about mental illness, ranging from erudite and scholarly discussions to views that are clearly uninformed. While much of this literature has focused on mental illness, less of it has looked at mental health and how to attain it.

There are numerous reasons for this. One reason could be that many people dissociate themselves from the realities of mental illness, preferring to believe it is something that happens only to others. Another reason may be that, for many, mental health is simply taken for granted, except when it is obviously compromised. Few people appear to take any active part in ensuring that they continue to enjoy good mental health. Despite the wealth of discussion that has taken place, it is still common for people to feel personal discomfort when discussing mental health and mental illness. This discomfort has probably been another factor that has, for many decades, limited the understanding and promotion of mental health, as well as treatment for those who experience dramatic and enduring changes to their mental health.

One of the objectives of this chapter is to differentiate states of mental health, mental health problems and mental disorder.

While the professional literature in the area of mental health and mental disorder has grown exponentially over past decades, it is unfortunate that the same literature is not read by the general public. The community's general lack of information about what constitutes mental illness, and about the prognoses of mental disorder, ensures that such illnesses are still surrounded by mystery, misinformation and **stigma**. The experiences of those who have the clinical conditions that are recognised as mental disorders often demonstrate how they can only too readily become marginalised from the rest of society (see Chapter 1). The rapid rise of the health consumer movement in recent times is one factor that is having a significant impact on community awareness of both the quality and outcomes of services provided for people with mental health problems and mental disorders. However, much remains to be done as entrenched attitudes are difficult to change.

One obvious strategy to remove some of the mystique associated with mental disorder, to reduce the stigma surrounding it, and to ensure that individuals who experience mental disorder are appropriately integrated into our communities, is to capitalise on the professional expertise of mental health practitioners and share their knowledge in appropriate ways with the rest of the community. Members of the health care professions have a significant responsibility to ensure that accurate information is available to the community, to challenge some of the deeply ingrained negative attitudes and stereotypes, and to play a key role in the design and delivery of strategies that will either prevent mental disorder occurring, or minimise its impact once it exists.

## MENTAL HEALTH

So what, then, is mental health? The World Health Organization defines *health* as 'a state of complete physical, mental and social well-being, not merely the absence of disease or infirmity'. In 1991 the Australian Health Ministers' (AHM) Conference provided a definition of mental health that will serve as a starting point for discussion. This definition asserts that mental health is

> ... the capacity of individuals within the groups and environment to interact with one another in ways that promote subjective well-being, optimal development and use of mental abilities (cognitive, affective and relational) and achievement of individual and collective goals consistent with justice.

In this definition, **cognitive** refers to all elements and processes involved in thinking, memory and recall; *affective* refers to emotional responsiveness; and *relational* to the abilities required to interact with others.

This is a broad definition and one that encompasses key ideas developed throughout this book. To possess good mental health, then, individuals must have several key capabilities that enable them to interact with one another, to use their mental abilities to maximum advantage and to be aware of the wishes and aspirations of others. The AHM Conference also produced a statement entitled *Mental health: statement of rights and responsibilities* which points out that:

> Good mental health is a resource for everyday life. It is a positive concept which embraces both inner individual experience and interpersonal group experience. To the individual, good mental health means happiness, competence, a sense of power over one's life, positive feelings of self-esteem and the capacities to love, work and play. Good mental health also allows individuals to deal with difficult life events.

This idealised view of mental health is often difficult to achieve. Exactly what constitutes 'difficult life events' is likely to vary considerably, depending on an individual's perspective and societal expectations. For example, in regions in which armed conflict is occurring, one's capacity to enjoy positive self-esteem, love, work and play is seriously impaired. Similarly, the transition from childhood through adolescence to adulthood and old age, while normative (common to all) and age-related (within the same age cohort), demonstrates the variety of events that can be experienced during these stages. For some people, these transitions are experienced as particularly difficult life events—but not by others. Many of the aspects of these idealised definitions of mental health are challenged by normative, age-related events and are thus difficult to achieve. Some life events are so far beyond the range of the day-to-day experiences of most people that they overwhelm the capacity to adapt.

**Mental health** is defined according to commonly held values. The definitions referred to above indicate that individuals are regarded as enjoying positive mental health when the behaviour they demonstrate is adaptive (that is, it causes no particular distress to themselves or others), and enables them to fulfil satisfactorily their culturally accepted daily activities, including communicating their needs clearly and without impediment. If, for some reason, events bring about a deviation from this ideal, and personal discomfort and distressing thoughts and behaviours interfere with everyday living, people are considered to have a mental health problem.

In addition to the ability to take maximum advantage of one's capacities for self-realisation, having good mental health confers a degree of flexibility that fosters adaptation. This flexibility enables individuals to tolerate uncertainty and to develop an awareness of their abilities and limitations, thus allowing adjustment to life events. Provided these fluctuations (which may be stressful) are relatively short-term, people can, and do, adapt satisfactorily. When disruptions to everyday life become protracted, good mental health is difficult to maintain. Mental health problems or clinically recognised mental disorders may then develop.

## MENTAL DISORDERS

In contrast with the definition of mental health, the term 'mental disorder' has a considerably more structured definition and a specific usage. In the correct clinical application, **mental disorder** is the term used to designate changes from normal mental functioning that are sufficient to become recognised as clinical disorders. It is only when these changes become persistent, repetitive, recognisable and exaggerated expressions of disordered thought, disturbed feeling and disruptive behaviour, that the presentation is correctly referred to as a *mental disorder*. In effect, mental disorder signifies an inability at that time to adapt, modify or change behaviour in response to changes in life events or environmental circumstances. While this definition and the structured concept of mental disorder are widely accepted, such an enlightened view has taken many centuries to evolve.

## STRESS AND MENTAL HEALTH

Difficult life events do occur, regardless of culture, age, occupation or gender. These difficulties are often fairly loosely referred to as 'stress' but, in fact, **stress** is the *reaction* to these events. The events themselves are more correctly termed 'stressors' (they trigger a stress response). How stress is defined is the subject of some controversy but, generally speaking, it is assumed that when the demands of life exceed a person's resources, a stress response occurs. Hans Selye (1974) defined stress as 'the non-specific response of the body to any demands made upon it'. Other authors indicate a more structured response and, in particular, focus on the processing that takes place in response to a stressor. For instance, one of the most distinguished authors on stress, Richard Lazarus (1971), defined stress as:

> ... a broad class of problems differentiated from other problem areas because [it] deals with any demands which tax the system, whatever it is, a physiological system, a social system or a psychological system, and the response of that system.

Lazarus added that 'the reaction depends on how the person interprets or appraises (consciously or unconsciously) the significance of a harmful, threatening or disabling event' (p.53). Responses to stress are presented in Table 2.1 and include the physiological, behavioural and emotional reactions that Selye referred to as the 'General Adaptation System'. Individual responses differ widely and the same stressor can trigger different responses in different people. The examples given in Boxes 2.1 to 2.3 demonstrate that some people can 'sail through life', apparently unaffected by events that others find overwhelming. The first example (Box 2.1) demonstrates the consequence of a common and automatic response to a fear-provoking situation.

## B O X 2 . 1 : *Hyperarousal*

Imagine that you were involved in a minor motor vehicle accident yesterday. No-one was hurt but you received a real fright. Imagine that today you are in a group of people who have started to cross an extremely busy, multi-laned metropolitan highway, and you are doing so on a marked pedestrian crossing close to a four-way intersection. You have checked your passage is safe and, with the others, you step out.

Cars in the first lane stop to allow you to cross. You start to move quickly and, as you pass the first lane, you see a car travelling at high speed in the second lane next to the stationary cars. The driver of the car is apparently unaware of your presence—until you step out. In the briefest second, without apparent conscious effort, you are aware of a real and imminent danger. You gasp! Your heart thuds! You run! You reach the pavement safely and stop to catch your breath.

The others in your group seem to have paid little attention to the danger. They wander down the street and disappear into a cafe. But you are aware of your heart pounding, beads of perspiration on your forehead, tension in your facial muscles. Your legs shake. You feel angry that your life was endangered. You yell in the direction of the now-receding car: 'Why don't you learn to drive?'

Almost as quickly as it started, the sensation of hyperarousal subsides. Your breathing returns to normal, your face regains some colour and you move off.

Then there are examinations. Some people seem oblivious to the stress of examinations, while others are preoccupied by it and find examinations so threatening that their performance is seriously affected (Box 2.2).

## Box 2.2: *Examination anxiety*

For most of the semester, a female student in an undergraduate university course has not been performing either to her own or her lecturer's satisfaction, and now her theoretical examinations are just weeks away. She has put in additional hours to improve her performance. She designed a plan of study in the weeks leading up to the examination and tried hard to follow this plan. Other things were distracting though—there were two birthday parties to attend, a new movie to see.

In the last week before the examination, she kept reading and re-reading her lecture notes, but none seemed to make much sense. In the few days immediately before the exam, her sleep pattern was disrupted by dreams of failure, and she had persistent difficulty falling asleep. When she woke early, all she could think of was how important this exam was to her career.

The night before the exam she slept very poorly, and woke later than intended. Tired, feeling frustrated and running late, she left for the exam venue. Her friends had already gathered outside the exam room and were chatting quietly. She hardly paid them any attention. Although she was late getting there, it seemed to her that it took ages before the door was opened; with a sense of reluctance she entered the room, sat down and turned over the examination paper.

As she scanned the pages, her heart sank. She couldn't understand several of the questions. She started to write down some answers, but couldn't concentrate, and soon put down her pen, staring blankly at her answer booklet. She was aware of the quiet rustling in the room, the sound of other students turning pages, sounds of pens on paper. She tried to focus on the questions, but became more anxious and worried that time was running out.

Time was up. They filed out. Her friends were animated in their discussion about the paper. It was difficult. Several hard questions. But wasn't this the answer? Wasn't that? She felt depressed and found herself thinking: 'I'm going to fail ... it's the lecturer's fault ... should have made it clearer what was required. I'm never going to succeed. I'm a failure at uni.'

The third example (Box 2.3) illustrates a further variation in response to a stressful event.

## B OX 2.3: *Interpersonal difficulties*

A third-year registered nurse had been rostered on late shift in a busy surgical unit of a regional hospital for several weeks. Towards the end of a particularly difficult shift, he accidentally contaminated several sterile dressing trays that were in use. The Unit Nurse Manager, who had witnessed the incident, called him over and reprimanded him loudly . The nurse was resentful at the criticism and felt embarrassed.

Over the next few days things went from bad to worse. The Nurse Manager seemed to be constantly finding things to complain about in his work—untidiness, lateness, inattention to detail, poor clinical notes—and seemed to find extra work for him to complete at the end of each shift. He often found himself leaving work later than his colleagues. He felt frustrated and increasingly resentful towards the Unit Manager. A few days later he decided to talk to the Nurse Manager about the event, to try to resolve the problem. His protestations were unheard.

Outside work, he and his girlfriend seemed to quarrel constantly, and they agreed not to see each other for a few days to let things settle down. He declined several invitations from his friends to join in social activities and felt increasingly despondent about his work and his life. His next performance appraisal was critical of his work. His thoughts became more negative and self-critical. He just couldn't shake off his despondency. He started missing rostered duty.

His friends became increasingly concerned for his well-being. They found him dejected and despairing about his future. He complained of tension headaches and considerable difficulty in maintaining a regular and satisfying sleep pattern. He became careless about his appearance and neglected his diet. He reluctantly agreed to see a doctor, who recommended that he undertake some counselling to help resolve the interpersonal difficulties he was experiencing.

People's interpretation and appraisal of a threatening situation depend on the context in which the stressor occurs, how they think about it (whether it is an imminent or delayed threat, as well as just how much of a threat it really is) and their sense of coping, or lack of it. In the example of hyperarousal (Box 2.1), the 'near miss' occurs close to the time of a minor motor vehicle accident, so you are likely to be hypervigilant around cars (a logical response to a fear-provoking situation); you experience the speeding car as a greater potential danger than other people exposed to the same situation, who seem largely unaffected by it.

In the second and third examples (Boxes 2.2 and 2.3), the responses indicate that it is unlikely that the actual events produced the stress response directly, but that cognitive appraisal (that is, the way we perceive and process information about an event) had an important role to play. The meaning assigned to a particular stressor often has negative emotional overtones (such as feeling overwhelmed) and is strongly associated with doubts about coping (King,

Stanley & Burrows 1987). Table 2.1 shows common stress responses, classified as physical, emotional and behavioural reactions, and it may be helpful to consider how many of each category are demonstrated in the three boxed examples. It should also be noted that psychological traits (such as personality attributes and emotionality), which define an individual's cognitive appraisal patterns may determine whether biochemical changes triggered by stressors are interpreted in a positive or a negative mental fashion (Clair, Oei & Evans 1992; Weir et al. 1993), resulting in further (de)escalation.

T A B L E   2 . 1 :   *Symptoms of stress*

| PHYSICAL | EMOTIONAL | BEHAVIOURAL |
|---|---|---|
| Increased blood pressure | Feeling down in the dumps | Tremulousness |
| Increased muscle tension | Anxiety—excessive worry about everything | Increased general activity |
| Tension-related headaches | Irritability—outbursts of temper and hostility | Pacing |
| Feeling worn out | | Fidgeting |
| Chronic fatigue | Frequent spells of brooding | Hand-wringing |
| Difficulty sleeping | Feelings of inadequacy | Abusive or aggressive behaviour |
| Frequent indigestion | Erratic, inexplicable behaviour | |
| (Increased) use of cigarettes, alcohol and other drugs | Inability to concentrate | |
| Excessive eating | Forgetfulness | |
| Increased startle reaction | Difficulty making decisions | |
| | Excessive daydreaming | |
| Increased psychomotor activity | Suspiciousness | |
| | Feelings of helplessness | |
| | Overinterpretation of events | |

Humans possess an inbuilt response to changes in the immediate environment, including situations which are unfamiliar to us, or which are perceived as dangerous or threatening in some way. It is likely that physical responses to stress are determined by innate genetic factors. Stress-initiated changes in the sympathetic division of the autonomic nervous system produce a cascade of physiological responses. These include changes in hormonal system activity, cardiovascular responsivity and muscle tension. All the changes that occur in response to stressors are variable: the physical responses (especially changes accompanying the release of the so-called 'stress hormones', such as adrenaline and noradrenaline); the emotional responses (in particular, cognitive or thinking responses); and the behavioural responses. Variation in responses can occur even in people experiencing the same degree of stress. For example, a recent study by Kenardy et al. (1993) reported that, even in individuals in whom clinical conditions of anxiety were diagnosed, there was marked variation in biological and psychological responses when they were exposed to the same stressors. This suggests that, in addition to biogenetic factors, psychological factors such as personality, conditioning to past experiences, coping skills and preparedness all have an impact. One person may have an increase in muscular tone that leads to tension headaches or backache; another may experience a stress-induced release of gastric acid, leading to decreased appetite and indigestion; a third may experience a hypersecretion of adrenaline from the adrenal medulla so that they feel 'jittery' and find it difficult to relax or get to sleep. These non-specific responses are, in fact, early warning signs that interventions aimed at buffering and resolving persistent stress are called for.

These inbuilt stress response patterns are common to all people, irrespective of whether or not they have a mental disorder. In the case of those with mental disorders, however, their responses may be coloured by the nature of the disorder. Whether people are predisposed to mental disorder or not, one aspect of the stress response that is frequently overlooked is that 'taxing of the system' is generally a temporary state of unbalance or disequilibrium; once the stressor is removed or resolved, things soon return to normal. In other words, the whole stress response is transient, subsiding once hyperarousal has diminished. Recognition of the short-term nature of the stress response provides a realistic perspective of the physical and psychological discomfort that accompanies it.

## ADAPTIVE AND MALADAPTIVE RESPONSES TO STRESS

Throughout life, people face many situations that produce stress and the presence of stress symptoms requires them to make some effort to cope. Unrelieved stress can lead to interruptions in adaptation and these interruptions may be experienced as mental health problems; in other words, disruptions in the interactions between the individual, the group and the environment produce a diminished state of mental health (AHM 1991). In response to poor adjustment to stress, some of these symptoms result in a number of psychological, behavioural and psychosomatic problems. Examples of the consequences of poor or maladaptive adjustment to stressors are provided in Table 2.2. Note the similarity of the responses to the reactions to stressors listed in Table 2.1. Many of the consequences of the maladaptive responses to stress in Table 2.2 are extensions of the reactions listed in Table 2.1.

*T*ABLE  2.2:    *Consequences of maladaptive adjustment to stressors*

| PHYSIOLOGICAL | PSYCHOLOGICAL | BEHAVIOURAL |
|---|---|---|
| high blood pressure | depression | behavioural avoidance |
| tachycardia | anger | social withdrawal and isolation |
| hyperventilation | job dissatisfaction | |
| dizziness | low self-esteem | smoking, alcohol and other drug use |
| paraesthesia (numbness) and tingling sensations | poor concentration | interpersonal disruptions |
| | poor decision making | |
| diaphoresis (sweating) | impaired memory | increased aggression and frustration |
| muscular rigidity | increased negative or self-critical thoughts | |
| headaches, stomach ulcers | | violent behaviour |
| | distorted, irrational ideas | loss of sexual interest |
| nausea | catastrophising (imagining the worst possible outcome) | |
| frequency of urination | | |
| diarrhoea | | |
| disrupted sleep patterns | exaggerating the effects out of true proportion | |
| | overgeneralising a few negative events to many life situations | |

How people cope with intense psychological needs and how they communicate their needs varies widely. Some respond with withdrawal, some with an increase in activity, some with emotional release. Responding with violence is one of the most immediate (albeit destructive) means of communicating an intense human need, as well as being a maladaptive and destructive coping behaviour. Violent behaviour (see Chapter 3) gives a sense of immediate and intense power and diminishes severe anxiety, at least temporarily (Moore, Dalziel & Burrows 1991). The kind of response that is likely to occur and its consequent effects on mental health are subject to factors other than personal attributes (see Chapter 5 for a discussion of these factors).

## *S*TRESS MANAGEMENT

There are many well-known stress management techniques which do, in fact, work, and there exists a rich body of literature to support their use. In order for them to work, however, they have to be learnt and applied. As with other personal expectations, people may expect stress management strategies to provide them with perfect **adaptation**. One of the dangers of having excessively high expectations of such techniques is that, if they fail to deliver, people may abandon them altogether, rationalising that 'they just don't work'. Such abandonment means that people obtain no benefit from the techniques at all. It is more realistic to recognise that, on the particular occasion the techniques were tried, they did not provide the relief sought. This does not mean they do not work but, rather, they didn't work as expected on that occasion.

Expectations that life will always be 'plain sailing' and stress-free are also unrealistic. Many life events are unpredictable and a view that we can 'control' stress is not helpful. Stress is inevitable and people may need to develop the capacity to tolerate occasional periods of increased stress. People should have appropriate strategies that enable them to reduce the unpleasant effects of stress to levels that are manageable.

It is common for people to want immediate relief from their distressing symptoms. Sometimes immediate symptomatic relief is possible, but it is useful to recognise that it is only symptomatic relief. The situations that generated the distress are most unlikely to be affected by relief of the symptoms. These are all key realisations in developing successful stress management strategies. The material presented in Chapters 5 and 11 highlights strategies that can be applied at a personal level in day-to-day life and also at a therapeutic level by mental health nurses in clinical settings. They are useful in managing responses to stressors and in helping to bring about a positive adaptation to stressful events (see also suggestions for further reading a the end of this chapter, where these strategies are referred to under 'stress management techniques').

## THE STRESS-VULNERABILITY MODEL

Vulnerability to stress, and the capacity to deal with stressors and adapt to them when they occur, are significant contributors to whether the response is ultimately adaptive or maladaptive. This perspective is referred to as the 'stress-vulnerability' model of adaptive and maladaptive responses to stressors (Falloon & Fadden 1993).

The stress-vulnerability model suggests that, in those predisposed, the symptoms of mental disorder are most likely to become evident at times when the combination of vulnerability and stress overwhelms the individual's capacity for adjustment and triggers the behavioural responses that are characteristic of that person's disorder.

From time to time, certain people experience major problems in relating to their environment, whether that environment is personal, social or cultural. A consequence of this unresolved disruption may be the development of mental disorder—a significant impairment in an individual's cognitive, affective and/or relational abilities which may require intervention and may be a recognised, medically diagnosable illness or disorder (AHM 1991). Acceptance of this definition of mental disorder implies that individuals can experience levels of maladaptation that are 'sub-threshold' or 'subclinical', and do not necessarily develop the clinical disorder. In order to qualify as having a disorder, the individual must enter a 'clinical range' of maladaptive responses which may become chronic and overwhelming (see Chapter 9). To justify a clinical diagnosis, very clearly defined criteria must be met. (To understand the scope and specificity of these criteria, refer to the *Diagnostic and Statistical Manual of Mental Disorders.*) These criteria include time factors such as how long the symptoms of disruption must be experienced before the diagnosis can be made.

Three recent studies have reported that stressful life events were precipitants of mental disorder. The studies showed that individuals with a diagnosis of panic disorder or depression had a higher frequency of life events that were 'more dangerous', severely threatening or involved severe loss than controls did (Finlay-Jones & Brown 1981; Roy-Byrne, Geraci & Udhe 1986; Faravelli, 1985). In those vulnerable to specific mental disorders, the stress response may precede the onset of the specific symptoms of the disorder. Case Study 2.1 describes the onset of panic disorder when the man was faced with a threatened separation from his wife.

## *C*ASE  STUDY  2.1:  *Onset of panic disorder*

David was a married research officer who had presented to his family doctor complaining of dizziness, headaches and tingling sensations in his fingers and toes. He had a negative result from a complete neurological examination, including both a normal CAT scan and a normal electroencephalogram. Despite these normal findings, David couldn't shake off the idea that the symptoms were the forerunners of an imminent stroke. His history indicated that his childhood had been dominated by a poor relationship with his father with whom he seemed to argue incessantly throughout his adolescence. His father suffered from hypertension and died of a stroke when David was 19 years old. In a subsequent argument with his mother, David was shaken when she accused him of contributing to his father's death by his rebellious behaviour.

Six months ago, David married, but since then the relationship with his wife has become tense and strained. His current symptoms actually started around the time of his marriage. He described how his first panic attack began after an argument with his wife during which she had yelled 'Your behaviour will kill me just as it did your father!' and stormed out. He later indicated to his doctor that this comment stirred painful feelings about his father and he was afraid that he would also lose his wife. He said his panic attacks also included shortness of breath, sweating, and a sense of impending disaster. He had become increasingly fearful of a recurrence of these attacks and the worry that he might actually die from a stroke, and was becoming more and more dependent on his wife to accompany him whenever he went out.

He was diagnosed as meeting the criteria for panic disorder, and treated accordingly.

There may be a predisposition (e.g. genetic, biological) that is a necessary element to mental disorder but, by itself, this predisposition may be insufficient to manifest within the clinical range so that a disorder can be diagnosed. Whatever the aetiology or predisposition, the addition of stressful life situations may be sufficient to push the individual beyond this threshold and into the clinical range. It is worth remembering, however, that stress does not inevitably lead to a mental illness. As Marks (1985) points out: 'stress ... a condition under which many of us work (and even play), does not necessarily have any adverse effect on the human mind or body' (p.16). It is often helpful to remind ourselves of this point.

Thus mental health and mental disorder exist on a continuum of adaptation to maladaptation and are influenced by biogenetic factors, personal vulnerability, personal attributes, coping abilities and coping strategies. General indicators of mental health are met when individuals have the capacity and the opportunity to interact in a meaningful way both within their own groups and with the environment in which those groups exist. This interaction promotes subjective well-being and optimal personal growth through the use of cognitive, affective and relational abilities.

Mental health problems arise when these abilities are impeded; when the impairment reaches defined thresholds at which persistent and repetitive distortions of thought, feeling and/or behaviour occur, the individual demonstrates the clinical characteristics of mental disorder. Environmental factors are important determinants of maladaptive responses to stressful events, but coping strategies that are adequate for the individual's day-to-day requirements can and do effectively assist management of stress responses.

## SUMMARY

- It is important to distinguish clearly between mental health and mental disorder. Mental health includes the capacity to get on well with other people in a way that promotes mutual well-being and the optimal development and use of mental abilities, including the cognitive processes involved in thinking, memory and recall.

- Mental disorder has a more structured definition and more specific usage than the concept of mental health. Mental disorder is the term used to designate changes from normal mental functioning that are sufficient and persistent enough to be recognised as clinical disorders.

- Stress is the reaction to life events that are experienced as difficult or powerful—more correctly referred to as stressors. Definitions of stress vary, but a useful rule of thumb is to assume that people are stressed when the demands of their lives exceed their personal resources.

- It is important for nurses to understand that stress is common, and that people with mental disorder have the same inbuilt responses to stress as everyone else. A frequently overlooked aspect of stress is its temporary effect; once the stressor has been removed, or the situation resolved, things quickly return to normal.

- Stress management techniques are effective methods of stress reduction, but they are not effective for everyone on all occasions. Excessively high expectations can lead to the opinion that the techniques 'just don't work', but stress is inevitable and people can learn to tolerate stress and to control their reactions to stressors.

# DISCUSSION QUESTIONS

1. What is positive mental health?
2. What distinguishes mental health problems from mental disorder?
3. How would you differentiate the term 'stress' from the term 'stressor'?
4. What accounts for the variability in biological and psychological responses of people exposed to the same stressors?
5. What are some of the techniques people can use to manage their reactions to stressors? (See further reading below.)

# EXERCISES

1. Keep a diary for a day and identify the factors that contribute to your mental health.
2. Analyse a situation in which you have felt stressed recently. Note your physical, emotional and behavioural responses to the relevant stressors and describe the coping strategies that worked best for you.
3. With a friend, discuss a situation that you both find stressful. Make a list of what it is about the situation that you both find stressful, taking careful note of similarities and differences. Compare the coping strategies you both use and their effectiveness. Next time you face the same situation try out some of the coping strategies used by your friend. Tell your friend how they worked for you. (See further reading below.)
4. Consider and explain any differences in the way you and your friend respond to situations you both find stressful.
5. Practise three different stress management techniques and demonstrate one of them to your group.

# FURTHER READING

- Standard texts on stress:
    King, M., Stanley, G. & Burrows, G. (1987) *Stress: Theory and Practice*, Sydney: Harcourt Brace Jovanovich.

Lazarus, R.S. (1971) 'The concept of stress and disease' in L.Levi (ed.) *Society, Stress and Disease*, London: Oxford University Press.

- Popular and accessible books on stress management techniques include:
  Bailey, R. (1989) *50 Activities for Managing Stress*, Aldershot: Gower.
  Benson, H. & Stuart, E. (1993) The Wellness Book: The Comprehensive Guide to Maintaining Health and Treating Stress-related Illness, New York: Simon & Shuster.
  Burns, R. (1992) *10 Skills for Working with Stress*, Sydney: NSW Business & Professional Publishing.
  Carnegie, D. (1994) *How to Stop Worrying and Start Living*, Sydney: Reed.
  Thompson, N. (1994) *Dealing with Stress*, Basingstoke: Macmillan.
  Wilkie, W. (1995) *Understanding Stress Breakdown*, Sydney: Millenium.

# REFERENCES

Australian Health Ministers' Conference (1991) *Mental health: statement of rights and responsibilities*. Report of the Mental Health Consumer Outcomes Task Force, adopted by the AHM, March 1991. Canberra: AGPS.

Clair, A.L., Oei, T.P.S. & Evans, L. (1992) 'Personality and treatment responses in agoraphobia with panic attacks', *Comprehensive Psychiatry* 33(5), pp.310–18.

*Diagnostic and Statistical Manual of Mental Disorders* (1994) (4th edn), Washington: American Psychiatric Press.

Falloon I.R.H. & Fadden, G. (1993) *Integrated Mental Health Care*, Cambridge: Cambridge University Press.

Faravelli, D. (1985) 'Life events preceding the onset of panic disorder', *Journal of Affective Disorders* 9, pp.103–5.

Finlay-Jones, R. & Brown, G.W. (1981) 'Types of stressful life events and the onset of anxiety and depressive disorders', *Psychological Medicine* 11, pp.803–15.

Henderson, A.S., Scott, R. & Kay, D.W. (1986) 'The elderly who live alone: their mental health and social relationships', *Australian & New Zealand Journal of Psychiatry* 20(2), pp.202–9.

Kenardy, J., Oei, T.P.S., Weir, D. & Evans, L. (1993) 'Phobic anxiety and panic disorder: cognition, heart rate and subjective anxiety', *Journal of Anxiety Disorders* 7, pp.359–71.

King, M., Stanley, G. & Burrows, G. (1987) *Stress: Theory and Practice*, Sydney: Harcourt Brace Jovanovich.

Lazarus, R.S. (1971) 'The concept of stress and disease' in L.Levi (ed.) *Society, Stress and Disease*, London: Oxford University Press.

Marks, F. (1985) 'Stress and the legal context', *Journal of Occupational Health and Safety—Australia and New Zealand* 1(1), pp. 16–20.

Moore, K., Dalziel, G. & Burrows, G.D. (1991) ' "Towards a gentler society": a series of questions: do you have the answers?' *Mental Health in Australia* 3(3), pp.52–6.

Roy-Byrne, P.P., Geraci, M. & Udhe, T. (1986) 'Life events and the onset of panic disorder', *American Journal of. Psychiatry* 143, pp.1424–7.

Selye, H. (1974) *Stress without Distress*, New York: New American Library.

Weir, D.N., Notowidjojo, F., Oei, T.P.S. & Evans, L. (1993) 'Cognitive concordance: impact of self-referent verbalisations on emotional and physiological arousal'. Presentation to World Federation for Mental Health, World Congress, Tokyo, August 1993.

# *C*overing up

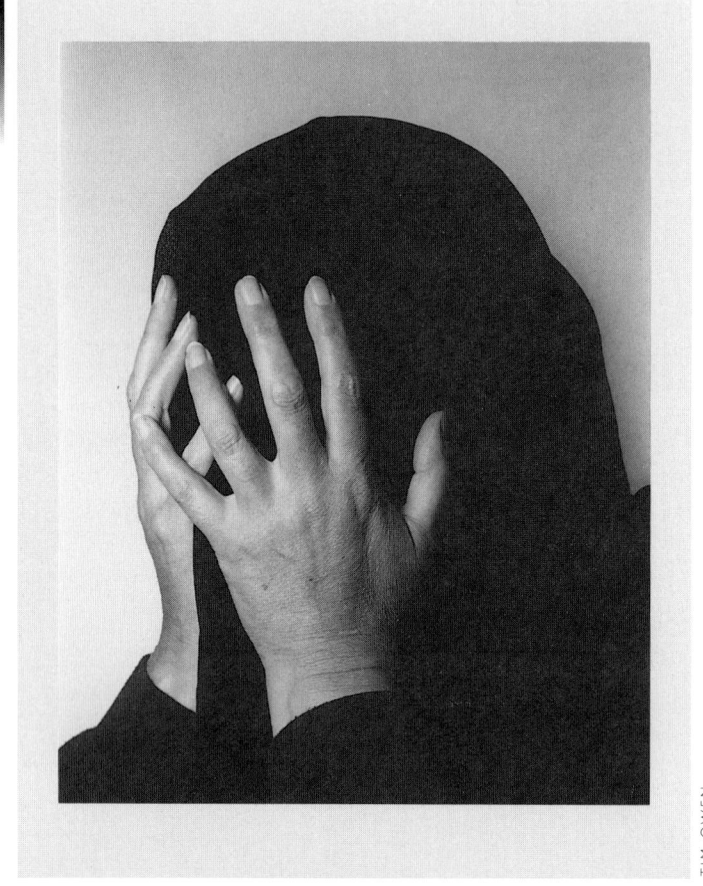

TIM OWEN

She could be anybody.
Domestic violence remains a hidden epidemic.

CHAPTER 3

# **V**IOLENCE AGAINST WOMEN

Marilyn Harris and Gail Hart

# CONTENTS

# LEARNING OBJECTIVES

This chapter will assist the reader to:

- appreciate the social, psychological and economic significance of violence against women;
- discuss the relationship between violence and gender inequality, indicating how violence is perpetuated by social, political and economic institutions;
- compare and contrast different explanations of violence;
- describe the cycle of violence;
- discuss the nurse's role in relation to violence in terms of prevention, advocacy, assessment and intervention;
- outline appropriate nursing interventions at individual, group and community level.

# INTRODUCTION

Australian and New Zealand societies both condemn and condone violence. On the one hand, people have a tolerance for violence as seen on television, in movies, or through the use of violent language by certain groups or individuals. On the other hand, violence is condemned as intolerable because of the suffering it causes. Nurses concerned with promoting mental health require an understanding of the nature of violence, including the historical, sociological and psychological factors that constitute it. The relationship between violence and issues of power and gender relations also needs to be understood, and will be addressed in this chapter.

Violence against women has been defined by a United Nations Declaration as

> ... any act of gender-based violence that results in, or is likely to result in, physical, sexual or psychological harm or suffering to women, including threats of such acts, coercion or arbitrary deprivation of liberty whether occurring in public or private life. (Canadian Panel on Violence against Women 1993, p.5)

Violence is linked to power. The persistence of violence against women is a manifestation of historically unequal power relations between men and women. At the same time violence operates as a social mechanism to perpetuate inequality.

Violence occurs on a continuum that ranges from verbal 'put-downs' to physical injury and death. Violence occurs across all types of family, social and domestic relationships (Flitcraft 1992). Violence is not limited to a particular social class, racial, religious or political group. It affects women of all ages. All women are vulnerable to violence simply because of their gender.

Eighty-seven per cent of all crimes are committed by men, and women and children are most at risk of physical and sexual assault, injuries and murder at the hands of men with whom they have been or are currently living with. (National Committee on Violence against Women 1993, p.15)

For many women the family home is a dangerous place as perpetrators of violence are often known to the victim—fathers, husbands, lovers.

It is vital that nurses acknowledge that they have a responsibility to understand violence, to act to identify abuse through appropriate assessment processes, and to intervene at the individual, family and group or community level in ways that will have positive outcomes for the future of our society.

# E XTENT OF THE PROBLEM

According to the National Committee on Violence (1990), as many as three in every ten families may be affected by violence. This estimate is comparable to figures from studies in the United States. In Queensland alone an estimated 24 000 women are seriously and chronically abused each year (Department of Family Services and Aboriginal and Torres Strait Islander Affairs 1991, quoted in Domestic Violence Resource Centre 1992). Yet wife battering is one of the most underreported crimes. One difficulty in obtaining accurate statistics on violence is that many victims choose not to report it. Instead they try to normalise abuse and keep it a private matter. Many women are unaware of the means of reporting violence, or fear retaliation for doing so.

An assessment of the incidence of wife abuse in Australia has not been made. However, several surveys have been conducted for specific purposes and provide a picture of violence, albeit a fragmented one. Alexander (1993) reported on a selection of results from Australian literature.

> From 1968 to 1986, 42.5% of all reported homicides in New South Wales were domestic killings, where the homicide victims were killed by members of their own family. Within the category of spouse killings, 73% of offenders were males … In Queensland, over 12 months from 1987 to 1988, 35 813 women's refuge bed-nights were provided for women and over 59 700 (bed-nights) for their children … From July 1991 to June 1992, over 4500 protective orders were made in Victoria in summary courts. While the cost of individual suffering related to violence is difficult to quantify, the economic costs to the Queensland community are estimated to be $108.6 million a year. (Alexander 1993)

Extrapolated to an Australian picture, the data suggests that the cost of **domestic violence** is $557 million a year and the cost of rape and sexual assault $63 million a year—a total of $620 million a year (NCVAW 1993). Violence against women and violence within families is widespread in our society and has consequences for people across all socioeconomic and cultural groups, occupations and educational backgrounds. Changing roles, social and economic pressure, alcohol, emotional tension and problems with children may be cited to explain individual cases of abuse. It must be acknowledged that these factors are not the cause of abuse, but that they may contribute to or become catalysts for episodes of abuse. Therefore, the issue of violence must be addressed at individual, family and community levels, and at the primary, secondary and tertiary levels of **prevention**, if Australia is to work towards a society free of violence and the suffering it causes.

## IMPACT ON HEALTH

Women who experience violence are more vulnerable to mental health problems. A Canadian study (Canadian Panel on Violence against Women 1993, p.11) found that women and children who had left a violent environment were five times more likely to exhibit psychological problems than a comparable group that had not experienced violence. These problems included severe **anxiety**, irritability, **depression**, confusion and memory loss. Almost half the women from violent relationships exhibited such problems. In contrast, less than 10% of the group that had not experienced violence reported such problems. The report of the National Inquiry into the Human Rights of People with Mental Illness (Human Rights and Equal Opportunities Commission (HREOC) 1993) noted that one-third of New Zealand women who had suffered domestic violence had also suffered mental health problems. Similar findings were reported in 1988 by the Queensland Domestic Violence Task Force.

Survivors of violent relationships are more likely to have higher **stress** levels and to suffer from **somatic** complaints. They have more time off work, difficulty concentrating, and reduced productivity because of injury and psychological trauma. Abuse accounts for one in every four **suicide** attempts by women (Flitcraft 1994). Women who are victims of violence are often misdiagnosed when they seek help and receive inappropriate treatment. They are institutionalised, medicated and restrained—sometimes for years—before an accurate diagnosis is made. The cost to the community is great; the cost to the women concerned is beyond calculation.

Table 3.1 shows the injuries sustained as a result of abuse. Note that related 'injuries', such as psychological problems, nervous breakdown and stress-related problems, are significant in the range of injuries that abused women experience.

TABLE 3.1: *Injuries sustained as a result of abuse (multiple response)*

| INJURY | FREQUENCY | % (table population = 661) |
|---|---|---|
| Bruising and bleeding | 403 | 61 |
| Psychological problems | 293 | 44 |
| Facial injury | 229 | 35 |
| Body injury | 177 | 27 |
| Head injury | 176 | 27 |
| Lacerations | 165 | 25 |
| Broken bones | 144 | 22 |
| Nervous breakdown | 105 | 16 |
| Loss of consciousness | 63 | 10 |
| Stress-related problems | 41 | 6 |
| Injuries to sexual organs | 37 | 6 |
| Obstetric problems | 18 | 3 |
| No injury | 32 | 5 |

VOICE BOX 3.1: *Breaking point*

After being in an abusive relationship for many years, suffering emotional, physical, sexual, social and financial abuse ... the women were able to leave the relationship with the help of women's refuges or other community support and move on to the independent living situation. It was during this period of independence, when the women were faced with the sole responsibility of providing and caring for their children and also faced with the years of abuse to their well-being and mental stability, that they experienced a mental and emotional breakdown.

These women had no previous history of mental illness. During this breakdown they were placed in a psychiatric hospital—separating them from their children. This placed the associated stigma on them of having been in a psychiatric unit. While the women were being treated in a psychiatric hospital their ex-husbands went to the Family Court and gained custody of the children on the basis that the mother was mentally unstable and unable to care for the children ... We believe that this illness was a short-term, 'one-off' occurrence directly related to years of abuse.

Voice Box 3.1 illustrates the deep trauma associated with violence and demonstrates how the victim continues to suffer even after the abuse ends. Importantly, it also illustrates how women are further victimised in the manner they are cared for by social welfare, health and legal institutions within our community. All forms of abuse have an impact on the mental health of those who are directly and indirectly involved. This indirect involvement may include children, other family members, friends who may witness the violence or the results of it, and other support people to whom the abused person discloses the abuse.

The role of the nurse and other health workers is crucial in helping women understand that any abuse is unacceptable. Violence destroys self-esteem; the lower a woman's self-esteem the less likely it will be that she will have the confidence to leave. The nurse's role is that of support and **advocacy** for women to facilitate their protection and personal growth. It is simply inappropriate that violence be managed as an illness. It is appropriate, however, that the mental health of women is addressed and, further, that the perpetrator be brought to justice through the courts.

## COMMUNITY ATTITUDES

There are harmful myths surrounding violence against women. One of the most damaging is the suggestion that the woman 'asked for it'. She teased and provoked him; she drank too much; she dressed seductively; she walked home alone; she went home with him; she didn't go home; she argued and disobeyed him; she never stood up to him. It can be argued that individual men exercise a choice to be violent and individual women exercise a choice to remain in a violent situation. Yet any explanation of violence against women which focuses on the choices and actions of individuals fails to account for the magnitude of the problem.

A national telephone survey revealed that almost half the population knew either a victim or a perpetrator of domestic violence, and that one person in five considered the use of physical force by a man against a female partner acceptable under certain circumstances. Verbal abuse, frightening a partner or threatening to hit, push or shove were all considered acceptable to some degree. One-third of this sample believed that domestic violence is a private matter and should be managed within the home (Public Policy Research Centre 1988). This attitude has significant consequences for women and children who are abused because the very institution that is considered appropriate to deal with the issue is also the place where violence is likely to occur.

While violence implies the use of physical force, violence may also be emotional, sexual or psychological. Emotional abuse includes teasing, criticising, isolating the woman from friends and family, and extreme jealousy. Sexual abuse is the use of force to secure sexual favours or the infliction of pain or injury during sex. Psychological abuse includes the threat of violence, attempts to control behaviour through fear or the destruction of property. Power over the victim is maintained by any of these means.

In some cultures hitting or punching a woman or child is common. An extreme example of violence against women which is culturally embedded is the custom of female circumcision. For many ethnic communities the conflict between 'family honour' and wider cultural beliefs of equality for women is causing heartbreak and violence (see Voice Box 3.2).

## VOICE BOX 3.2: *Father's honour*

Her face was bruised and swollen. Her nose broken. Her Syrian-born father had caught her smoking. She was 14. He displayed no remorse; quite the opposite. He refused to let his daughter see a doctor because he felt the injury should stand as a reminder of her sin. He was quite calm when he discussed the incident with the Community Services Officer who came to investigate at the prompting of a concerned schoolteacher. Over tea and biscuits the officer tried to draw him out on alternative forms of conflict resolution. 'What would you do if your daughter fell pregnant?' he asked. 'Kill her,' the father said. 'But if you killed her you'd go to jail,' the officer advanced. The father collected himself. 'I would rather go to jail a proud man than have my family live in shame.'

It is important that nurses are sensitive towards, and understanding of, cultural differences. Misunderstanding or ignoring a client's cultural beliefs and practices may contribute to feelings of alienation and prevent the development of trust and rapport. It can be difficult for Australian-born women who are victims of violence to seek help. For migrant women the barriers may be even greater. Not only are they protesting against the actions of an individual, usually a family member, they are protesting against the beliefs and practices of their community.

Nurses must be alert to attitudes and practices that allow violence. As a health care professional there is a responsibility to take action to eliminate such attitudes or practices, whether they occur on a personal or institutional level. Nurses can help individuals, families and larger communities to identify the cultural, social and economic conditions that restrict both men and women from making changes that would support less violent solutions to conflict (see Voice Box 3.3).

$V$*OICE BOX 3.3: Why didn't you seek help?*

Why didn't you seek help? I did. Early in our marriage I went to a clergyman who, after a few visits, told me that my husband meant no real harm, that he was just confused and felt insecure. I was encouraged to be more tolerant and understanding. Most important, I was told to forgive him for the beatings just as Christ has forgiven me from the cross. I did that, too.

Things continued. Next time I turned to a doctor. I was given little pills to relax me and told to take things a little easier. I was just too nervous. I turned to a friend, and when her husband found out, he accused me of either making things up or exaggerating the situation. She was told to stay away from me. She didn't, but she could no longer help me. Just by believing me, she was made to feel disloyal.

I turned to a professional family guidance agency. I was told there that my husband needed help and that I should find a way to control the incidents. I couldn't control the beatings—that was the whole point of seeking help. At the agency I found that I had to defend myself against the suspicion that I wanted to be hit, that I invited the beatings. Good God. Did the Jews invite themselves to be slaughtered in Germany?

I did go to two more doctors. One asked me what I had done to provoke my husband. The other asked if we had made up yet.

I called the police one time. They not only did not respond to the call, they called several hours later to ask if things had 'settled down' ... I could have been dead by then!

## THE CYCLE OF VIOLENCE

Women stay in abusive relationships because they hope that the relationship will eventually improve, they want to keep the family intact, or they are financially dependent. The experience of abuse damages self-esteem. Women who have experienced abuse often become isolated and alienated from friends and family. Sometimes the alienation occurs when they share their experience and are met with disbelief and suspicion. Sometimes the attempt to keep secret the violence in their life isolates them from a range of supports.

Violence within a relationship rarely happens only once. Usually a cyclical pattern of abuse develops—a build-up of tension, then a violent episode followed by a 'honeymoon period'. Tension builds up as the woman is attacked with insults, accusations or threats. She tries to calm the situation but the tension erupts into violence, involving sexual assault, injury or death to the woman. An external event or the emotional state of the man is more likely to trigger an incident than the woman's behaviour. After the incident the man is remorseful and seeks forgiveness. He may threaten suicide. He promises it will never happen again. He persuades her that she will be responsible for his welfare and the break-up of the family should she leave. If she stays, the honeymoon period is quickly concluded and another cycle of violence begins.

Abusive relationships within the context of marriage can start at any time. Sometimes abuse begins in a dating relationship. It may also begin after marriage, during pregnancy, after the birth of a child or after years of marriage. Abuse may occur only occasionally or it may be a daily experience. Often the abusive partner will apologise and promise to change, but few stop without outside intervention. Pressures of work, financial responsibilities, the influence of alcohol and the woman herself may be cited as excuses. It is important to remember that there are no acceptable excuses. Violence is a crime.

The cycle of violence as developed by Walker (1979) describes the consistent pattern of violence in which many people live. The cycle begins with a build-up of tension through disagreement without resolution: the tension-building phase. A standover phase occurs where fear and control are apparent. The victim becomes submissive to the control and anger until the perpetrator demonstrates self-righteous rage: the tension-relieving explosive phase. Tension is released and a remorse phase of justification, minimisation and guilt sets in. Pursuit and promises, helplessness and sometimes threats of suicide occur. This comprises the buy-back phase. As things settle, hope begins to rise and a honeymoon phase begins through a mutual dependency. The cycle is one of alternating denial and hope: denial in the controlling phase and hope in the calm phase. While this cycle describes violence for a single relationship, violence is also an intergenerational matter. Widom (1993) found that people arrested for delinquency, adult crimes and violent behaviour were more likely to have been abused or neglected as a child.

## ROLE OF NURSES

The first activity for nurses working in any setting with clients who are experiencing the effects of abuse is to examine their own attitudes to violence. King and Ryan (1989) give an account of myths that form the basis of beliefs held by some people—beliefs which either blame the victim of violence or prevent the nurse from cueing into signs that abuse exists, thereby preventing appropriate intervention. It must be remembered that nurses, too, are products of cultural values where victim blaming is commonplace. Fear is a common reaction of those who are faced with the situation of trying to help individuals protect themselves from abuse. The fear may be covertly demonstrated as a distancing from, or avoiding the plight of individuals or families experiencing abuse. What nurses need is an attitude that upholds gender equity, characterised by equality in interactions between individuals and groups.

### Prevention and advocacy

Nurses frequently come into contact with women who have experienced violence. Women may be admitted on the basis of their injuries, but sometimes hospitalisation for other reasons such as childbirth may offer an opportunity for a woman to share her experience of violence and seek support and counselling. A recent Australian study (McMurray & Moore 1994) of the problems faced by victims of spouse abuse when hospitalised has important implications for mental health nursing practice. The women in the study experienced disengagement and loss of status, disempowerment and lack of control, **stigma** and social isolation, and a sense of being misunderstood. They needed understanding and sensitive nursing care. They needed the opportunity to share their experience with someone who could listen with compassion and without judgment. Instead, the clients described the nurses as cold and impersonal. The nurses failed to ask enough questions to encourage the women to relate their story. They were not interested in the social context in which the abuse occurred.

Nurses can listen **empathically** and offer reassurance and information about support services. Women need to be reassured that they are not responsible for the assault. They need reassurance that leaving is an appropriate response and that assistance in developing an emergency plan to avoid future assault is available. Information and advice about child protection agencies, sheltered accommodation and legal support is also helpful, even when the woman is not yet ready to make major life changes. In this way, nurses can provide a boost to a woman's self-esteem and sense of self-worth.

## Assessment and intervention

It is important to bring the issue of abuse into the open for women who may feel ashamed, guilty or fearful of further abuse. Always make sure a private area is available to talk with women and always ensure that your exploration with the woman is done separately from the male partner. Perpetrators of abuse may have threatened the woman to maintain secrecy about the violence. Questioning a woman in front of a perpetrator may put the woman in further danger. Eye contact is important (although this may not be so in some cultures). **Screening for abuse should form part of any health assessment**. Explain to the woman that nurses have a general concern for the health of women and one of the major health risks is violence perpetrated against women in many different settings, including the home.

Women should be encouraged to respond to abuse assessment questions, but the woman will choose when she will talk, and how much of her personal experience she will share. The nurse needs to take care to develop a trusting relationship to make disclosure easier. The client needs to be aware of the cycle of violence, to know that violence usually escalates and is repetitive in nature. Providing an environment that is comfortable and allowing a trusting relationship to develop will optimise the likelihood of the woman being able to tell her story. Remember, you may be the first person to whom she has acknowledged her experience of abuse. All clients should be offered literature on referral resources and community services for abused women.

Even if the information is not used by that individual, it may be useful to family, friends or work colleagues.

The art of assessment to identify abused clients requires both a framework for assessment and a sensitivity to the information and cues being given by members of the family. Women need to be asked directly about their experience of abuse. It may be all that is needed to encourage a woman to disclose abuse to you. Unless the invitation is made, the burden of responsibility for exposing violence is left to the woman herself. Many women who experience abuse will have low self-esteem and will choose not to risk further humiliation if a trusting relationship with a health professional does not exist. King and Ryan (1989) provide questions which may be helpful when talking to women (Table 3.2).

TABLE 3.2: *Questions to use to uncover violence*

| DIRECT | INDIRECT |
|---|---|
| • Is somebody hurting you?<br>• Did someone hurt you?<br>• You seem frightened by your partner; has he hurt you?<br>• Have there been times during your relationship when you and your partner have had physical fights?<br>• Are you now in a relationship with a person who has hit (pushed, shoved, punched, kicked) you?<br>• Do you feel that your partner controls your behaviour too much? | • I see many women in my practice who come to me with injuries (or complaints) like yours. Some of them are being hurt by someone they are close to.<br>• I ask all my women clients if they are in a relationship or have an association with a person who is abusing or controlling them.<br>• Many women in our society experience abuse from men in their lives; is anything like that happening in your life? |

These questions not only invite clients to share their experiences, but they also demonstrate that the nurse has an empathy for women who may find themselves in a situation of wanting to disclose abuse and get help. A general screening approach may also help people to be more informed about the issue, enabling them to help others.

As well as direct and indirect questioning there are other indicators of abuse to look for. They include any one or more of the following: low self-esteem; submissiveness, nervousness, anxiety or flinching when touched; feeling withdrawn, depressed or excessively tired; physical injuries with inconsistent, vague or implausible explanations; personal time organised to ensure partner's needs are met; low stress tolerance; abuse of drugs or alcohol to 'escape'; extreme isolation—no friends, lack of telephone or family contact; sudden unexplained absences from work.

Should you be in a position to observe interactions between couples where one party is perpetrating violence against the other, the following behaviours may be evidenced by the violent partner: extreme jealousy and possessiveness; inconsistently very caring or over-solicitous; speaking for the other. Conversely, the victim may keep constant eye contact with her partner and/or change behaviour patterns in his absence (Women's Centre 1988). Observations and questions such as those described need to become part of a broad assessment to provide information that indicates abuse exists or that the woman or family is at risk.

## Intervention at the individual level

When a woman discloses abuse, always listen and believe her story. She may be comforted by telling her she is not alone. Allow her to express her feelings and validate them. Try to focus her energies on the immediate crisis, expressing concern for her safety and that of her children. She will need to know that help is available. The idea that no one deserves to be beaten, and that it is not her fault, should be reinforced. She may be embarrassed and humiliated by the abuse. The nurse should recognise and understand the woman's ambivalence. There may be cultural values which affect her behaviour and she may believe some of the myths about violence. It can be helpful to help her separate the myths from the truth about abuse. Remember that the effects of isolation, control, and crisis situations inhibit decision-making abilities. Work at building a rapport with her that is based on trust, remembering to address the problems that she identifies as immediate concerns.

The aims of continuing care will be to increase independence and self-esteem and to increase decision-making and assertion skills. Difficulties may arise for the nurse as a result of believing some of the myths about violence, or from a temptation to rescue a victim of violence. One helpful tactic is to think of the client as a **survivor** of violence rather than a victim. Seeking help is an active and two-way process. Learned helplessness may be a survival strategy of the health worker who fails to support women who disclose abuse.

Strategies in counselling women should focus on a caring approach that entails confronting the issue of violence for the client and defining the problem. The client is the expert and, given a range of alternative choices, will be able to decide on appropriate goals. An equal power relationship must be maintained, with health workers taking responsibility for their own point of view. A range of actions may be considered by the survivor—involving the police, counselling for practical and emotional assistance, making decisions, receiving support. She may also plan to leave home and, should this be the case, information on safety planning and the availability of emergency accommodation will be helpful. Legal advice may also be in the woman's interest for issues such as criminal action protection orders, getting the perpetrator to leave, child custody, access, and property disputes.

If a child confides an experience of violence or abuse, remain calm and find a private place to talk. Reassure the child that it is all right to tell someone. Do not push for information but reassure the child that support and protection are available. Do not confront parents or make promises you cannot keep. Seek advice while being sensitive to confidentiality. Resist the temptation not to get involved. Above all, believe the child.

## Intervention at a group level

Structured groups help to break down isolation, provide opportunities for women to talk about their experience and empower them through support. The group will be able to guide a woman through a range of issues that need to be dealt with: practical issues; feelings such as guilt, shame or fear; and developing assertiveness and self-esteem.

**Support groups** may also be helpful to children who are directly or indirectly affected by abuse, or are at risk of abuse. The themes of such groups include developing children's self-esteem and teaching them to value themselves. Teaching children that abuse is unacceptable in any form and under any circumstance are also major themes. Groups need to create a safe and positive atmosphere for children, to enable them to identify and express feelings in a non-violent way, and to help them sort out ambivalent feelings. The group should provide opportunities for children to learn facts about domestic violence and child abuse, and to alleviate their sense of responsiblity for their parents' problems. Groups also enable children to expand their knowledge and awareness of their rights and responsibilities. Developing problem-solving skills and building personal support systems need to be included to enable children to function effectively in their own environment.

## Intervention at the community level

The Duluth model (Pence & Paymar 1993) advocates a coordinated community response to the issue of violence in society. The model encompasses the development of common goals for multi-agency intervention, policies and procedures for intervening agencies, the development of a coordinating and monitoring project, and a process for interagency information sharing, as well as strategies that aim to reduce victim blaming in the system. Nurses have a role in strengthening existing networks and creating new ones to develop community-based facilities that address the needs of the community in regard to the prevention of violence at the primary, secondary and tertiary levels.

The Family Violence Team from the Doveton-Hallam-Endeavour Hills Community Health Centre, Victoria, won a Violence Prevention Award in 1992 for the Family Violence Program for Perpetrators and Survivors of Abuse. This program provides an example of a multifaceted, multidisciplinary and intersectoral approach to the needs of that community to prevent violence and alleviate the suffering from it. The program base is the Leeside Rotary House Project (Victoria), which provides accommodation for perpetrators of violence instead of moving the families who are the victims. The perpetrators are encouraged or ordered to take responsibility for their violent behaviour by entering a rehabilitation program, the Men's Violence Program. A men's support group also exists to help men while they are waiting to begin more formal courses to address their violent behaviour (Pence & Paymar 1993). As well, a skills development and support group is conducted for women who are, or have been, in destructive relationships, and special weekends are organised for women who wish to develop their ability to care for themselves and their children. On a broader community scale, a family violence education and information program has been implemented. Sexual abuse was identified as a problem in the area, so a course has been developed to help survivors heal from this trauma. This program consists of an eight-week course followed by a support group for the participants (Australian Institute of Criminology 1993).

Nurses should be aware of specialised services available to survivors of violence in order to provide appropriate referrals and ensure ongoing support. In addition, all nurses should be confident to provide appropriate assessment and counselling on an individual basis. Nurses can also play a role in breaking the silence surrounding violence by lobbying for more effective means of prevention and improved services.

## SUMMARY

- Violence against women is endemic in our society.
- Nurses have a responsibility to understand violence, to act to identify abuse through appropriate assessment processes and to intervene at the individual, family and community level in ways that have positive outcomes for the future of our society.
- Women who experience violence are more vulnerable to mental health problems. Studies show that women who have left a violent environment are five times more likely to exhibit psychological problems than women who have not experienced violence.
- The cycle of violence is an important concept in understanding the pattern of violence in which many women live. Typically the cycle begins with a build-up of tension, and includes standover, tension-release, buy-back and honeymoon stages.
- If abuse is disclosed, always listen and believe the person. Work at building support based on trust, and address the problems identified as immediate concerns.
- Aim to think of women who have been abused as survivors, not victims.

*C A S E   S T U D Y   3 . 1 :*   *'Promise you won't say anything'*

Jenny Hines is the CNC of a busy neonatal intensive care unit. She is well liked by her colleagues and has a reputation for being an excellent clinician and good manager. She has been married for less than twelve months to the Chief Radiographer at the hospital. She is delighted to learn that she is pregnant and shares the news with her workmates. Over the next month she misses six days of work and sometimes appears distracted and anxious. Then she suffers a miscarriage and has an additional week off work. A colleague visits her at home with a gift of flowers to offer condolences and support on behalf of the rest of the staff.

Jenny is understandably teary and distressed, but the colleague is unprepared for the story she relates. Jenny explains that her husband was very angry about the pregnancy. The evening of the miscarriage he returned home late after drinking with some friends, was verbally abusive, then shoved her down a long flight of stairs and kicked her in the abdomen. Afterwards he was apologetic and caring. He took her to the hospital, sought leave from work to care for her and made her promise to tell no one of the incident. She is unsure what she should do. She has visited her local GP, who prescribed medication to reduce her anxiety. Her husband is urging her to leave her job.

Before there is time to respond, Jenny's husband appears. Jenny's manner changes immediately and she explains to her husband that she has just been catching up on the gossip at work. As the colleague is leaving, Jenny whispers an urgent request: 'Please forget what I told you. It would hurt me more than losing the baby if anyone at work should know the truth. He's promised to change. I think we can work things out if I give up work'.

## Exercises

1.  From the above case study identify all the data indicating that Jenny Hines may be a victim of domestic violence.

2.  As a nurse, how might you establish rapport with Jenny in order to make a thorough assessment? Outline the questions you would ask. In your role as an advocate, what information would you offer Jenny?

3.  As a friend and colleague, what role (if any) do you have in making an assessment and offering appropriate intervention? Is there a conflict between the responsibilities of a colleague and those of a nurse? If so, how could such conflicts be resolved?

## *D* ISCUSSION QUESTIONS

1.  Why do women stay in abusive relationships?
2.  How is violence against women perpetuated by the media?

3. Can violence ever be considered culturally appropriate?

4. Why do nurses and other health workers often demonstrate unsympathetic attitudes towards women who are victims of violence?

# EXERCISES

1. Review a daily newspaper over a period of two weeks and collect any articles relating to violence against women. How are social values reflected in the style of reporting and the priority given to news items?

2. What services, including refuges, are available to women and children who experience violence in your community? Can these services be accessed by public transport? What costs are involved? Are the services accessible in the evenings and at weekends? How easy was it for you to find this information?

3. Outline the advantages and disadvantages of providing refuges for the men who are violent rather than for women and children who are victims of violence.

4. Arrange to have a women's shelter worker or a women's support group come and talk to your class.

5. You have a close friend or relative whom you suspect is being abused by their spouse. What do you do?

# FURTHER READING

- Campbell, J. (1989) 'A test of two explanatory models of women's responses to battering', *Nursing Research* 38(1), pp.18–24. This paper explores two models of responses to violence—grief and learned helplessness—and reviews the models' utility for nursing practice.
- Campbell, J. & Humphreys, J. (1994) *Nursing Care of Survivors of Family Violence*, St Louis: Mosby. This work offers a summary of the explanations of violence.
- Walker, Alice (1992) *The Color Purple*, New York: Bantam. A moving account of women's lives.

# OTHER RESOURCES: MOVIES

- *Once were Warriors* (1994). Powerful film depicting violence within a Maori family. Directed by Lee Tamahori.
- *The Accused* (1988). Film about a rape case that explores community attitudes to violence against women. Directed by Jonathan Kaplan.

# REFERENCES

Alexander, R. (1993) 'Wife battering—an Australian perspective', *Journal of Family Violence* 8(3), pp.229–49.

Australian Institute of Criminology (1993) *The Australian Violence Prevention Awards 1992*, Canberra: AIC.

Canadian Panel on Violence against Women: Final Report (1993) *Changing the Landscape: Ending Violence, Achieving Equality*. Minister of Supply and Services, Ottawa, Canada.

Human Rights and Equal Opportunities Commission (1993) *Human Rights and Mental Illness: Report of the National Inquiry into the Human Rights of People with Mental Illness*, vols 1 & 2, Canberra: AGPS.

Derouard, M., Marz, C. & Cava, M. (1993) *The Road beyond Violence against Women: A Public Education Manual for Nurses*, North York, Ontario: North York Public Health Department.

Domestic Violence Resource Centre (1992) *Factsheet No. 2: Statistics on Domestic Violence*, Brisbane: Domestic Violence Resource Centre.

Flitcraft, A. (1992) 'Violence, values, and gender' (editorial). *Journal of American Medical Association* 267(23), pp.3194–5.

Flitcraft, A. (1994) 'The AMA Guidelines one year later', National Committee on Violence Against Women Newsletter (1994) *NCADU Voice Special Edition Domestic Violence is a Health Issue*, Washington DC: NCADU, p.3–5.

King, C. & Ryan, J. (1989) 'Abused women: dispelling myths and encouraging intervention', *Nurse Practitioner* 14(5), pp.47–58.

Legge, K. (1994) 'Living two lives', *The Australian Magazine*, September 3–4, pp.20–7.

McMurray, A. & Moore, K. (1994) 'Domestic violence: Are we listening? Do we see?' *Journal of Advanced Nursing* 12(1), pp.23–8.

National Committee on Violence (1990) *Violence: Directions for Australia*, Canberra: Australian Institute of Criminology.

National Committee on Violence against Women (1993) *The National Strategy on Violence against Women*, Office of the Status of Women, Department of Prime Minister and Cabinet. Canberra: AGPS.

Pence, A. & Paymar, M. (1993) *Education Groups for Men who Batter—The Duluth Model*, New York: Springer Publishing Co.

Public Policy Research Centre (1988) *Domestic Violence Attitude Survey*, Canberra: Office of the Status of Women, Department of Prime Minister and Cabinet.

Queensland Domestic Violence Task Force (1988) *Beyond these Walls*, Brisbane: Qld Government Printing Service.

Walker, L. (1979) *The Battered Woman*, New York: Harper & Row.

Widom, C. (1993) 'The cycle of violence'. Paper presented at the Second National Conference on Violence, Canberra.

Women's Centre (1988) *Why does she stay?* San Joaquin County, Stockton, California.

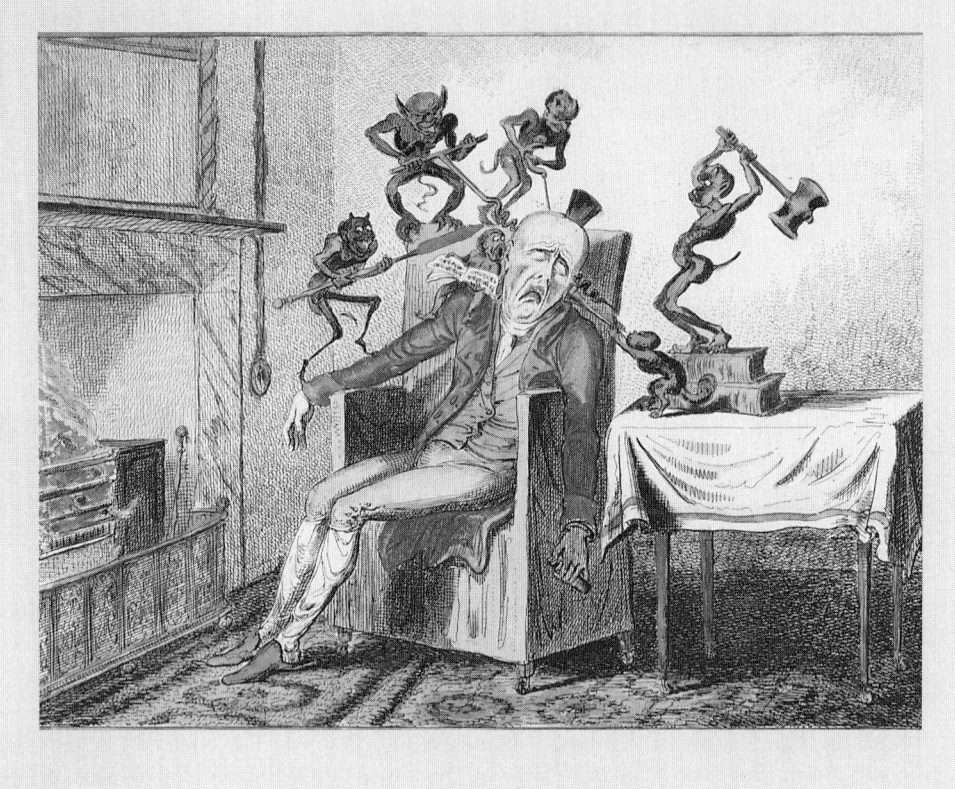

GEORGE CRUIKSHANK

The immediate, if sometimes only fleeting, experience of pain and suffering are part
of the everyday lives of so many people with chronic illness.

## CHAPTER 4

# CHRONIC ILLNESS

Anne Dewar and Jennie Barr

## *C*ONTENTS

# LEARNING OBJECTIVES

This chapter will assist the reader to:

- understand demographic trends relevant to the mental health of people with chronic illness;
- identify the impact of chronic illness on people's lives;
- describe mental health changes that may result from chronic illness or from the use of prescription drugs;
- discuss possible explanations for the association between chronic illness and mental health problems.

# INTRODUCTION

An ageing population and advances in technology have led to an increase in the presentation of chronic illness and **disability** in Australia and New Zealand. The chronically ill and the disabled have become major health care consumers in these countries, increasing demands on social resources, the health care system and caregivers. In line with these trends, nurses are increasingly caring for clients with chronic illness in all practice settings. This chapter discusses the prevalence and seriousness of mental health problems attendant on chronic illness. It aims to provide nurses with an awareness of the problem, and strategies to ensure that the nursing care of people with chronic illness does not neglect the promotion of mental health in this high-risk group of clients.

# DEMOGRAPHY OF CHRONIC ILLNESS AND DISABILITY

Recent surveys show that 66% of the Australian population report that they have a long-term illness or disability (McLennan 1990) and 37% of the New Zealand population report that they have been told by a health professional that they have a long-term illness or disability (New Zealand Public Health Commission 1993). Disability increases with age: 3% of children 0 to 4 years are disabled compared with 64% of people aged 75 years and over.

The main categories of chronic illness and disability for both Australia and New Zealand are: asthma; high blood pressure; diabetes; hearing and sight loss; physical disability; psychiatric/psychological problems; and intellectual handicap. Rates of these conditions vary between countries and it is extremely difficult to make valid comparisons because there is no internationally standardardised method of collecting statistical data on disease rates. When assessing for changes in rates of illness or disability, it is best to compare within a country so that an accurate determination of increase or decrease in conditions can be made.

# EFFECTS OF CHRONIC ILLNESS ON PSYCHOLOGICAL WELL-BEING

The experience of chronic illness involves adjustment to losses: loss of function (paralysis, deafness or blindness) and/or loss of independence or mobility. These losses create an emotional challenge for the client and can lead to mental health problems such as **anxiety**, mood alteration, **depression** and, possibly, **suicide**. Anxiety and mood alteration are the most common mental health problems associated with chronic illness. However, not all people with a chronic illness or disability develop such problems. In fact, the relationship between **mental disorder** and physical illness is complex and difficult to predict. It is also difficult to appreciate how chronic illness is perceived by the sufferer. Voice Box 4.1 offers insight into how the person with a chronic illness feels.

## $V$OICE BOX 4.1: *The experience of chronic illness*

The illness becomes a part of you, it may not always be seen or felt but its always there. Just as you begin to feel its all over and you're on top of the world it strikes back knocking you to the ground again. It's not the symptoms so much … oh, they get you down too but rather it's how the symptoms affect other parts of your life. I used to do a lot of knitting but now the pain in the fingers is so great that I had to give it up. I love to cook for the family but I can't manage the big saucepans on the stove with my hands. My daughter cooks for me on the weekend now and meals-on-wheels delivers meals for me during the week. People fussed over me at the time telling me that it was better this way, at least I'd eat but they missed the point, I felt like I was losing something … I don't know, a part of me, my independence, something like that.

I know I have to keep going, I have to keep active but even walking is hard sometimes with the pain in the hip. It means I can't go out like I used to … I miss my friends, they used to visit, you know, but I guess they got sick of always having to come here. I get so down sometimes, the doctor tells me it's common for people in pain to be depressed. He was trying to be nice I guess but it didn't make me feel better. I've got the pain not him. I'm on so many pills, pills for this, pills for that. That's enough to make anybody feel down. Still, life is okay. I've learnt to do things differently, I take it slowly now.

Having an illness can make you lonely though. You don't like to whinge but sometimes you need to talk about it. People don't want to talk about the illness. I guess they don't know what to say but they don't have to say anything really. I know there are no answers or cures but I just want people to listen. Sometimes I wish people would look at me, there is so much focus on the illness and what I can and can't do, but nobody asks me if I'm okay, or whether I mind if I can't cook anymore.

The experience described in Voice Box 4.1 indicates how depressive symptoms may be experienced by a person with a chronic illness. Estimates are that 20–50% of psychiatric patients have an undiagnosed medical illness (Koranyi 1979; Hall et al. 1981; Wise & Taylor 1990), with at least 25% of this group requiring drug treatment for the psychiatric disorder (Nickel, Brown & Smith 1990; Wise & Taylor 1990). Mental health problems can develop in a medically ill patient due to a psychological reaction to the physical illness (Mayou, Seagroatt & Goldacre 1991) or the mental health problem may have existed prior to the onset of physical symptoms. Mental health problems can also arise from the disease process itself, or as a result of treatment, particularly drug treatment. Furthermore, mental health problems can present as somatic complaints. Thus, the picture is difficult to unravel and it is not always possible to determine the coexistence of more than one illness. For example, when a person suffers fatigue, it is difficult to ascertain whether this is a symptom of an illness or a psychological reaction to illness. Mood changes, too, may be either a symptom of illness or a reaction to illness.

Long-term illness can have an unpredictable course with exacerbations of symptoms and intervals of relative wellness. Additionally, the impact of chronic illness on lifestyle may be significant, due to continuous interventions such as special diets, medications, injections, dialysis or other invasive procedures. The demands of the illness, together with the requirements of daily life, must often be managed with decreasing physical and emotional resources. Factors particular to specific diseases can also contribute to depression; for example, nocturnal symptoms and the amount of distress experienced during an asthma attack have been associated with depression in people with asthma (Janson-Bjerklie, Ferketich & Benner 1993).

Physical problems that commonly accompany chronic illness are sleeplessness, limited mobility, pain and fatigue. Sleeplessness, which often compounds the symptoms of an illness, can occur because of incontinence, pain or anxiety. Limited mobility and subsequent dependence is a major stressor (see Chapter 2). Pain, a frequent symptom of a diverse range of health problems, may involve modifying or discontinuing valued activities. Responses to pain include frustration, fear, anger, helplessness and dependence. Fatigue, a common symptom of many chronic physical and psychiatric conditions, has been associated with negative moods (Small & Graydon 1993). In one study, 50–80% of people with a psychiatric disorder were found to have persistent and disabling fatigue (Price et al. 1992). These physical symptoms can have a profound impact on the person's emotional well-being.

Changes in **body image** too can result from illness or disability. It must be remembered that body image is formed both by people's *perceptions* of how they look, as well as their actual appearance. As social worth is often attached to the ability to perform tasks and functions, and to physical appearance, those unable to adjust to disfigurement, disability or reduced functioning are at greater risk of developing psychological complications (Drench 1994). Changes in body image threaten the self-concept, which in turn increases feelings of being different and of rejection. Nurses must be aware that such feelings can lead to withdrawal from social contacts and reluctance to engage in conversation. Therefore, it is vital for nurses to create opportunities for chronically ill clients to express freely their concerns about disfigurement, disability and loss of function.

## *M*ENTAL HEALTH CHANGES ASSOCIATED WITH CHRONIC ILLNESS

There are several mental health problems that can be associated with chronic illness. They include depression, anxiety, mania and medication-induced psychosis.

## *Depression*

The relationship between chronic illness and **depression** is complex, as many factors other than the presence of illness influence the onset and course of depression. Certain sociodemographic factors such as living alone, low income, low educational status, old age, and changes in personal or professional roles can predispose even a well person to depression (Badger 1993). Depression is prevalent in the general population and is not always detected or treated (see Chapter 5). A proportion of people with depression will become physically ill and the subsequent effects of the disease may compound any existing emotional problems. As well, individuals suffering from chronic illness may also experience distressing life events or losses, such as the death of a significant other, or divorce, and these can precipitate depression.

Depression is more prevalent among disabled people than among the non-disabled. However, controversy exists regarding the significance of severity of illness or disability to the severity of depression (Friedland & McColl 1992). Level of disability does not always correlate with depression. Seriously disabled people have been found not to be depressed and much less disabled people have reported severe depression. For example, in a study of patients with spinal cord injuries, Schulz and Decker (1985) found that rates of depression were not significantly higher in disabled people. Estimates of the frequency of major depression in studies of spinal cord injury vary, but generally researchers agree that the level of depression is not high—15–20% (MacDonald, Nielson & Cameron 1987; Cairns & Baker 1993).

Depression has been associated with increased mortality in children suffering from asthma (Janson-Bjerklie et al. 1993). Both depression and anxiety have been reported in middle-aged males suffering from cardiac disease. Studies of myocardial infarction in this population have found that depression may continue for as long as eight years after the event (Nickel et al. 1990). In the older person, depression can result not only from the diseases commonly experienced by this age group, but also from the many stressful life events that occur in later life, such as retirement, loss of spouse, decrease in income and changes in daily activities (Badger 1993). (See Chapter 12.) Pain has also been associated with depression in the older person. Individuals experiencing a combination of stressors may become more prone to psychological problems and psychiatric illness. Therefore, it is important to be particularly vigilant for behavioural and mood changes in chronically ill clients and older people, as these groups of clients have an increased risk of depression.

## Neurological conditions

Depression has been associated with many neurological conditions. It can present as a neurological symptom, or as an exaggeration of a neurological symptom (Caplan & Ahmed 1992). A further contributing factor to depression in this group is the cognitive disturbance that may be associated with neurological conditions. These disturbances can reduce the person's ability to access resources and sources of support (Caplan & Ahmed 1992). Parkinsonism, multiple sclerosis (MS) and cerebrovascular accidents (CVAs) carry a particularly high incidence of depression. For example depression in CVA victims has been reported to range from 25% to 50% of all victims (Graff-Radford & Biller 1992; Acorn & Andersen 1990; Caplan & Ahmed 1992).

The aetiology of depression in these conditions is not clearly understood because of the complex neurochemical, anatomical and psychological factors involved (Acorn & Andersen 1990; Habermann-Little 1991; Bunting & Fitzsimmons 1991; Caplan & Ahmed 1992). Symptoms of depression, such as mood disturbances, fatigue, decreased ability to participate in activities, slowing of actions and changes in behaviour, may either be part of the disease process itself (Caplan & Ahmed 1992) or a psychological reaction to functional losses and pathological changes. The symptoms experienced will depend on the site of neurological lesions and the functions of the affected lobes.

It is important for the nurse to understand the pathological processes involved in neurological conditions and the corresponding changes in function, behaviour and mood that can occur. Left frontal lobe cerebrovascular lesions are associated with a higher incidence of depression, while the more severe depressions correlate with lesions close to the left frontal pole. Right hemisphere and parietal lobe lesions, on the other hand, produce decreased awareness of deficits and a lack of concern, which may reduce the incidence of depression (Caplan & Ahmed 1992). Cerebral involvement has been linked to a greater incidence of depression in people with MS (Acorn & Andersen 1990).

## Treatment factors in depression

Although differentiating between depressive symptoms due to disease processes and depression related to the stressors and losses of illness is a medical responsibility, the nurse can assist. This differentiation is important because the two conditions are treated differently. Symptoms associated with changes related to the disease process require treatments relevant to the condition. Depression associated with an emotional reaction can be treated with medication and other forms of treatment such as counselling. Nursing responsibilities include assessment of client reactions and changes in mood. Such observations should be recorded and reported.

## Measurement of depression

Caution must be used in assessing depression in a chronically ill person. Many instruments commonly used to measure depression contain somatic items such as fatigue, decreased physical activity and loss of appetite, which can indicate depression and/or a physical illness. It has been suggested that instruments with somatic indicators should not be used to assess the presence of depression in people with a known physical illness (Marks & Millard 1990), or should be used with caution, to prevent confusion and ensure proper treatment.

## Effects of depression

Depression in association with chronic illness can result in greater disability, poorer functioning and higher morbidity (Badger 1993). Anxiety and depression affect quality of life by interrupting the activities of daily living. As a result, adherence to a drug regimen and the ability of the individual to access and utilise social support may be affected. In the process of adapting to the demands of an illness, an individual may become set apart from others. A sense of isolation can compound psychological problems and lead to a reduction in social support. For example, depression following a CVA has been associated with inadequate social support, and decreasing functional ability has been associated with a decreasing number of social supports (Lambert et al. 1990).

Social support from partner, family, friends and health professionals is related to psychological well-being because it provides a buffer against the associated stressors and promotes adaptation to illness (Primomo, Yates & Woods 1990). Research into the association between social support and well-being has concluded that there is a positive relationship between psychological well-being and satisfaction with both social supports and the number of social supports (Barerra 1991; Olsen & Sabroe 1991; Krol, Sanderman & Suurmeijer 1993). Despite the recognised benefits of social support, dependence on caregivers can be stressful, particularly when this involves role changes for both the chronically ill person and the carer. Such **stress** is compounded when care is long-term.

## Anxiety

Anxiety is a reaction to a perceived threat and is a common response to illness (Brunner & Suddarth 1988). **Anxiety**, experienced in a physiological, psychological and behavioural manner, is defined as a sense of self-doubt, apprehension and dread (Brunner & Suddarth 1988; Murray & Huelskoetter 1991). (See Chapters 2, 9 and 10.) Anxiety can occur with any illness, but has been particularly associated with cardiovascular conditions, endocrine disorders, asthma and chronic obstructive airways disease.

An anxiety disorder may compound the symptoms of an existing chronic illness. If the symptoms of anxiety are secondary to a medical illness, the person will need to be supported until these symptoms abate. This usually occurs as the primary illness improves. During this process, the nurse should offer opportunities for the person to express feelings such as fear and frustration, and assist the client through attentive listening.

Pharmacological treatment may be prescribed for anxiety—benzodiazepines, short-acting barbiturates and clonidine. Nurses can complement pharmacological treatment through reassurance, education about anxiety and its symptoms, and by teaching the patient relaxation techniques (see Chapters 11 and 15).

As certain medications have the potential to cause anxiety, the nurse must be alert for the various signs and symptoms of anxiety, such as increased heart and respiratory rate, increased perspiration, restlessness, irritability, sleeplessness and other behavioural changes (see Chapter 9). The nurse can also suggest the possibility of a change in medication. Drugs reported to have caused anxiety include:

- cardiac inotropic agents
- thyroid and antithyroid agents
- corticosteroids
- neuroleptics
- nonsteroidal anti-inflammatory compounds
- bronchodilators
- salicylates
- antihistamines

*Note: Readers are advised to refer to a comprehensive drug handbook to familiarise themselves with the drug groups identified in this chapter. Specific drugs, their therapeutic range, indications, contraindications and possible side effects should be noted.*


## Mania

**Mania** is a disturbance in mood which can present with elation, hyperactivity, agitation, and accelerated thinking and speaking (Kah & Kupper 1993). Occasionally, a medically ill person becomes manic. It is important to differentiate between bipolar disorder and secondary mania, which is associated with a medical illness or caused by the medication used in the treatment. From reported case studies, people who are vulnerable to mental disorder may be predisposed to secondary mania. Medical conditions which have been reported to be associated with mania include epilepsy, multiple sclerosis, infections, tumours, and endocrine and neurological disorders (Matsumoto & Ueyama 1994; Salazar-Calderon-Perriggo, Oomen & Sobonya 1993).

Where secondary mania is present, changes in medication could be considered; otherwise, the treatment should be the same as that for primary mania (see Chapters 9 and 11). Drugs reported to have caused mania include:

- thyroid and antithyroid agents
- corticosteroids
- neuroleptics
- antianxiety agents
- histamine antagonists
- tricyclic antidepressants
- alcohol

## Medication-induced psychosis

Several drugs are known to affect a person's mental status. Steroids are known to have caused significant mental health changes (Klein 1992; Travlos & Hirsch 1993; Wysenbeck, Leibovici & Zoldan 1990). The mental health side effects of steroids can persist for as long as 150 days after the cessation of the drug (Travlos 1993). Headaches, sleep disturbances, restlessness and increased motor activity have been reported in patients who have taken steroids. Elderly patients and those with a pre-existing mental illness are more susceptible to mental health reactions to steroid therapy (Goldstein & Preskorn 1989). In a study of 150 patients who were diagnosed with steroid-induced **psychosis,** 17% displayed suicidal behaviour (Braunig, Bleistein & Rao 1989).

There are isolated reports of non-prescribed drugs, such as sinus medication, being associated with changes in a person's mental status (Brown 1990; Nurses' Drug Alert 1990). These reports have noted psychological reactions which have been associated with the abuse and overuse of these drugs. It is recommended that, during the assessment of people with psychotic symptoms or other changes in mental status, all medications—both prescription and non-prescription drugs—and the dosage should be noted. If medication is to be withdrawn, medical supervision is required.

Nurses should be alert to the possibility that toxic levels of certain drugs can cause acute psychosis. Patients can be educated about the overuse of prescription and non-prescription medications. Although the number of reports of non-prescribed drugs associated with psychosis is small, the idiosyncratic nature of individual responses to drugs and dosages requires nurses to be alert to the possibility of mental status changes in any individual taking either prescription or non-prescription drugs. Drugs reported to have caused psychosis include:

- antiparkinson agents
- corticosteroids
- antibiotics
- antihypertensive agents

## SUICIDE AND CHRONIC ILLNESS

Patients with chronic debilitating diseases are at risk of **suicide**. Increased suicide rates have been found in association with cancer, Huntington's chorea, epilepsy, musculoskeletal disorders, peptic ulcer and HIV/AIDS (Blumenthal 1990, p.529). Statistics on suicide rates are difficult to obtain as the cause of death is not always accurately determined; for example, death due to suicide in the terminally ill may be attributed to the disease. However, a Swedish study estimated that 25–70% of adult suicide victims suffer from physical illness (Allebeck & Bolund 1991, p.529). It is not the diagnosis of the illness that leads to suicide, but the concerns about physical deterioration and social losses that cause depression and intense emotional distress (Allebeck & Bolund 1991). Suicide has been linked to chronic illness sufficiently often for nurses to be vigilant in identifying symptoms of depression and anxiety, and to heed warning signs that may indicate suicide intent (Valente, Saunders & Cohen 1994; Garden, Garrison & Jain 1990).

In older clients the combination of advancing age and chronicity increases the risk of suicide because of the concomitant losses in this age group. In young people who suffer from a chronic illness the risk is also high. Diseases with an increased risk of suicide in the younger age group are HIV/AIDS, epilepsy (Blumenthal 1990) and schizophrenia (Caldwell & Gottesman 1992). When assessing suicide risk, the nurse should consider not only the disease but the condition of the individual, the accompanying losses, the degree of impairment and the individual's response to these factors.

## NURSING ASSESSMENT

Nurses must be able to identify symptoms of anxiety and depression and be alert for the onset of these symptoms, particularly in those most at risk (see Chapter 9 for guidance on how to conduct a mental status examination). The nurse must also be ready to use strategies that will lessen the impact of these reactions. Assessment is particularly important when working with the older person, who may suffer from more than one chronic illness and experience concurrent losses.

Baseline nursing assessments should incorporate a personal and family history (see Chapter 12), taking careful note of any episodes of depression and/or anxiety. The type of depressive episodes, frequency and pattern, and type of symptoms should be noted (Acorn & Andersen, 1990, p.212). Assessments should include problem-solving techniques and methods of managing stress (see Chapter 11). Determining support networks, including type and even number of social supports, and subsequent satisfaction with that support, is also important in a nursing assessment.

### Joint goal setting

Nursing care of people with a chronic illness requires accurate assessment and joint planning and implementation of interventions that are satisfactory to clients. To develop strategies that will enhance well-being, nurses should focus on the needs from a client perspective. The goals set should be based on achievable aims; they should reflect the personal and cultural beliefs of clients, and be suited to their lifestyle. The value of this process is enhanced by involving clients as much as possible in setting goals for their own care.

## NURSING INTERVENTIONS

Nursing interventions must be directed towards minimising the impact of the illness. Fatigue, for example, can be addressed by treating pain, promoting sleep, and establishing means of conserving energy. The person will require skills in managing both the physical condition and the emotional impact of the illness. If clients have a neurological condition with depressive symptoms, their education should be tailored to their decreased function. Clients who are depressed and have cerebral involvement may also have verbal, visuospatial and attention deficits, so particular strategies that allow for these deficits must be developed (Acorn & Andersen 1990). These nursing strategies help to prevent and overcome **learned helplessness**.

### Stage theories of adjustment

Elisabeth Kübler-Ross (1969) identified a five-stage process of adjustment to loss. These stages are frequently described as denial, anger, bargaining, depression and acceptance. Stage theories assume that people who have suffered a loss, or are terminally ill, will progress through clearly defined stages, albeit at different rates, with movement back and forth between stages. Unfortunately, the popular conception of progression through these stages has resulted in unrealistic expectations being placed on patients to comply with stage theories (Friedland & McColl 1992). Failure to progress through these stages has even been considered an indication of poor adjustment and a forewarning of difficulties in adaptation later on. This notion has been criticised by Wortman and Silver (1989) who have argued that depression is not inevitable in adjustment to loss.

Recent research has also been critical of the notion of stage theories of adjustment (Cairns & Baker 1993; Friedland & McColl 1992), as it is difficult to determine a generalised concept of normal reactions to illness and disability. The expectation that they will conform to stages of adaptation is a burden for patients. Instead of attempting to label and categorise patients into stages, the focus of adaptation should be on nurses accepting emotional expressions as genuine and relevant (Cairns & Baker 1993).

### Adjustment

Determining the meaning of any losses to clients is essential and should be thoroughly assessed, but the nurse should be careful to avoid making assumptions about the appropriate amount of distress associated with any loss. The nurse should also keep in mind that clients' subjective assessments of their physical limitations are a more valid indicator of health impairment than any objective assessment (Badger 1993).

To help clients adjust to the effects of their illness, nurses must accept the full range of emotions experienced by patients, including mood swings and anger, in the knowledge that people respond to chronic illness in different ways. Nursing interventions help to reduce the stress experienced by people with chronic illness, but sick and disabled people still experience the stress associated with negative life events, including divorce and bereavement. Sensitivity to the patient's thoughts and feelings offers opportunities for the nurse to encourage more positive thoughts that will assist the client to rebuild confidence and self-esteem.

If a change in lifestyle is required, the person will need support and encouragement. The nurse may need to suggest the development of new skills that will aid the transition. Such changes impact on significant others such as family and friends, so the nurse may also need to support the people significant to the patient.

The client will require skills in managing the emotional impact of the illness as well as the physical condition. This process includes recognition that times of feeling 'down' are normal, and that fatigue drains emotional reserves. Teaching strategies to conserve energy can decrease fatigue and give patients a sense of control over their symptoms. For example, people can plan daily activities around times of maximum energy or choose to do those things that provide the greatest personal satisfaction.

The unpredictable nature of many chronic illnesses makes people believe that their illness is beyond their control (Taal et al. 1993). Perceptions of reduced control may cause anxiety and depression (Bandura 1986). Feeling depressed and anxious may in turn decrease motivation to meet the demands of the illness (Badger 1993). Taal et al. (1993) found that to improve the self-management of disability and pain it was important to strengthen the client's **self-efficacy**. Strengthening clients' beliefs in their ability to control symptoms can improve their capacity for self-management and facilitate adjustment. However, feeling that one should be in control of a condition when this is not possible may increase stress (Doan & Gray 1992).

## Valuing client knowledge

The knowledge held by clients regarding their chronic illness should be highly valued because they develop familiarity with their condition (Cooper 1990; Schaffer 1991). This experiential knowledge involves specific details of the illness, such as how it reacts to different stimuli, and previous successful management strategies. Chronically ill people utilise this knowledge to make decisions about their treatment and self-care that enable them to participate actively in the day-to-day management of their condition (Barr 1993). The personal knowledge of the client is an important resource for the nurse to draw on when making clinical decisions, planning care and working with the person.

## Family focus

The person with a chronic illness must always be considered in the context of the family. Chronic illness tests the ability of families to adapt to the long-term needs of their relative (see Chapter 12). Both the predictability of illness outcome and its impact on life span will be important factors in determining the response of families (Bloch et al. 1995, p.153). Gradually, families develop the capacity to accept that their family member may regress physically or mentally; they learn how to give support to ward off the stresses evoked by illness, and how to tolerate their relative's expressions of his or her feelings and fears. Families are also instrumental in mobilising resources to support people with chronic illnesses and disabilities, and in enlisting their sense of personal responsibility and basic trust (Bloch et al. 1995, p.161). Mental health nurses can assist families with these roles by understanding that family members need to be listened to, and need help to cope with their anxieties, if relatives with chronic illnesses and disabilities are to be supported and enabled to remain as independent as possible. To summarise, nurses should adopt the following approach to maximise the mental health of clients with a chronic illness.

- Work to minimise the impact of illness.
- Support and encourage the client.
- Teach energy-conserving strategies.
- Value client knowledge.
- Strive to improve the client's self-management and self-efficacy.
- Adopt a family focus to care, assisting and supporting the family in their support of the client.

Chronic illness taxes the emotional resources of the people affected and their significant others. Preserving well-being when faced with symptoms that do not remit, and when deterioration is a likely course, is very difficult. Many people become prone to psychological distress and deteriorating mental health. Some even choose suicide as a way out. Assessing the person's needs, reactions to illness, and coping resources is a major component of nursing care. Providing comfort, **empathy**, support and understanding are helpful nursing interventions. Often the nurse becomes an important source of support and encouragement. Vigilant monitoring of changes in the client's mood, an understanding of pathophysiological disease processes, and knowledge of the side effects of prescription drugs assist the nurse to meet complex health needs in challenging situations. The role of the nurse extends to supporting the families and friends of people with chronic illnesses and disabilities.

## SUMMARY

- A chronic illness can result in mental health complications such as anxiety, mood alteration, depression, and possibly suicide.

- There are two possible explanations for a chronically ill person presenting with a mental disorder. Firstly, a mental illness may have been pre-existing, or the person has presented with the somatic symptoms of a mental disorder. Secondly, the two conditions may be unrelated, or the psychiatric condition may be due to the subsequent emotional and psychological impact of a physical illness.
- Mental disorders can arise from the disease process itself, or result from medical treatment, particularly the administration of certain drugs.
- Mental health problems do not always occur in conjunction with chronic physical illness.
- As chronically ill people are at risk of mental health changes, nurses need to be alert for indications of these changes.

## *C*ASE STUDY 4.1: 'Everything is so hard'

Ms Jones is a 35-year-old married mother of two boys, aged 10 and 12. After almost two years of experiencing poor coordination and visual disturbances she was diagnosed a year ago as having multiple sclerosis. Since the time of diagnosis her condition has deteriorated. She has the use of her upper limbs but not her legs, and is in a wheelchair. Ms Jones has been admitted to hospital for an exacerbation of her symptoms. She feels very tired and irritable.

You have been assigned to care for Ms Jones. She states: 'I thought that once I knew what was wrong with me I would be OK emotionally, but lately I am up and down all the time. I get upset and angry at the children. I wonder if I really am going mad. I get so frustrated being stuck in a wheelchair because I can't do all the things that I want to do. Some days I am so exhausted that I can't do a thing'.

Ms Jones says that her husband, family and friends are very supportive and help her with the housework and shopping, and that the boys are very independent. But she feels that she should be able to do the housework because she sees it as an important part of her role as wife and mother.

## Exercises

1. Review the literature on the relationship between multiple sclerosis and depression.
2. Devise a care plan for Ms Jones with particular attention to her mental health needs.
3. Suggest possible problem-solving and coping skills that Ms Jones may find useful.
4. Refer to Chapter 12 and apply the family assessment model to a hypothetical family member with a chronic illness.

## CASE STUDY 4.2:   *Hobson's choice*

Mrs Helen Black is 69 years of age. Helen has had chronic obstructive airway disease for 43 years. During winter she is prone to bronchitis. This causes considerable problems with the stability of her asthma and she often requires systemic steroids. In the past three years, Helen has been admitted to hospital for unstable asthma, and during these periods she has sustained a number of fractured ribs from spasmodic coughing. Osteoporosis has been diagnosed as the cause. This presents a significant problem for Helen, as steroids are contraindicated for people who have osteoporosis, yet such treatment has been a lifesaving measure for her.

Following a serious bout of unstable asthma which required hospitalisation, Helen returned home with a prescribed course of oral steroids. Four weeks later the community nurse noted that Helen appeared apathetic, moody and unmotivated. Life seemed too much of an effort, and Helen refused her shower. 'What's the point? I can't be bothered with it all,' she said, and she appeared sad and distressed.

The nurse identified depressive symptoms and referred Helen to her general practitioner. Following diagnosis of depression, Helen, the doctor and the community nurse discussed her steroid regime. Helen decided to continue with the course of steroids, even though it was possible they were the cause of her depression. The doctor prescribed a short course of antidepressants (doxepin 75mg/day) to help her.

### Exercises

1. What are some of the other possible explanations for Helen's depression?
2. Describe the caring strategies that could be used to complement Helen's drug regime.
3. Devise a care plan for Helen with particular attention to her mental health needs.

## DISCUSSION QUESTIONS

1. Discuss the association between mental illness and at least three physical conditions.
2. Identify possible mental health changes associated with chronic illness and the ways in which a chronic illness can impact upon a person's life.
3. What is causing the increased presentation of chronic illness in Australia and New Zealand? What are the implications for the delivery of health care in the two countries?

# EXERCISES

1. Familiarise yourself with the examples of drugs mentioned in this chapter. Identify the indications and contraindications for their use, the dosage usually prescribed, and possible adverse reactions.

2. In small groups, or in pairs, draw up an inventory of losses and adaptations that have occurred in the case of a person with a chronic illness (and his or her family) that you know personally. Describe the mental health challenges the person has faced in coping with the illness.

# FURTHER READING

- Morse, J. & Johnson, J. (1991) *The Illness Experience*, Newbury Park: Sage Publications. For an account of the subjective experience of chronic illness and its wider family and social impact.

- For an account of survival and adaptation, read Sara Henderson's *Strength to Strength*, Sun Books 1995.

# REFERENCES

Acorn, S. & Andersen, S. (1990) 'Depression in multiple sclerosis: critique of the research literature', *Journal of Neuroscience Nursing* 22(4), pp.209–14.

Allebeck, P. & Bolund, C. (1991) 'Suicides and suicide attempts in cancer patients', *Psychological Medicine* 21(4), pp.979–84.

Badger, T. (1993) 'Physical health impairment and depression among older adults', *Image: Journal of Nursing Scholarship* 25(4), pp.325–30.

Bandura, A. (1986) *Social Foundations of Thought and Action: A Social Cognitive Theory*, Englewood: Prentice Hall.

Barr, J. (1993) 'An illumination of a lived experience: persons who live with asthma and are hospitalised for an unrelated condition'. Unpublished honours thesis, Deakin University, Victoria.

Barrera, M. (1991) 'Social support interventions and the third law of ecology', *American Journal of Community Psychology* 19(1), pp.133–8.

Bloch, S., Hafner, J.M., Harari, E. & Szmukler, G. I. (1995) *The Family in Clinical Psychiatry*, Oxford: Oxford University Press.

Blumenthal, S. (1990) 'Youth suicide: risk factors, assessment, and treatment of adolescent and young adult suicidal patients', *Psychiatric Clinics of North America* 13(3), pp.511–56.

Braunig, P., Bleistein, J., & Rao, M. L. (1989) 'Suicidality and corticosteroid-induced psychosis', *Biological Psychiatry* 26, pp.209–10.

Brown, T. (1990) 'Organic affective psychosis associated with the routine use of non-prescription cold preparations', *British Journal of Psychiatry* 156, pp.572–5.

Brunner, L. & Suddarth, D. (1988) *Medical-surgical Nursing*, Philadelphia: Lippincott Company.

Bunting, L.K. & Fitzsimmons, B. (1991) 'Depression in Parkinson's disease', *Journal of Neuroscience Nursing* 23(3), pp.158–64.

Cairns, D. & Baker, J. (1993) 'Adjustment to spinal cord injury: review of coping styles contributing to the process', *Journal of Rehabilitation* Oct.–Dec., 30–3.

Caldwell, C.B. & Gottlesman, II (1992), 'Schizophrenia—a high risk factor for suicide clues to risk reduction', Suicide and Life Threatening Behaviour, 22(4), pp.479–93.

Caplan, L. & Ahmed, I. (1992) 'Depression and neurological disease: their distinction and association', *General Hospital Psychiatry* 14, pp.177–85.

Cooper, M. (1990) 'Chronic illness and nursing's ethical challenge', *Holistic Nursing Practice* 5(1), pp.10–16.

Doan, B. & Gray, R. (1992) 'The heroic cancer patient: a critical analysis of the relationship between illusion and mental health', *Canadian Journal of Behavioural Science* 24(2), pp.253–66.

Drench, M. (1994) 'Changes in body image secondary to disease and injury', *Rehabilitation Nursing* 19(1), pp.31–6.

Friedland, J. & McColl, M. (1992) 'Disability and depression: some etiological considerations', *Social Science Medicine* 34(4), pp.395–403.

Garden, F.H., Garrison, S.J. & Jain, A. (1990) 'Assessing suicide risk in stroke patients: review of two cases', *Archives of Physical Medicine and Rehabilitation* 71(12), pp.1003–5.

Goldstein, E.T. & Preskorn, S.H. (1989) 'Mania triggered by steroid nasal spray in a patient with stable bipolar disorder', *American Journal of Psychiatry* 146, pp.1076–7.

Graff-Radford, N. & Biller, J. (1992) 'Behavioral neurology and stroke', *Psychiatric Clinics of North America* 15(2), pp.415–23.

Habermann-Little, B. (1991) 'An analysis of the prevalence and etiology of depression in Parkinson's disease', *Journal of Neuroscience Nursing* 23(3), pp.165–9.

Hall, R.C.W., Gardner, E.R. & Popkin, M.K. (1981) 'Unrecognized physical illness prompting psychiatric admission: a prospective study', *American Journal of Psychiatry* 138, pp.629–35.

Janson-Bjerklie, S., Ferketich, S. & Benner, P. (1993) 'Predicting the outcomes of living with asthma', *Research in Nursing and Health* 16, pp.241–50.

Kah, S. & Kupper, N. (1993) 'Mood disorders: depressive and bipolar disorders' in B.S. Johnson (ed.) *Adaptation and Growth: Psychiatric-Mental Health Nursing*, Philadelphia: Lippincott Company.

Klein, J. (1992) 'Adverse psychiatric effects of systemic glucocorticoid therapy', *American Family Physician* 46 (5), pp.1469–74.

Koranyi, E.K. (1979) 'Morbidity and rate of undiagnosed physical illnesses in a psychiatric clinic population', *Archives of General Psychiatry* 36, pp.414–19.

Krol, B., Sanderman, R. & Suurmeijer, T. (1993) 'Social support, rheumatoid arthritis and quality of life: concepts, measurement and research', *Patient Education and Counseling* 20, pp.101–20.

Kübler-Ross, E. (1969) *On Death and Dying*, New York: Macmillan.

Lambert, V.A., Lambert, C.E., Klipple, G.L. & Mewshaw, E.A. (1990) 'Relationship among hardiness, social support, severity of illness, and psychological well-being in women with rheumatoid arthritis', *Health Care for Women International* 11, pp.159–73.

MacDonald, M. R., Nielson, W.R. & Cameron, M.G.P. (1987) 'Depression and activity patterns of spinal cord injured persons living in the community', *Archives of Physical Medicine and Rehabilitation* 68, pp.339–63.

McLennan, W. (1990) *Disability and Handicap in Australia, 1988*, Canberra: Australian Bureau of Statistics.

Marks, S.F. & Millard, R.W. (1990) 'Nursing assessment of positive adjustment for individuals with multiple sclerosis', *Rehabilitation Nursing* 15(3), pp.147–51.

Matsumoto, K. & Ueyama, K. (1994) 'Central nervous disease and manic state', *Nippon-Rinsho* 52(5), pp.1306–10.

Mayou, R., Seagroatt, V. & Goldacre, M. (1991) 'Use of psychiatric services by patients in a general hospital', *British Medical Journal* 303, pp.1029–32.

Murray, R. & Huelskoetter, M. (1991) *Psychiatric/Mental Health Nursing*, California: Appleton and Lange.

New Zealand Public Health Commission (1993) *Our Health Our Future, Hauora pakari, Koiora Roa*, Public Health Commission, Wellington.

Nickel, J., Brown, K. & Smith, B. (1990) 'Depression and anxiety among chronically ill heart patients: age differences in risk and predictors', *Research in Nursing and Health* 13, pp.87–97.

Nurses' Drug Alert (1990) 'Psychosis associated with sinus medications', *Nurses' Drug Alert* Dec, 91–2.

Olsen, O. & Sabroe, S. (1991) 'Age and the operationalization of social support', *Social Science and Medicine* 32 (7), pp.767–71.

Price, R., North, C., Wessely, S. & Fraser, V. (1992) 'Estimating the prevalence of chronic fatigue syndrome and associated symptoms in the community', *Public Health Reports* 107 (5), pp.514–22.

Primomo, J., Yates, B.C. & Woods, N.F. (1990) 'Social support for women during chronic illness: the relationships among sources and types of adjustment', *Research in Nursing and Health* 13, 153–61.

Salazar-Calderon Perriggo, V., Oommen, K. & Sobonya, R. (1993) 'Silent solitary right parietal chondroma resulting in secondary mania', *Clinical Neuropathology* 12(6), pp.325–9.

Schaffer, S.D. (1991) Current approaches in adult asthma assessment, education and emergency management', *Nurse Practitioner* 16(12), pp.18–34.

Schultz, R. & Decker, S. (1985) 'Long-term adjustment to physical disability: the role of social support, perceived control, and self blame', *Journal of Personality and Social Psychology* 48, pp.1162–72.

Small, S. P. & Graydon, J.E. (1993) 'Uncertainty in hospitalized patients with chronic obstructive pulmonary disease', *International Journal of Nursing Studies* 30(3), pp.239–46.

Taal, E., Rasker, J., Seydel, E. & Wiegman, E. (1993) Health status, adherence with health recommendations, self-efficacy and social support in patients with rheumatoid arthritis', *Patient Education and Counseling* 20, pp.63–76.

Travlos, A. & Hirsch, G. (1993) 'Steroid psychosis: a cause of confusion on the acute spinal cord injury unit', *Archives of Physical Rehabilitation* 74, 312–15.

Valente, S.M., Saunders, J.M. & Cohen, M.Z. (1994) 'Evaluating depression among patients with cancer', *Cancer Practice: A Multidisciplinary Journal of Cancer Care* 2(1), pp.65–71.

Wise, M. & Taylor, S. (1990) 'Anxiety and mood disorders in medically ill patients', *Journal of Clinical Psychiatry* 51(1) (Supp.), January, pp.27–32.

Wortman, C.B. & Silver, R. (1989) 'The myths of coping with loss', *Journal of Consulting and Clinical Psychology* 57(3), pp.349–57.

Wysenbeck, A., Leibovici, L. & Zoldan, J. (1990) 'Acute central nervous system complications of pulse steroid therapy in patients with SLE', *Journal of Rheumatology* 17:12, pp.1695–6.

# PART III

# NEEDS

THERE ARE MANY WAYS of thinking about mental health needs. Chapter 5 adopts an epidemiological approach and discusses the prevalence of mental illness in Australia and New Zealand. An important distinction is made between mental health problems and serious mental disorder. The lack of comprehensive data on mental health and illness is also discussed.

The relationship between Aboriginality and mental health is taken up in Chapter 6. The chapter shows how it is the social conditions in which Aboriginal people live, rather than anything about Aboriginality itself, that predisposes towards the diagnosis of mental illness. Indigenous peoples should be given priority when mental health problems are addressed in any society, but they are not the only people who experience mental health problems related to their perceived difference. Migrants, too, face particular challenges in maintaining their mental health in an alien cultural environment. Chapter 7 takes up this theme by looking at the relationship between mental health and ethnicity. The fallacy of regarding all people from a particular cultural background as the same is corrected.

Chapter 8 describes how the health sectors of Australia and New Zealand respond to mental health needs. Service delivery models are discussed in the context of changing mental health policies.

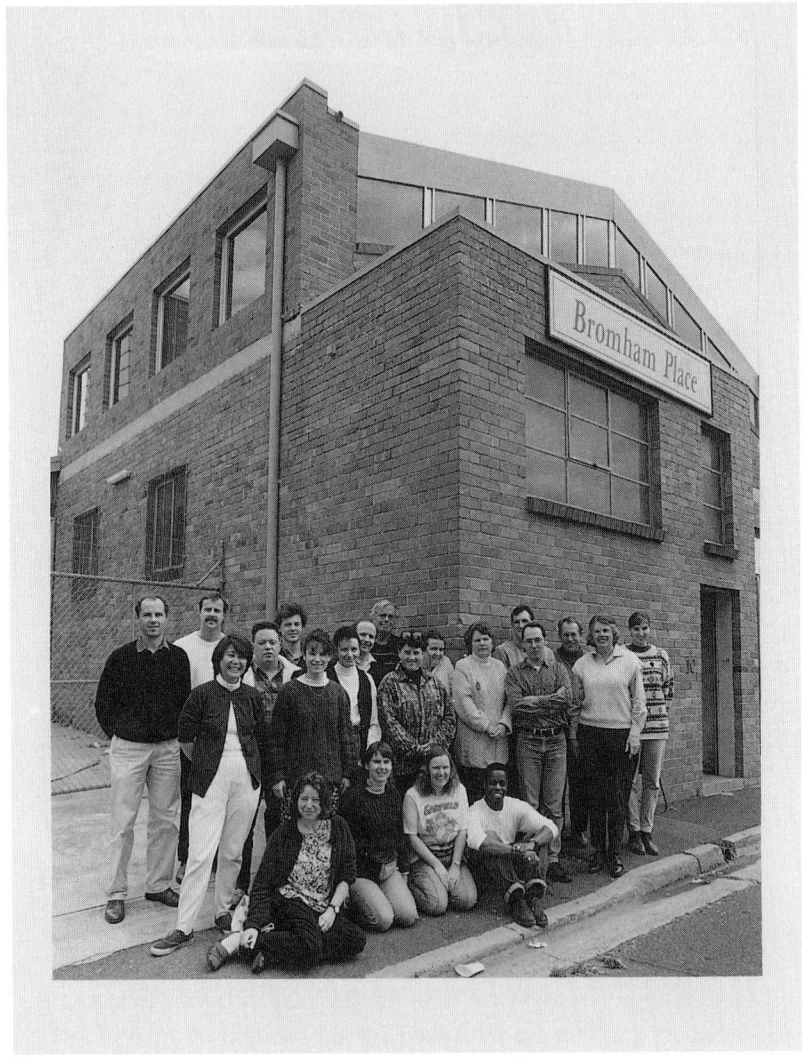

*Bromham Place* – Richmond, Melbourne
Australia's first clubhouse centre for vocational rehabilitation
for people with a psychiatric disability

## CHAPTER 5

# MENTAL HEALTH NEEDS

Michael Clinton and Sioban Nelson

## CONTENTS

# LEARNING OBJECTIVES

This chapter will assist the reader to:

- outline mental health needs in Australia and New Zealand;
- explain why some people are at greater risk of mental illness than others;
- interpret selected demographic and epidemiological data;
- distinguish between two levels of mental health need;
- estimate the prevalence of serious mental illness;
- apply a simple model of prevention in mental health.

# INTRODUCTION

What are the mental health needs of people in Australia and New Zealand? To answer this question this chapter will make a number of points about the interrelationship between social structures and health. Predictions of health status and risk of illness can be made by examining the health patterns of a population. However, it must be emphasised that regardless of the individual risk from genetic, biological, social, cultural, economic or behavioural factors the health of any particular individual cannot be predicted from epidemiological studies. Neither can the outcome of a mental health problem for any one individual be known. Some people suffer extreme adversity without residual problems, while others sustain long-term damage to their physical health and psychological outlook. Some individuals suffer one episode of serious mental illness and recover fully; others experience repeated episodes. What is known is the risk load or vulnerability of social groups. In other words, while aggregate trends are known, the factors are too complex to make predictions in individual cases. This is not to say that clinical predictions based on the detailed case history of an individual client cannot be made, but that is the science of diagnosis and prognosis, not epidemiology.

How then can sense be made of the relationship between epidemiological data and social structures? To examine aggregate trends in mental health, social, cultural, economic and mental health needs must be understood from within the social context of a given society. While there is evidence that schizophrenia occurs throughout the world, independent of cultural or economic variations (Sartorius, Jablensky & Shapiro 1977), other mental health problems are less ubiquitous. For example, adolescent suicide, the prevalence of depression, or drug and alcohol dependence are widely variable across countries, cultures and communities, and particular subgroups within society carry the highest burden of these problems. Later chapters deal with the mental health problems associated with specific age groups (Part V). This chapter will provide the framework for understanding the wider social significance of these problems.

# DEMOGRAPHY AND EPIDEMIOLOGY

**Demography** and **epidemiology** provide the framework for understanding mental health needs in Australia and New Zealand. Broadly speaking, demography is the study of human populations and epidemiology is the study of the factors that determine the distribution of diseases. More specifically, demography is the statistical description and analysis of human populations, and epidemiology is the study of the distribution of the factors that influence the patterns of sickness and health in a community. Demographic and epidemiological data are needed to identify mental health needs. These data provide the means of estimating the number of people with mental health problems and hence the means of planning of mental health services.

To determine the extent of mental health problems in Australia and New Zealand it is first necessary to establish what is meant by mental health problems. As is emphasised throughout this text, mental health is a broad concept encompassing a wide range of nursing responsibilities, from health promotion to the care of people with severe mental illness. The issue of precise definition, however, must be addressed for the purposes of statistical analysis, as each health problem must be defined and measured if epidemiological data is to be useful. For example, the distinction between planning for the needs of those with severe mental illness, and planning measures to optimise mental health, will be shown to be important when issues of **prevention** are discussed later in this chapter.

Meanwhile, mental health needs must be understood as operating on two levels. First, there are the needs of the groups of people with mental illness, identified from epidemiological data. Second, there are the needs of people who experience challenges to their mental health from such life experiences as changing schools, leaving home, going to university, entering the workforce, getting married or entering into a long-term relationship, having children, parenting, changing jobs, moving house, and so on. These mental health needs are difficult to quantify because comprehensive data is unavailable in a form that can be easily used to plan services. Significant trends, however, can be found by an examination of census data and household surveys. In this way, changes in lifestyle, living and working conditions and patterns of spending provide insight into the way Australians and New Zealanders live. The mental health implications of trends such as the increasing number of households that do not represent the nuclear family constellation of mother, father and dependent children, or the increase in utilisation of paid child care, or the amount of time people spend watching television or videos are subject to much debate and research. Where a correlation between these behaviours or trends and mental health problems is demonstrated by research, policy moves can be made to implement preventive measures. Whether this happens or not depends on the significance of the problem and the strength of the political will to act.

## Data analysis

How then is the data for research and policy and service development analysed? In discussing demographic and epidemiological features of a population, it is useful to examine groupings in society based on such factors as age, sex, race/ethnicity, and so on, to establish whether health trends are associated with the demographic characteristics of particular groups. This section examines some of these categories and demonstrates their relevance to understanding mental health needs in Australia and New Zealand.

## Age

The age structure of a society is a major determinant of the mental health services that should be provided. This is because age is a particularly important indicator of need. For example, once the number of people aged over 65 years is known, the number of people likely to suffer from **dementia** at various levels of severity can be estimated; this age group is also heavily represented in **depression** statistics (Kay, Henderson & Scott 1985; Osgood 1985), and **suicide** rates for men (Osgood 1985). Adolescence is another significant age group for mental health because it is in this age group that first episodes of serious mental illness generally occur (Rey 1992).

## Gender

The issue of gender is relevant to both epidemiological analysis and health planning. The health profile of men and women differs, particularly across age groups. So, too, does the pattern of health behaviours; for example, far more women than men seek treatment for ill health (AIHW 1992). In terms of mental health, different age/gender configurations have differing prevalence rates for the many disorders. Post-partum depression is obviously gender and age group specific. Currently, the suicide rate for men is far higher than that for women, particularly the young male suicide rate. In fact, deaths by suicide exceed motor vehicle accident deaths in Australia (AIHW 1994). However, an often overlooked figure is the attempted suicide rate, and hospital admissions for injuries from self-harm—figures dominated by young women (AIHW 1994; Davis 1992, p.95). Women tend to figure highly in the neurotic and affective disorders, too (NHMRC 1993), although the aetiology is unclear and subject to much debate (Pilgrim & Rogers 1993), whereas men predominate in the alcohol and drug addiction rates (Gove 1984). Thus mental health problems, no less than general health problems, are patterned by gender and age. An understanding of these features of health problems is essential to attune service delivery to the specific groups in the population with the highest need.

## Race and ethnicity

The relation between health and race and **ethnicity** is a complex one. Research has found that a number of communities, such as Aboriginal people and Torres Strait Islanders in Australia (AIHW 1994), Maori and Pacific

Islanders in New Zealand (Abbott & Kemp 1993), the Afro-Caribbean community in Britain (Pilgrim & Rogers 1993) and the Afro-American community in the United States (Reiger et al. 1988), demonstrate poor health status in comparison with most other groups in the community. How can this be explained?

The simple fact is that socially disadvantaged sectors of the community—people who experience poverty, high rates of violence and drug and alcohol abuse, high unemployment, and so on—also experience lower life expectancy, and higher infant mortality rates. However, the aetiology of these poor outcomes is controversial, especially in mental health. There are two main theories: social drift and social causation. *Social drift theory* argues that those who are sick with mental illness *become* poor as a result of their illness (Gerdard & Houston 1953). *Social causation theory* emphasises the importance of **stress** combined with lack of opportunity (Ciompi 1989). Ciompi argues that stressors (including genetic/biological predisposition), experienced without the buffering effects of economic resources, education and employment opportunities, and access to quality health services, produce poor health outcomes—mental and physical. It is not only that socioeconomic status is a predictable correlate of mental disorder: the outcome is poorer for those with fewer resources (Pilgrim & Rogers 1993). Thus, a significant factor in the poor health status of racially/ethnically disadvantaged groups in society is their socioeconomic disadvantage (Feinstein 1993). Such disadvantage is characterisistic of indigenous peoples, including Aboriginal Australians and Maori New Zealanders.

Another significant feature of Aboriginal, Torres Strait Islander and Maori populations is their demographic profile. For example, 40% of the Aboriginal population is less than 15 years of age, whereas the general population has less than 25% in this age group (Hunter 1992). The total population of New Zealand in 1991 was 3 373 926. People of Maori background made up almost 9% of the population, people of Pacific Island background 5%, and people of other racial or ethnic backgrounds a little over 82%. Maori children, however, comprise 25% of all children in New Zealand, and Pacific Islander children 9% (Core Services Committee 1992).

Like race, ethnicity must also be understood as bearing a complex relationship to health. As argued in Chapter 7, the health of migrant individuals depends on their circumstances before migration. Of particular significance is whether they are refugees or immigrants, whether victims of torture or war. Of further importance is the manner in which transition to life in Australia is made; for example, the questions of wider community support, employment, and skill recognition are particularly relevant to the individual's adjustment to the stressful process of migration.

Thus it can be seen that race and ethnicity are significant in terms of the *social factors* that contribute to mental health status, rather than carrying any intrinsic significance to mental health. The cultural-specific aspects of mental health for people of minority ethnic and racial backgrounds are examined in Chapters 6 and 7.

# T HE EXTENT OF THE PROBLEM

It follows that there is a complex effect of stressors on individuals with specific biographical profiles: age, sex, genetic load, family circumstances, and so on. To understand the implications of these effects it is necessary to examine the prevalence of mental health problems in Australia and New Zealand by reviewing selected data. However, the limitations of this data betray the traditional division between psychiatry and the health specialties. Historically, mental illness has been synonymous with psychiatric disorder. People suffering from psychiatric disorders were cared for in psychiatric institutions. Therefore, the data on serious mental illness is readily available on psychiatric inpatients. Comprehensive data on the mental health of communities is found less easily. For instance, the Australian Institute of Health and Welfare report, *Australia's Health 1994*, does not include mental health in its coverage due to this lack of comprehensive data (AIHW 1994).

But there are two further areas of concern: the need for data to guide mental health promotion, and the need to understand the concerns of people experiencing serious mental illness. Until recent times these two cohorts have been kept separate statistically, so they will be dealt with here as directed by the available data. In order to examine both the prevalence of mental health problems and serious mental illness, evidence from three sources will be presented: the Bridges-Webb et al. (1992) study on morbidity in general practice in Australia; the Christchurch epidemiological study of psychiatric morbidity; and data on serious mental illness in Australia and New Zealand. In this way the discussion of prevalence moves from the general (why people visit GPs), to the specific (what are the mental health problems and services used in one identified community), to the specialist (rates of serious mental illness and admissions to psychiatric inpatient facilities).

## Prevalence of mental health problems

The prevalence of mental health problems within the general community, and the type of problems that every nurse must expect to encounter, can be found by looking at the primary health care survey, 'Morbidity in general practice', by Bridges-Webb et al. (1992). One question asked in this study was why people consult their GPs. A summary of expenses can be seen in Table 5.1. It was found that 'psychological' problems ranked sixth as a reason for consultation (Bridges-Webb et al. 1992, S43). The GPs often managed more than one problem for each encounter and psychological problems were the sixth most frequently encountered individual problem. Specifically, anxiety, depression and sleep disorders accounted for 5.9% of all encounters (S26).

TABLE 5.1: *Why people consult GPs (reasons for encounters across body systems)*

| INTERNATIONAL CLASSIFICATION OF PRIMARY CARE (ICPC) CHAPTER | PERCENTAGES OF ENCOUNTERS | PERCENTAGE OF ALL PROBLEMS (N = 145 799) |
|---|---|---|
| Respiratory | 18.8 | 16.7 |
| Cardiovascular | 10.4 | 12.5 |
| Skin | 13.0 | 12.4 |
| Musculoskeletal | 12.2 | 12.0 |
| Digestive | 7.4 | 7.1 |
| Psychological | 5.9 | 6.6 |
| General | 7.3 | 6.6 |
| Endocrine | 4.1 | 4.9 |
| Female genital | 4.7 | 4.9 |
| Ear | 4.0 | 3.6 |
| Reproductive | 3.4 | 2.8 |
| Neurological | 2.7 | 2.7 |
| Eye | 2.2 | 2.3 |
| Urological | 2.0 | 2.0 |
| Blood | 1.2 | 1.3 |
| Social problems | 0.7 | 0.8 |
| Male genital | 0.8 | 0.7 |

The rate of consultation for 'psychological problems' by general practitioners is by no means insubstantial if one considers two points. First, these overall figures cross all age groups and all problems from prescription renewals to the common cold. Second, these figures underrepresent mental health problems due to the separate and parallel operation of mental health services for patients with a history of serious mental illness (see Chapter 10). This state of affairs is slowly changing and the model for the future is that of shared care, with GPs attending to the primary care needs of people with severe mental illness (National Health Strategy 1993). However, for the purposes of the Bridges-Webb et al. study, the routine follow-up and care of those with serious mental illness is not represented.

But how many people in the community at large have 'psychological' problems? The Christchurch epidemiological study (Hornblow et al. 1990) completes much of Bridges-Webb's picture. Recent research in the series of epidemiological studies modelled on the US Epidemiological Catchment Area (ECA) study (Reiger et al. 1988) in Canada, New Zealand and Puerto Rico has demonstrated remarkable uniformity across populations. In these successive large studies, lifetime prevalence for specific communities was estimated. These studies present a picture of mental disorder that differs from the one derived from data on hospital populations (Kosky 1992, xiii). A surprising finding was that women had a 30% lifetime incidence of mental health disorder, while the rate for men was 36%. The active rate for both disorders was 20% for both sexes. This finding goes against the belief of many that women are overrepresented in studies of mental disorder (Gove 1984).

Similarly, the age of onset of mental health problems was found to be far earlier than had been assumed—the median age was 16 years (Rey 1992; Hornblow et al. 1990). This has caused some authors to raise questions about the target age for intervention programs (Rey 1992). Furthermore, it appears that people with serious mental illness do indeed consult their GPs—about 27% (Hornblow et al. 1990)—but not about their mental illness. In fact, the amount of medical management of mental illness received by those diagnosed with severe mental illness is very small: Andrews estimates it at only 3% (1991).

## Prevalence of serious mental illness

But what about severe mental illness? Although there is much disagreement about the definition of **serious mental illness,** the US National Advisory Mental Health Council developed a definition in 1993. This same definition has been cited in the Australian First National Mental Health Report (FNMHR 1993).

> Severe mental illness is defined through diagnosis, disability and duration and includes disorders with psychotic symptoms such as schizophrenia, schizoaffective disorder, autism, as well as severe forms of other disorders such as major depression, panic disorder and obsessive compulsive behaviour.

In the US ECA study, the lifetime incidence of one or more of the 30 major psychiatric disorders was one in three, and one in five had an active disorder at time of interview (Rey 1992). Henderson's (1993) estimates of the prevalence rates in Australia are given in Table 5.2.

*T A B L E  5 . 2 :  Estimates of one-year prevalence of mental disorders in Australia: people aged 20 years and over*

| | |
|---|---|
| Schizophrenia | 1.00% |
| Major depression | 3.70% |
| Alcoholism:  men | 11.90% |
| women | 2.16% |
| Generalised anxiety disorder | 1.72% |
| Somatization disorder | 3.98% |
| Anti-social personality | 1.20% |
| Severe cognitive impairment (55+) | 3.30% |

These estimates for Australia closely reflect New Zealand and US epidemiological patterns and clearly demonstrate the extent of the problem in the community.

## Admission rates

The extent of the treated problem gives some measure of severity. The reasons for admission to psychiatric facilities, particularly first admission, are an indication of the acuteness and severity of mental health problems. The admission rates within Australia vary considerably and are subject to a number of factors. For example, people in rural and remote communities may have high admission rates because local services are unable adequately to diagnose and treat those suffering from acute episodes of mental illness. However, programs are being developed to improve the support for staff in remote locations. Interview and case conferences via telecommunications links are easing the pressure for evacuation for admission to acute facilities (see Chapter 16). In the Northern Territory, programs exist that manage patients well in their own communities without the need for evacuation to Darwin or Alice Springs. Similarly, admission rates vary throughout Australia and areas of New Zealand depending on the community resources available, the features of the mental health acts governing care (i.e. whether community treatment orders (CTOs) exist (see Chapters 8 and 16)) and, crucially, the availability of acute beds.

With these limitations in mind, the New Zealand admission rates for first admissions, for public patients, do give an indication of the range and severity of the mental disorders. As the pie chart in Figure 5.1 clearly shows, the overwhelming problem for treatment is alcohol abuse. Maori people are overrepresented in the figures for schizophrenia, and alcohol dependence and

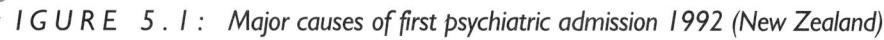

FIGURE 5.1: *Major causes of first psychiatric admission 1992 (New Zealand)*

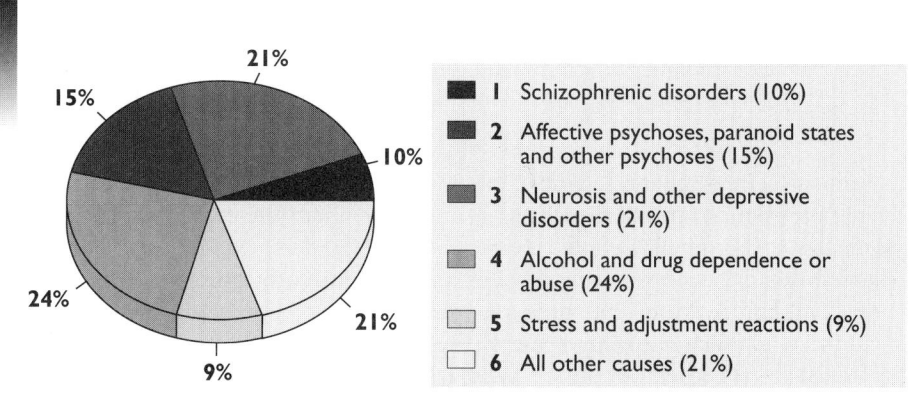

15%  
21%  
10%  
21%  
9%  
24%

1  Schizophrenic disorders (10%)

2  Affective psychoses, paranoid states and other psychoses (15%)

3  Neurosis and other depressive disorders (21%)

4  Alcohol and drug dependence or abuse (24%)

5  Stress and adjustment reactions (9%)

6  All other causes (21%)

abuse (NZ Health Information Service 1993). The alcohol and drug dependence figures are similar in Australia for Aboriginal people and Torres Strait Islanders. The diagnosis of schizophrenia, however, is problematic and the prevalence rates for this disorder among Aboriginal people and Torres Strait Islanders is difficult to determine (Human Rights and Equal Opportunities Commission 1993). In both countries it seems that the most common route of referral for Aborigines and Maori is through the justice system. In New Zealand the Maori are the group most frequently admitted under the Criminal Justice Act and, together with Pacific Islanders, they are overrepresented in involuntary admission rates (Abbott & Kemp 1993). The pattern is similar for referral from law enforcement agencies for first admissions (see Table 5.3).

*T A B L E  5 . 3 :  Involuntary and law enforcement admissions in New Zealand*

| INVOLUNTARY ADMISSIONS | |
| --- | --- |
| Pacific Islanders | 45.0% |
| Maori | 36.0% |
| Other | 24.0% |
| **ADMISSIONS VIA LAW ENFORCEMENT AGENCIES** | |
| Pacific Islander | 29.0% |
| Maori | 18.3% |
| Other | 8.1% |

Comparable figures do not exist for Australia. However

> ... the Human Rights and Equal Opportunities Commission heard evidence that in Criminal Justice System provided a common referral point for Aboriginal people who required mental health care (see Chapter 6)(HREOC 1993).

Admission rates are interesting data. However, they may reveal less about the overall prevalence rates of the disorders and more about the custodial nature of psychiatry. Aboriginal people, Torres Strait Islanders, Maori and Pacific Islanders require access to the services and preventive measures that protect their communities from experiencing such high admission rates, particularly involuntary admissions. What some of these preventive measures could be will be discussed in the next section.

# **P** *REVENTION*

Having argued both the complexity and the pervasiveness of mental health problems, it can be seen that preventive measures for mental health problems must be broad in their scope. Primary prevention sets out to alter forces in the community that are thought to influence mental health adversely. Secondary prevention involves activities to reduce the prevalence of mental illness in the community. Tertiary prevention involves effective rehabilitation services (Caplan 1969, 1989).

Preventive programs encompass:

- the need for measures that enhance people's resilience in order to equip them to withstand adversity;
- the need to intercept vulnerable individuals through psychosocial programs that assist people who are experiencing problems; and
- the need for early intervention programs that actively treat those who are suffering from a mental disorder at the first possible opportunity; the aim is to limit the damage done to their educational, professional and social circumstances as a result of the debilitating effects of severe mental illness.

**Primary prevention** covers a range of approaches: education, service provision and legislation:

- *education*, to increase public awareness of mental health problems and work to destigmatise mental disorder;
- *service provision*, to enable individuals and groups to access services that have a preventive role;
- *legislation*, which may include diverse aspects of law such as equal employment opportunity legislation, anti-race discrimination legislation, and land rights legislation for Aboriginal Australians and Maori New Zealanders.

Thus, aspects of prevention may include interventions, such as legislation, which are not intended as overt mental health interventions. Their effect, however, is to counter threats to the psychological well-being of specific groups of citizens and, in this sense, they constitute an important mental health prevention measure.

In **secondary prevention, disability** is minimised by early diagnosis, **crisis intervention** and effective treatment. Care is provided by the primary health care worker, and serious episodes are either prevented or managed before a crisis point is reached. **Tertiary prevention** involves the provision of rehabilitation services as community-focused interventions. These are enhanced at the individual and group level by informal social support from relatives, friends, work groups and more formal counselling services.

## *A model of prevention*

Puckett (1993) argues that preventive mental health involves three loosely related processes: identifying people at risk, assessing their needs, and arranging appropriate support. A simple model of these processes is shown in Figure 5.2.

F I G U R E  5 . 2 :  *Preventative mental health: a simple model*

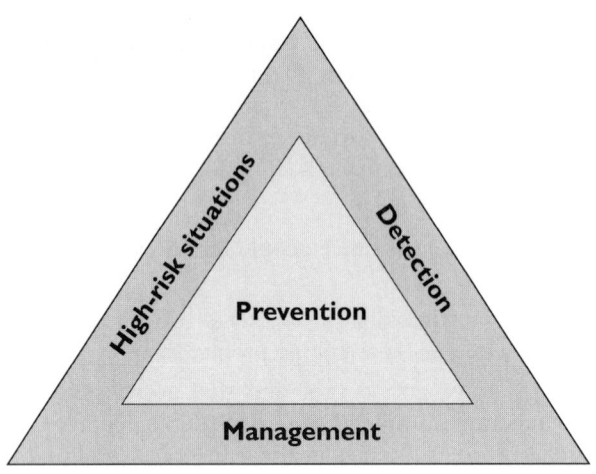

| HIGH-RISK SITUATIONS | DETECTION | MANAGEMENT |
|---|---|---|
| **Children** | | |
| Underprivileged families: (health, size, poverty, criminality), resettled families, migrant and itinerant families, single parenthood | Gynaecologists, obstetricians, midwives, nurses (Plunket Society, NZ), general practitioners, social workers, preschool and school personnel, family planning services, family counselling services | Social and welfare agencies, non-professional and voluntary groups, day nurseries, kindergarten, child minders, in-home services, crisis intervention programs, specialist services |
| **Adolescents** | | |
| Underprivileged families, living away from home, difficult school or work situations, dropouts from school or work, gang membership | Parents, peers, teachers, youth workers, social workers, school nurses, vocational guidance services, clergy, police, general practitioners | Parents, peer support groups, youth clubs and advisory services, student counselling services, career counselling services, religious groups, sports groups |
| **Adults** | | |
| Loneliness, menopause, bereavement, retirement, unemployment (transitions), family history of mental illness or handicap, excessive work load, ethnic minorities | General practitioners, hospitals, public health nurses, relatives, friends, mental health services, lawyers, employment services, employers, clergy, community leaders, occupational health services, social services, community organisations | Voluntary groups, social services and support groups, specialised mental health services, family counselling, legal services, personnel specialists, trade unions, ethnic organisations |
| **The Aged** | | |
| Isolation, chronic illness, sensory and other handicaps, recent bereavement, acute illness and sudden hospitalisation, discharge from hospital, previous mental illness, financial stress | Family, neighbours, friends, peer groups, social services, voluntary organisations, general practitioners, hospitals | Clubs, day care centres, day hospitals, telephone services, in-home services, respite care, part-time employment, comprehensive diagnostic services, legal services, retirement villages |

High-risk situations can be identified by age group and those most at risk can be detected by a range of individuals and services. An equally wide range of services and individuals is involved in minimising the risk of people under stress developing mental health problems or serious mental illness. This triple-process model is helpful in pointing out the range of people and organisations well placed to assist people at risk to receive help, and the diverse ways in which people at risk can be supported. The model is applied to older people in Box 5.1.

B *O X  5 . 1 : Preventative model applied to older people*

| | |
|---|---|
| RISKS | loss or bereavement ■ social isolation ■ depression ■ suicide ■ dementia ■ burden of care |
| NEEDS | social contact ■ information ■ respite care ■ interpreters ■ diagnosis and treatment |
| SERVICES | community facilities (particularly culturally appropriate facilities) ■ counselling ■ education ■ respite care ■ trained primary health care workers to diagnose and treat mental disorders |

However, there is not always a clear and direct relationship between high-risk situations and their management. More effort is required to ensure that those in need receive the most support, and that resources are not used on those who have the personal resources to manage without assistance. Furthermore, in a primary prevention program it is imperative that an individual's competence is not undermined by the support process, nor must the **stigma** attached to mental health problems and/or difficulty in coping be allowed to interfere with the personal **autonomy** of individuals. Primary prevention programs that did not guard against this possibility would end up doing more harm than good, by creating the idea that people in general are ill-equipped to manage life's tribulations and adversities. A primary prevention program must therefore be available through everyday health care services, yet be targeted to reach the populations at greatest risk.

## Young people

Adolescent and child psychiatry has been singled out as the area in need of prevention programs and increased service resources (Rey 1992; Kosky 1992; Raphael 1993; Human Rights and Equal Opportunities Commission 1993). There are several reasons for this. First, the ECA studies found that the median age of onset for mental disorder is 16 years (Rey 1992). This fact alone emphasises the importance of early intervention programs. The opportunity to limit the course of an episode of mental disorder, to maintain the individual within school, to prevent the sequelae of unemployment and poor education that attend serious mental disorder is one that must not be lost. Second, this age of onset applies across the spectrum of mental health problems, from psychotic disorders such as schizophrenia and depression to other mental health problems such as substance abuse.

Preventive programs targeted towards young people aim to reduce behaviour that increases an individual's vulnerability to mental disorder by encouraging self-protective behaviours, and enhancing the individual's resilience to adversity. The negotiation, or avoidance, of problems such as substance abuse, depression, parental conflict, unprotected sexual activity (HIV and teenage pregnancy), conflicts with the criminal justice system, and (un)employment prospects determines to a great extent the course a young person will take in adult life. It is therefore critical to mental health prevention programs that young people are helped to develop the resilience to deal with these issues. In addition to this, however, there must be services for those who confront these issues in a vulnerable state. There is evidence that young people who come from backgrounds of substance abuse or violence (NZ Public Health Commission 1993; Davis 1992; Mathias 1992), and young people in rural or isolated areas, whose prospects of employment are grim (Hunter 1992; Human Rights and Equal Opportunities Commission 1993) have a higher risk of developing a mental disorder. An intervention program that reduces the vulnerability of these at-risk groups is what is required.

One example of a primary intervention program that aims to close this gap between members of a vulnerable group and the rest of the population has been devised by Gerald Caplan. His eight-year program/research has provided outreach to all divorced families in the city of Jerusalem. The aim of the program is to intercede with divorced families to prevent the development of mental health problems in children. According to Caplan (1994), this group of children carries a threefold risk of developing mental health problems in comparison with children whose families have not divorced. The manner in which the separation is achieved is significant for the outcome for the children. If the separation involves an escalation of the discord, if the children are the focus of dispute, and if the separation results in poverty for the children (NHMRC 1993), the mental health effects are likely to be more significant. This applies particularly to children who have experienced or witnessed parental violence (Davis 1992). Given the increasing divorce rate in most countries of the west, the Caplan program is an example of a global measure that attempts to intercept these children by a purely preventive program, to facilitate the process of separation, and to help parents to guide their children through the divorce. Caplan argues:

> What must be used is a model of repeated interventions from time to time, as needed, whenever parents and children become involved in current difficulties produced by the incapacity of a broken family to cope with changing life circumstances and tensions linked with such developmental

crises in the growing children as upheavals of adolescence. The program of intervention in such cases should be geared to crisis approach, so that minimal efforts are expended when the times are ripe. The expectations of the interveners and of parents and children should be that over the years crises are inevitable, and that when they occur the caregivers are prepared to lend a helping hand on a short-term basis to ensure that parents and children master their temporary difficulties and then continue on their own. (Caplan 1994, p 376)

This model is of key relevance to mental health nurses. The importance of information, intensive support and ongoing access to services frames the supportive and preventive role as one that is sensitive and reactive to client needs.

Secondary prevention programs are aimed at reducing the morbidity and chronicity of those who develop a mental health problem. There is increasing evidence that early prevention is the key to preventing mental illness and psychiatric disability. Early intervention with adolescents and in early adulthood is particularly required (Kosky & Hardy 1992). One model program for working with people, particularly young people, when they first develop psychosis is the Early Psychosis Prevention and Intervention Centre (EPPIC) in Melbourne, run by Associate Professor Patrick McGorry. McGorry argues that the care of young people with a first episode of psychosis is critical. He says that the usual form of treatment in an inpatient unit, with patients who suffer from longstanding mental disorders and perhaps severe levels of chronicity, is extremely traumatic and contributes to secondary morbidity in its own right (McGorry 1992). This program aims to intercept individuals early in their first episode of psychosis:

- to reduce secondary morbidity;
- to reduce the frequency and severity of relapse;
- to reduce disruption to vocational and development performance; and
- to prevent family dysfunction and promote family well-being.

(EPPIC, 1993).

In this secondary prevention program psychosis is approached as a condition that can be managed. The emphasis is on the prevention of morbidity, rather than solely on the treatment of symptoms. In both Caplan's program and the EPPIC, specific groups have been targeted, with a clear aim, for a range of interventions. Where such aim and focus is absent, there are several concerns about the efficacy of prevention programs.

## Problems with prevention

There is considerable agreement about the existence of risk factors for mental disorders. However, it is not possible to use this awareness to predict mental disorder in an individual. Consequently, there is a need for global interventions that address the high-risk groups generically, to be followed through by resources that enable health professionals to intervene with individuals identified as having specific needs. As noted earlier, the needs of people at risk of mental illness, and of those facing the normal tribulations of everyday life, should be distinguished when considering preventive mental health strategies. Priority should be given to early intervention and treatment strategies, especially in childhood and adolescence, because these are more likely to have an impact on the prevalence of mental illness.

Preventive mental health strategies may assist people facing the stresses of adult life, especially in the later years. However, with some notable exceptions such as crisis intervention, bereavement counselling, and psychological support for people with physical illness (Raphael 1980), there is no conclusive evidence that such strategies produce positive results (Huxley 1990). Arguably, the only real primary prevention measures in psychiatry have been the lessening of psychiatric complications of syphilis and vitamin deficiency, lowered rates of birth injury, and the elimination of lead from house paint (Raphael 1980). The addition of vitamin B to alcoholic beverages is another example of successful primary prevention (Raphael 1980).

Therefore, preventive strategies are best thought about along the two dimensions shown in Figure 5.3. Intervention in childhood and adolescence and early treatment influence the course of mental illness. However, the effect of preventive strategies used with people in good mental health is difficult to demonstrate. The effectiveness of measures can only be confidently asserted

**FIGURE 5.3:** *The two dimensions of preventive mental health strategies*

**Dimension 1**

| Mental health | early intervention produces positive results | Mental illness |

**Dimension 2**

| Mental wellness | preventive strategies do not generally yield long-term positive results | Enhanced mental wellness |

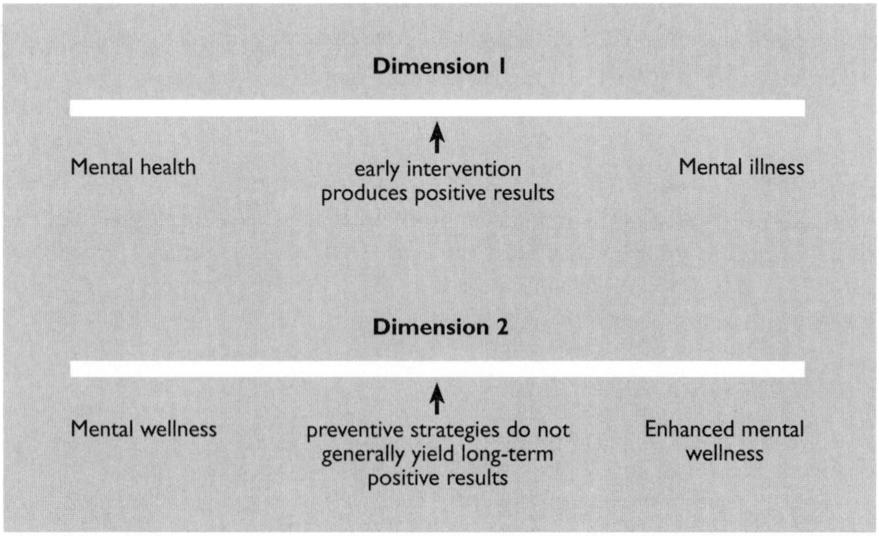

through a process of 'incorporating them into systems' where they will be accessible to those in need (NHMRC 1993, p.17). The implications for planning services and mental health nursing practice are clear. More resources should be targeted at interventions with high-risk groups, and more early treatment programs should be established and rigorously evaluated. The efforts of mental health nurses should be concentrated on the support of the most vulnerable groups of clients. The NHMRC publication, *Scope for Prevention in Mental Health*, outlines models for defining prevention, for evaluating the efficacy of a program and for determining whether the program is indeed warranted (NHMRC 1993). This last point is particularly crucial. It must be clearly established that the benefits of an intervention outweigh any possible problems that it may cause. Programs to enhance personal resilience must not paradoxically reinforce the notion that individuals are unable to cope with life's vicissitudes.

From the service planning point of view it is important to have data on the effectiveness of preventive mental health programs, because a choice has to be made about the relative importance of prevention and treatment services. As expenditure on health care increases and resources are redirected to support new and expanded community services, better outcomes will be expected of preventive services. Seminal work by Lalonde (1974) in Canada has displaced hospitals as the prime focus of health care and stressed broader concerns about the health of populations. Unfortunately, the increased emphasis on lifestyle factors in illness prevention has encouraged an incipient tendency to blame the victim (Davis & George 1988). While lifestyle is an important determinant of health, without caution the new concern with healthy lifestyle promotion can lapse into an ideology of 'healthism' in which health becomes an amorphous end in itself, rather than a means to an end. Therefore, care needs to be taken not to blame members of disadvantaged groups for any failure on their part to respond to well-intentioned preventive mental health programs. As argued throughout this chapter, mental health status is influenced by social as well as individual factors. Thus, only limited success will be achieved by preventive mental health programs until issues of institutionalised inequality and powerlessness are addressed.

It has been emphasised that these patterns must be understood along two dimensions. The first dimension is the spectrum of mental illness, varying from short episodes of self-limiting conditions to much more serious and potentially chronic illness. The second dimension varies with subjective experiences of stress. The two dimensions are important for understanding the concept of prevention, which has been introduced with a simple model applied to the needs of older and younger people, two groups with equally important but very different needs. The implications for mental health nursing practice are clear. The attention of mental health nurses should be directed mainly to meeting the needs of the most vulnerable groups in society. In the field of prevention this means emphasising the contribution that can be made to maintaining and improving the mental health of young people.

# SUMMARY

- The mental health needs of a community are complex and reflect demographic and social characteristics. Therefore, aggregate trends in mental health needs must be understood from within the context of a given society, and from the perspective of social, cultural and economic trends.

- Some people have a high risk of suffering a mental illness. Such risk is related to age, gender, genetic load, family circumstances and so forth, but to understand the implications of these factors it is necessary to consider data aggregated for social groupings.

- Mental health prevention measures need to be targeted to reduce the vulnerability of at-risk groups. However, the measures adopted must not undermine personal responsibility and effectiveness.

- Priority should be given to early intervention and treatment strategies, especially in childhood and adolescence, because these are most likely to have an impact on the prevention of mental illness.

- From a service planning point of view, it is important to have data on the effectiveness of preventive mental health programs because choices have to be made about the relative importance of prevention and treatment services when resources are allocated. It is particularly important that mental health nursing resources are allocated to communities and clients in greatest need.

- Care must be taken not to blame members of disadvantaged groups for any failure on their part to respond to well-intentioned mental health programs. Only limited success will be achieved until issues of institutionalised inequality and powerlessness are addressed.

# DISCUSSION QUESTIONS

1. What are the major mental health needs in Australia and New Zealand? Which of these needs do you think should be given highest priority? Why?

2. Why are some people at greater risk of developing a mental illness than others?

3. Why is it important to distinguish between two levels of mental health need?

4. How would you account for variations in the patterns of admission to psychiatric facilities?

5. What factors are important in explaining the prevalence rates of serious mental illnesses among *either* Aboriginal Australians (see Chapter 6) *or* Maori New Zealanders?

6. Can serious mental illness be prevented? If so, how? If not, why not?

# EXERCISES

1. Analyse the mental health needs of members of an identified age group in Australia or New Zealand.

2. Next time you undertake clinical experience in a mental health setting, analyse the social characteristics of the clients.

3. Interview three or four friends and identify the stressors they experience in their lives and how they cope with them. Predict how these stressors may change during the next ten years.

4. Critically analyse any model that seeks to account for the causation of *either* schizophrenia *or* depression (see Chapter 2).

5. Devise a plan to assist the mental health sector to become more sensitive to the cultural needs of *either* Aboriginal Australians *or* Maori New Zealanders.

6. Use the simple model of prevention presented in this chapter to design a prevention strategy to address a selected mental health need.

# FURTHER READING

- *Australia's Health 1994.* This biennial work gives a comprehensive report on Australia's health sector. The work includes extensive appendices of data and an excellent overview of the main issues confronting the provision of health care. Mental health data is lacking. Canberra: AGPS.

- NHMRC (1993) *Scope for Prevention in Mental Health.* This monograph is available from the NHMRC free of charge. The publication gives a comprehensive analysis of prevention in psychiatry, both from the perspective of mental wellness and the prevention of disorder.

- Ministry of Health (1993) *Mental Health Data 1992.* This publication is a collection of New Zealand data on mental illness, based on inpatient data sets.

# REFERENCES

Abbott, M.W. & Kemp, D.R. (1993) 'New Zealand' in D. Kemp (ed.) *International Handbook on Mental Health Policy*, New Zealand: Greenwood Press.

Andrews, G. (1991) 'Costs of psychiatry revisited', *Schizophrenia Bulletin* 17(3), pp.389–94.

Australian Institute of Health and Welfare (1992) *Australia's Health.* Canberra: AGPS.

Australian Institute of Health and Welfare (1994) *Australia's Health 1994*, Canberra: AGPS.

Bridges-Webb, C., Britt, H., Miles, D.A., Neary, S., Charles, J. & Traynor, V. (1992) 'Morbidity in general practice', *Medical Journal of Australia*, 157 (Supp.) Oct. 19, S1–S55.

Caplan, G. (1969) *An Approach to Community Mental Health*, London: Tavistock.

Caplan, G. (1989) 'Recent developments in crisis prevention and the promotion of support services', *Journal of Primary Prevention* 10(1), pp.3–25.

Caplan, G. (1994) 'Organization of preventive psychiatry programs', *Community Mental Health Journal* 29(4), pp.367–95.

Ciompi, L. (1989) 'The dynamics of complex-biological psychosocial systems: four fundamental psychobiological mediators in the long-term evolution of schizophrenia', *British Journal of Psychiatry* 155 (Supp.5), pp.15–21.

Core Services Committee (1992) *Core Services and Disability Support Services for 1993/1994*, Wellington: National Advisory Committee on Core Health and Disability Support Services.

Davis, A. (1992) 'Suicidal behaviour among adolescents: its nature and prevention' in R. Kosky, H. S. Eshkevari & G.Kneebone (eds) *Breaking Out. Challenges in Adolescent Mental Health in Australia*, pp.89–105. Canberra: AGPS.

Davis, A. & George, J. (1988) *States of Health: Health and Illness in Australia*, Sydney: Harper & Row.

Department of Health and Human Services (1994) *First National Mental Health Report 1993*, Canberra: AGPS.

Early Psychosis Prevention and Intervention Centre (1994) 'Service Plan'. Unpublished document.

Feinstein, J.S. (1993) 'The relationship between socioeconomic status and health: a review of the literature', *The Milbank Quarterly* 71(2), pp.279–322.

Gerdard, D.L. & Houston,L.G. (1953) 'Family setting and the social ecology of schizophrenia', *Psychiatric Quarterly* 27, pp.90–101.

Gove, W. (1984) 'Gender differences in mental and physical illness: the effects of fixed roles and nurturant roles', *Social Science and Medicine* 19(2), pp.77–91.

Grant, C. & Lapsley, H.M. (1993). *The Australian Health Care System*. Australian Studies in Health Service Administration No 75. Sydney: University of NSW.

Hornblow, A.R., Bushell, J.A., Wells, J.E., Joyce, P.R. & Oakey-Browne, M.A. (1990) 'Christchurch psychiatric epidemiology study: use of mental health services', *The New Zealand Medical Journal* 12(103), pp.415–17.

Human Rights and Equal Opportunities Commission (1993) *Human Rights and Mental Illness. Report of the National Inquiry into Human Rights of People with Mental Illness* Vols 1 & 2. Canberra: AGPS.

Hunter, E. (1992) 'Aboriginal adolescents in remote Australia', in R. Kosky, H. S. Eshkevari & G.Kneebone (eds), *Breaking Out. Challenges in Adolescent Mental Health in Australia*, pp.76–87. Canberra: AGPS.

Huxley, P. (1990) *Effective Community Mental Health Services*, Avebury: Aldershot.

Kay, D.W., Henderson, A.S. & Scott, R. (1985). 'Dementia and depression among the elderly living in a Hobart community: the effect of the diagnostic criteria on the prevalence rates', *Psychological Medicine* 15, pp.771–88.

Kosky, R. (1992) 'Introduction', in R. Kosky, H.S. Eshkevari & G. Kneebone (eds), *Breaking Out. Challenges in Adolescent Mental Health in Australia.* Canberra: AGPS.

Kosky, R. & Hardy, J. (1992) 'Mental health: is early intervention the key?' *Medical Journal of Australia* 156, pp.147–8.

Lalonde, M. (1974) *A New Perspective on the Health of Canadians.* Information Canada, Ottawa.

McGorry, P. (1992) 'The concept of recovery and secondary prevention in psychotic disorders', *The Australian and New Zealand Journal of Psychiatry* 26, pp.3–17.

Mathias, J. (1992) 'Cycles of violence and abuse', in R. Kosky, H.S. Eshkevari & G. Kneebone (eds), *Breaking Out. Challenges in Adolescent Mental Health in Australia.* Canberra: AGPS.

NHMRC (1993) *Scope for Prevention in Mental Health*, National Health and Medical Research Council, Canberra.

National Health Strategy (1993) *Help where Help is Needed*, National Health Strategy Issues, Paper No. 5 Melbourne.

New Zealand Health Information Service (1993) *Mental Health Data 1992.* Wellington: Ministry of Health.

New Zealand Public Health Commission (1993) *Our Health Our Future. Hauora Pakari, Koiora Roa.* Wellington. Public Health Commission.

Osgood, N.J. (1985) *Suicide in the elderly*, Rockville, M.O., Aspen.

Pilgrim, D. & Rogers, A. (1993) *A Sociology of Mental Health and Illness*, Buckingham: Open University Press.

Puckett, A. (1993) *Community Mental Health*, Sydney: Harcourt Brace & Co.

Raphael, B. (1980) 'Primary prevention: fact or fiction', *Australian and New Zealand Journal of Psychiatry* 14, pp.163–74.

Raphael, B. (1993) Scope for Prevention in Mental Health, National Health and Medical Research Council.

Reiger, D.A., Boyd, J.H., Rae, D.S., Myers, J.K., Kramer, M., Robins, L.N., George, L.K., Karno, M. & Locke, B.Z. (1988) 'One month prevalence of mental disorders in the US based on five epidemiological catchment sites', *Archives of General Psychiatry* 45(11), pp.977–86.

Rey, J.M. (1992) 'The epidemiological catchment area (ECA) study: implications for Australia', *The Medical Journal of Australia* 156, pp.200–3.

Sartorius, N., Jablensky, A. & Shapiro, R. (1977) 'Two year follow-up of the patients included in the World Health Organisation pilot study of schizophrenia', *Psychological Medicine* 7, pp.529–41.

# Land

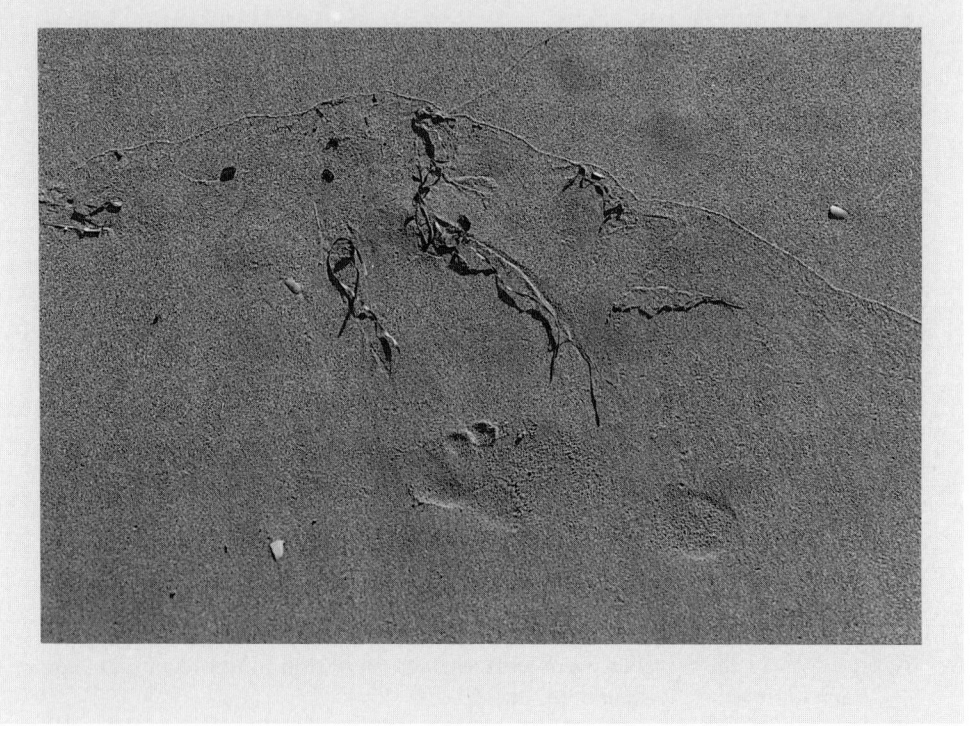

DAVID HOULDER

The land has spiritual significance for indigenous peoples.
To break this bond is an assault on mental health.

## CHAPTER 6

# **A**BORIGINALITY AND MENTAL HEALTH

Gracelyn Smallwood

## CONTENTS

# LEARNING OBJECTIVES

This chapter will assist the reader to:

- consider the cultural values implicit in western concepts of mental health and illness;
- appreciate how colonisation has impacted on the mental health of Aboriginal and Torres Strait Islander peoples;
- understand that Aboriginality in itself is not a risk factor for mental illness;
- appreciate cultural identity as a primary factor in mental well-being;
- recognise the importance of culturally safe care;
- understand the crucial importance of integrating nursing skills within traditional networks when working with Aboriginal communities;
- appreciate the need to reinforce the cultural identity of Aboriginal clients and their families.

# INTRODUCTION

The mental health care of people of Aboriginal and Torres Strait Islander background is the subject of this chapter. In this area, perhaps more than any other, mental health can only be a useful concept when considered in its historical and social context. The effects of the last 200 years of Australia's history, and the impact of very recent policies, continue to influence the mental health of Australia's indigenous peoples. To take this position on mental health is not to deny the medical model of psychiatric disorder, but to show that as an approach to individual assessment, it is of limited utility in situations that in far too many cases are well beyond the control of the individuals in question. It is at this juncture that social and medical inter-pretations of mental disorder and its treatment strain against each other. When the risk indicators that weigh against the individual are socially determined, the details of personal biography then become critical events that project the individual towards alcohol and drug abuse, the criminal justice system, and the asylum.

The inclusion of this chapter in a mental health nursing text does not signify that Aboriginality has specific attendant risks of mental disorder. On the contrary, being an indigenous Australian is not in itself a risk factor for mental illness. It is, however, a risk factor for poor health, shortened life expectancy, imprisonment, drug and alcohol abuse, violent death, poverty, low standards of education and *the diagnosis of behaviour as psychotic*. As these risk factors constitute mental health risks, it follows that Aboriginal peoples require prevention programs and high-quality mental health services as well as broadly based social and economic reforms, if the problems listed above are to be adequately addressed.

   Nurses working in the field of Aboriginal and Torres Strait Islander health must, therefore, be aware of the complex interplay between social, economic and political forces as they come to bear on health, particularly mental health. Aboriginal and Torres Strait Islander health is *exemplary* of these forces, rather than exceptional.

   Cultural identity is a primary factor in well-being. For the dominant culture the reinforcement of cultural identity is the norm. In this way culture becomes invisible; members of the non-dominant culture become defined as 'the other'. For the groups thus defined, the task to re-establish and maintain an identity separate from the dominant culture is inseparable from the struggle for survival. The integrationist schemes of colonial administration to eradicate the Aboriginal and Torres Strait Islander cultures through the removal of children and the attempted destruction of families were doomed to fail. Aboriginal people, even the pale-skinned children, taken from their families with no knowledge of their background did not become 'white'. The scale of misery caused by this policy is recorded in the tragedy of one such family in Box 6.1. The past ten years have witnessed the odyssey of many of these people home to their cultural identity, to their community. It is estimated, however, that there are 100 000 people of Aboriginal descent who do not know their families or communities (Edwards & Read 1989). The mental health issues implicit in these stories must be appreciated and understood by mental health nurses.

## Box 6.1: *Devastated lives*

In the 1960s this family of five children were forcibly removed from their home and placed in a number of children's homes. The pale-skinned children were fostered out to white families. This is the story of their lives thus far.

*Child 1* (9 years) spent seven years in the home, then he was sent to a farm till he was 18. He died of liver disease secondary to alcohol.

*Child 2* (7 years) was fostered to a white family. She ran away at 16 and was battered to death at the age of 22.

*Child 3* (6 years) was in the home for ten years. At 14 she was sent to a farm where the station owner physically and sexually assaulted her for 12 months. When she became pregnant she was returned to the home, then the unmarried mothers' home. Her child was taken from her. She has two children in care at present and is struggling to get them back.

*Child 4* (3 years) spent time in a number of institutions. He developed an alcohol problem, attained sobriety with the help of AA and now suffers from depression.

*Child 5* (6 months) was fostered to a number of white families, each time her name was changed. She was returned by one family to the Youth and Community Services Office for being 'strange' and was fostered out again. She is now in her 30s and is struggling with a number of problems.

The forces that have made the mental health of Aboriginal and Torres Strait Islander peoples a struggle are those of history, economics and politics. But what of the forces that have enabled Aboriginal and Torres Strait Islander peoples to survive? An indestructible sense of land, of ancestry, of community, of family, of laughter and strength has endured for 200 years and grows stronger as the struggle for self-determination defines the future. Land, culture and community are vital to the health and well-being of indigenous people in a profound way that is not easily understood by the migrants of the last 200 hundred years. The mental health nursing care of Aboriginal and Torres Strait Islanders must be underpinned by a respect for these values and for the autonomy and self-determination of their communities. Working in partnership with Aboriginal and Torres Strait Islander communities requires non-indigenous nurses to provide expertise as requested, and to be aware of their limitations. Community development principles demand that priority be given to the training of indigenous mental health nurses, and to helping communities to evaluate their mental health needs and develop mental health programs. It is only in this way that self-determination can have a solid community base, and a solid community base provides the road to mental health for Aboriginal and Torres Strait Islander people.

# COLONISATION

Through life every person faces many crises. However, indigenous people living under the dominance of western culture have extra crises to face. It has to be understood that the Australian indigenous population lived for over 50 000 years in harmony with themselves and their environment. When Captain Cook first encountered Aboriginal people he described them as fit and healthy; indeed, fitter than his own men. Since the colonisation of the country in 1788 there has been a major transition from holistic, healthy hunter–gatherer communities to a situation of unhealthy lifestyles. Many Aboriginal people have suffered:

- loss of land, culture and identity;
- loss of self-esteem;
- institutionalisation;
- discrimination and isolation;
- abuse, violence and murder.

Indigenous Australians have been declared 'fourth world' people (developing countries are designated 'third world'). 'Fourth world' is a term applied to countries where indigenous peoples are enslaved under colonial powers, enduring the plight of 'dispossession and ill health' (Reid & Trompf 1991, pp.xiii–xv). In fact, a representative of the World Council of Churches described Central Australian Aboriginal communities as worse than fourth world.

The report, *Human Rights and Mental Illness*, by Human Rights Commissioner Brian Burdekin, clearly highlights the need for culturally appropriate mental health services for Aboriginal and Torres Strait Islander peoples (HREOC 1993). The Commissioner interviewed many Aboriginal and Torres Strait Islander witnesses, who spoke of the effects of colonisation which had left a legacy of grief and loss still profoundly felt to this day.

In their submission to the Human Rights and Equal Opportunities Commission, the Central Australian Aboriginal Congress said:

> Our people were forced from their country and into missions or government settlements. This loss involved economic, spiritual and cultural disruption. There were massacres of our people as recently as the 1930s. Forced settlement came with handouts of food, white flour, sugar and tea. We were denied access to our natural sources of food—then a policy of assimilation was imposed on us and our children were taken away and families split up. (Central Australian Aboriginal Congress and Anyinginyi Congress Aboriginal Corporation, joint submission, (HREOC 1993)

## MENTAL HEALTH

> There is a need to identify more clearly the nature of mental health problems amongst Aborigines. (NAHS 8.16.1 1989, p.172)

A survey conducted by the Victorian Aboriginal Health Service in 1987 found that 65% of respondents had been separated from a parent during childhood, 47% had been separated from both parents (29% and 7% are the respective figures for non-Aboriginal peoples), and 21% had been in an institution as a child (Swan 1991, p.1).

The traumatic breakdown of Aboriginal communities is supported by the files of the South Australian Aboriginal Childcare Agency:

> ... of 55 children and natural parents who contacted Aboriginal Child Care Agencies in regard to adoption into non-Aboriginal families, 52 were experiencing, or had experienced, severe emotional stress and disturbance. This stress was in relation to identity crisis, and inability to locate natural family members due to Government regulations on adoptions. Twenty of the cases had severe drug or alcohol problems relating to their family, and identity issues. Anxiety, over-eating, and inability to care for their own children were other associated problems which came to our notice. Departmental files on adoption of Aboriginal children are not accessible to Aboriginal Child Care Agencies. (Ashka 1985, cited in Reid & Tromp 1991, p.32)

Over the past few years several Aboriginal and Torres Strait Islanders have been found in mental institutions or about to be sent to one. In my own practice I have come across people who have been diagnosed as mentally disturbed when, in fact, it was simply a matter of the staff being unable to communicate with

Aboriginal or Islander clients, particularly elderly clients with limited English. An Aboriginal field officer is an important resource to ensure accurate clinical assessment.

Similarly, any Aboriginal Legal Service would be able to cite numerous cases where indigenous offenders have not understood court proceedings and have simply answered 'yes' to all questions, believing this is what was required of them. They are put into gaol, totally confused, separated from family, friends and 'country' (traditional lands), and further alienated from mainstream society and authority figures.

Alcohol and drug abuse is common in indigenous people who are suffering from varying degrees of mental distress. Quite often they are simply dismissed as drunks and not given any counselling appropriate to their mental condition. Recommendation Number 70 of the Royal Commission into Aboriginal Deaths in Custody (RCADIC) states:

> That organisations developing policies and programs addressing Aboriginal alcohol issues must:
>
> a) Recognise the inadequacy of single factor explanations (such as the disease model of problematic alcohol use) of the cases of alcohol dependence and misuse among individuals, and
>
> b) Take into account the fact that multiple explanations are necessary to explain the causes of alcohol misuse and related problems *at the community level*. It is therefore inappropriate to focus too strongly on any one explanation to the exclusion of others. (RCIADIC 1991, 2.332)

The Western Australian Branch of the Royal Australian and New Zealand College of Psychiatrists presented evidence that Aboriginal people are massively overrepresented in involuntary admissions to psychiatric hospitals and within the corrective services system.

> Being Aboriginal carries a threefold increase of involuntary psychiatric admission to state hospitals, and being a metropolitan Aborigine carried a five-fold increased risk of compulsory admission. In comparison with non-Aboriginal patients, Aboriginal patients have a seven-fold greater chance of an alcohol or organic brain syndrome diagnosis being made. (HREOC 1993)

In Queensland, a survey conducted in 1991 found that 70% of Aboriginal and Torres Strait Islander inpatients were diagnosed as having schizophrenia or substance abuse disorders, in comparison to 42% of non-Aboriginal patients. These apparent disparities in diagnosis are due to culturally inappropriate methods of assessment.

Indigenous mental health workers can make a huge difference in many of the fields outlined above. However, there is a real need for a formalised course for *all* those who work, in any capacity, with Aboriginal and Torres Strait Islander people. Unless this is formulated, implemented and stringently adhered to, we will continue to see the same problems recurring.

Aboriginal and Torres Strait Islander people with mental health disorders sometimes have to be admitted to general hospitals. In these institutions they are confronted by cultural forces which affect their recovery. The problem is that non-indigenous health professionals do not understand the cultural mores of indigenous people. Former Commissioner of ATSIC, Sol Bellear, is quoted as saying: 'The mental health profession must understand, not merely pay lip service to the diversity of cultures in this country. They should show a willingness to train and if necessary re-train in cross-cultural understanding.'

# CROSS-CULTURAL CARE

Every employment advertisement for Aboriginal and Torres Strait Islander organisations and for those government departments dealing with Aboriginal and Torres Strait Islander peoples includes the following standard statement:

> Applicants must have demonstrated knowledge and understanding of Aboriginal and/or Torres Strait Islander cultures and the ability to communicate effectively with Aboriginal and/or Torres Strait Islander people.

A great deal is said about cross-cultural training for non-indigenous medical professionals, paraprofessionals, educators, the police, the judiciary and public services. But what is this cross-cultural training that everyone is being encouraged to undertake? Certainly, the expected outcomes are to be applauded—a greater understanding and sensitivity towards indigenous clients, their culture, beliefs and their law. This commitment to cross-cultural communication is based on a belief in cultural relativism that respects the differences between cultures and seeks to accommodate them. However, successful cross-cultural communication depends on more than commitment.

Structural obstacles to cross-cultural interaction have been identified in the guide to bridging cultures in Aboriginal health, *Binangoonj*. In addition to the impact of colonialism and racism, other factors such as the institutional constraints of health care services often mitigate efforts at cross-cultural interaction. *Binangoonj* specifically identifies the institutional nature of health care administration, which isolates patient care from family and community care, professional demands which may override client or caregiver needs, and the biomedical model of health which focuses on curative rather than holistic interventions (Eckerman et al. 1992, p.124).

The primary health care approach to nursing provides an extremely useful model to apply when working with Aboriginal and Islander communities. This approach works towards genuine community participation and empowerment through the effective use of intersectoral and interdisciplinary collaboration. The focus on social justice and social causes of illness is particularly pertinent to Aboriginal and Islander communities (see Chapter 16).

Health care workers require training in communication skills appropriate for work with the Aboriginal community. For example, Eckerman et al. (1992) outline a number of obstacles to cross-cultural communication which operate at the nurse–client level. These include difficulties, involving not just the use of words, but gestures, facial expressions, the context in which communication takes place, Aboriginal perceptions of the professional, and professionals' perception of their role.

## Communication

Aboriginal people have culturally specific communication conventions. Many of these are subtle and require skill and practice for the non-indigenous nurse to negotiate. For example, open-ended questions such as 'How are you feeling?' may well receive a null response—Aboriginal patients may feel more comfortable with a statement such as 'You are not feeling well', which they can affirm or deny (Eckerman et al. 1992, p.125). Tone of voice and the approach taken are also important to Aboriginal people, and communicate whether nurses are prepared to take time to find out what is happening with their clients, or if they are too busy. If nurses inadvertently communicate the message that they are busy, then they are unlikely to receive any response to questions. Aboriginal and Islander peoples can be extremely adept at reading body language and just as much attention should be paid to *how* the nurse says something, as to what is actually said (Menere 1992).

One feature of Aboriginal and Islander communication that has particular importance in the field of mental health is described by Holland (1995) as the 'blank wall effect'. A nurse may find herself confronted with an Aboriginal client who expresses no emotion, refuses eye contact and either declines to answer questions or anwers in monosyllables. This attitude is commonly encountered when clients are vulnerable or powerless, and particularly if they have been subjected to racist treatment by staff.

The 'blank wall effect' presents a number of challenges for the nurse, especially the mental health nurse. First, the phenomenon must be distinguished from negative affect (a psychiatric symptom, discussed in Chapter 10); second, the nurse must endeavour to establish goodwill and obtain the confidence of the client. This is difficult when the client has chosen to disengage. It is important that the nurse remains open and friendly towards the client and endeavours to break down what may be the experience of cultural isolation for the client. Aboriginal health workers are an invaluable resource for the nurse and should be utilised. In addition, it may be possible to move the client to a room with people from the same 'mob' or 'country'. The nurse should at all times be advised by Aboriginal health workers or community members and respect the cultural sensibilities of Aboriginal and Islander peoples.

Understanding the interpersonal relationships that exist in Aboriginal communities is also important. The care of an individual occurs within the context of the extended family, and it may not be clear to the non-indigenous nurse who are the key people to consult over care and discharge plans.

## Aboriginal understanding of health

For Aboriginal people health and sickness are often understood in terms of relationships between people. This approach impacts not only on Aboriginal understanding of the disease process, but also of treatment. *Binangoonj* gives a number of case studies that demonstrate how the role of professionals may be interpreted as central to the course of the illness. For example, if a patient in your care becomes sicker, then that patient and his or her family may avoid your care in the future. Thus, even with the best of intentions, a lack of understanding between cultures works against the needs of Aboriginal peoples. The only appropriate premise for an Aboriginal health service is to base it firmly on the community's view of health and sickness. To do this, the service must become part of that community.

## Professional perceptions

The view that health care workers treat everyone the same, regardless of their race or culture, is now challenged by ideas on cultural safety. This view, developed in New Zealand and proposed by some Aboriginal health workers (Eckerman et al. 1992), argues that, on the contrary, people should not all be treated the same. The supposed 'neutral' position on race or culture is a reinforcement of the dominant culture. Nurses do not treat everyone the same— they treat everyone as if they were Anglo-Celts. Ramsden (1990) argues that an altruistic ideal that denies the differences between people ignores very real distinctions and people's different needs, and in fact constitutes harmful practice. The principles of cultural safety enshrine the importance of culture to health, and cultural appropriateness to care. As is argued by the National Aboriginal Health Strategy (1989):

> Mental health services are designed and controlled by the dominant society for the dominant society. The health system does not recognise or adapt programs to Aboriginal beliefs and law, causing a huge gap between service provider and user ... As a result, mental distress in the Aboriginal community goes unnoticed, undiagnosed (and misdiagnosed) and untreated (or wrongly treated). (NAHS 8.16, p.172)

In order to provide cross-cultural care to Aboriginal and Torres Strait Islander peoples, the mental health nurse must develop an understanding of and respect for the interrelationship between culture and healing that is central to Aboriginal mental health.

## CULTURE AND HEALING

> For 200 years non-Aboriginal Australia has made many mistakes on our behalf, and there is no western model that can address the Aboriginal situation. Aboriginal people must be empowered by education and resources to control decisions affecting our lives, including mental health services. It is

clear to Aboriginal people that those with unfinished business have low self-esteem and those with high self-esteem don't self-mutilate. (Pat Swan 1991)

Christianity has played, and is still playing a major role in our cultural beliefs in traditional healing. The colonial notion when missionaries arrived was that traditional healings and ceremonies were paganistic, and that our healers were demonically possessed. Our bush remedies were also seen as satanic. The practice of promoting not only a western Christian philosophy but of acceptance of western medical healing was promoted. Sadly, this control by western ideologies still exists throughout the present system and although churches, schools, health institutions say in theory that they want to assist our cultural heritage, it is extremely difficult for them to change their narrow concept of the ways of healing and teaching.

Many Aboriginal and Torres Strait Islander people believe that the western medical model of mental health services applied to Aboriginal and Torres Strait Islander peoples is ethnocentric and definitely perpetuates stereotypes of Aborigines as deviant.

The western model treats the symptoms of mental illness as medical disorders. It does not cater for Aboriginal and Torres Strait Islander spiritual beliefs, therefore, if things are not tangible or confirmed with scientific evidence, Aboriginal and Torres Strait Islander clients are usually misdiagnosed as being 'crazy' or 'womba'. They are certainly mistreated, which can cause enormous problems leading to **suicide**.

It is imperative that nurses collaborate with our traditional healers, who are men and women of great wisdom and spiritual power, which has been passed down from generation to generation. It is vital that we respect the methods of our men and women of great wisdom who are our traditional healers (see Box 6.2). The way forward is for health workers to work with traditional healers, complementing each other in the healing process. In order to achieve this partnership, however, nurses must have cross-cultural awareness. This cross-cultural awareness is also essential for nurses to be able to deal with the enormous number of mental health problems that are the present-day consequences of past colonial practices.

The following case histories (Box 6.2) highlight some of the problems that indigenous people face when dealing with psychiatric services imbued with western assumptions.

## BOX 6.2: *Spiritual healing*

### Case 1

An indigenous female had lost 8 kilos within 3 months. She was regularly feeling tired and nauseous, with vomiting and diarrhoea. Her stomach became very swollen, as if she were pregnant. She was admitted to the gynaecology ward of

*continued ...*

the hospital where a scan was performed. Her abdomen was the size of a 40-week pregnant woman. After the scan, and other western medical testing, the client was diagnosed within 24 hours as having a massive tumour that was growing rapidly in her womb. The patient was transferred to the nearest large hospital with the likelihood of dying within the week.

The client urgently requested a traditional healer to give treatment as well as western intervention. The gynaecologist had no problems in allowing the traditional healer to treat this client before transferring her to a major hospital for an urgent hysterectomy.

The healer treated the client internally and externally. When she was operated on, the tumour had actually decreased in size within the three days, and was removed without any complications. The healer treated the client after her return from hospital. She is now completely well and has returned to work.

### Case 2

Three teenage Aboriginal girls were constantly misbehaving and seeing spiritual images in their home. Their mother had taken them to a doctor who could find no evidence of western sickness. All three described things moving in the home, and spiritual images antagonising them regularly. After the results of all medical tests were found to be normal, the mother contacted a traditional healer to assist.

The healer treated the girls for removal of sorcery as their home had been contaminated by articles found on the roof and in their bedrooms. The healer 'smoked' the building (a traditional exorcism). Mother and girls are convinced that they had been 'caught' or 'puri purried', and since the traditional healer has treated them they no longer see any of the spiritual images. The girls are back to living their normal healthy lives.

### Case 3

A 39-year-old Torres Strait Islander male woke up one evening and couldn't move his right side. The man, who was strong and healthy, became very lethargic and sick. He was admitted to hospital where all medical tests were normal. Doctors were puzzled as to the cause of his condition and could not treat with specific therapy except with broad spectrum antibiotics, although tests showed no infection.

The client's family requested a traditional healer, who immediately diagnosed him as having been 'purried'. Since treatment from the healer, the client is back to a normal life and is very strong and healthy.

### Case 4

A 50-year-old non-indigenous woman had a breast removed some three years ago for cancer. She was told her prognosis was very poor as doctors were unsure if all the cancer was removed. She did not want radium therapy and strongly believed in alternative holistic approaches to healing. She requested the assistance of a traditional healer, who treated her before and after her surgery. Today the woman is employed and enjoying a healthy life. Her regular follow-ups reveal no cancer.

## Partnership

The western medical model can complement Aboriginal and Torres Strait Islander cultural values if both cultures are respected, and accepted equally. It is of great importance that mental health nurses work closely with the community and integrate their skills within traditional networks. A clear example of the effectiveness of this approach is provided by Neil McCloud, the community nurse consultant for East Arnhemland. According to McCloud (1993), 'success is more likely in East Arnhemland Aboriginal mental health, when mental health issues remain community owned and recognise and utilise local resources'. In the case history in Box 6.3, McCloud relates the importance of mobilising traditional networks as part of his mental health nursing practice.

## BOX 6.3: Working with the community

... some months ago I was in a particular community trying to locate a man visiting from one of the coastal communities. This man has a history of self-mutilation and serious suicide attempts by self-immolation. All these acts had taken place in highly public areas of his community. This man is of mixed descent having a Yolgnu (Aboriginal) mother and balinda (European) father. I am aware that he was teased by his Yolgnu peer group regarding his mixed descent. My role was one of ongoing counselling and **crisis intervention**.

We were sitting on the front verandah but unable to get into any meaningful conversation due to continual interruptions either by people calling from the road in Yolgnu Matha or by the telephone ringing. At the risk of being impolite I finally asked if my visit was interrupting Yolgnu business. This young man confided that on the previous night, when under the influence of alcohol, he had placed a curse on the community shop. Consequently the shop was unable to open. The elders were very angry with him and he was under pressure to appear before community council members to explain his actions. Unfortunately, this man had the power to place the curse on the shop but he had not yet been given the words or ceremony to remove it.

The grandfather of this man is an important traditional land owner and elder. His stature in the community is such that he is often asked to complete or assist in ceremonies. In this case my intervention was simple; this man was trapped and as such remained a high risk to himself. By removing him from the community and explaining the situation to his grandfather we were able to work as a team to resolve this crisis. His grandfather removed the curse and placated the community. In later discussion we reviewed his grandson's case history together and identified a joint approach involving traditional and western interventions.

The grandfather identified that his grandson perceived he lacked identity and as such had no self-respect. With identity would come self-respect.

*continued ...*

The grandfather would give him that identity in ceremony. My work continues with this person mainly in crisis intervention, problem solving and impulse control.

Last week I watched this man play a significant role by dance in a funeral ceremony. This indicates a change in his community stature and reinforcement of his self-respect and dignity.

It is the role of the nurse to recognise and work within community networks, alongside traditional healers, and to support the Aboriginal health workers as the key facilitators of this process. The aim is to 'complement traditional mental health with additional western mental health skills, allowing these skills to be utilised within community structures ... [to] demystify mental health services and make them more accessible to Aboriginal people' (McCloud 1993).

## Urban solutions

Not all Aboriginal people have access to traditional healers or live in traditional communities. For urban Aboriginal and Torres Strait Islander people the issues may well be the same, but local solutions are required. The tragic, but sadly far from exceptional, fact is that many of the 'stolen' children have experienced periods in institutions (see Box 6.1). Overall, Aboriginal people experience high rates of incarceration via both the juvenile justice system and the prison system. They also experience high levels of intervention from corrective services, parole officers, police officers, social workers and welfare officers. It is difficult to see how admission to another institution (a psychiatric facility), and the management of another set of professionals (mental health nurses), often with police involvement, would be a helpful strategy in the management of a mental health problem experienced by an Aboriginal person. What then is an appropriate approach to take? One model is that developed in Victoria by the Aboriginal Mental Health Network (VAMHN), which emerged out of the Victorian Aboriginal Health Service. This Unit has taken a number of steps to make mental health services more appropriate to the care of Aboriginal and Torres Strait Islander peoples.

One of the problems identified by the VAMHN is that, for Aboriginal people, admission to a psychiatric facility generally compounds their sense of isolation. As health services are regionalised they may be the only Aboriginal inpatient in the facility. The VAMHN has responded to this problem by establishing a supra-regional inpatient facility as a Koori treatment unit (McKendrick et al. 1992). In this way Aboriginal patients are able to have their cultural identity affirmed, as opposed to threatened, if inpatient treatment is required.

Secondly, Aboriginal people cannot be treated in isolation from their community and their extended families. Part of the process of a Koori Unit is to involve the family in the care given to the client. A residential centre in Fitzroy provides clients with the chance to undergo treatment or receive care among Aboriginal mental health workers, with a great amount of involvement from their families (McKendrick et al. 1992). Thus, model programs such as the Koori Unit allow for culturally appropriate care to be the *first* priority in the care of Aboriginal and Torres Strait Islander people suffering from mental health problems.

Similar moves are underway in New South Wales where a Primary Community Mental Health Development Program has been developed as a joint venture between Aboriginal communities, Aboriginal independent medical services, Aboriginal Health Education officers/workers and health professsionals (Richards, Shields & Holland 1993).

The programs outlined above are underpinned by the belief that the answer to the mental health problems facing Aboriginal Australians is to be found as much in empowerment and self-determination as in the orthodox approaches of modern psychiatry and the assumptions of non-indigenous health professionals. Single-factor explanations of the medical model must be widened to recognise the need for culturally safe and culturally appropriate forms of care. Preparation for cross-cultural care should therefore be mandatory, because without it health professionals will continue to undermine the cultural identity of their indigenous clients. Western assumptions about mental health and illness must now be complemented by Aboriginal understandings; and the skills of mental health workers must be complemented by the wisdom and spiritual power of traditional healers, and incorporated into the traditional networks of Aboriginal communities. Similarly, mental health services in urban areas must become more attuned to reinforcing the cultural identity of indigenous clients.

## SUMMARY

- The mental health of Aboriginal and Torres Strait Islander peoples can only be considered in the historical and social context.
- Aboriginality does not cause mental illness.
- Cultural identity is a primary factor in mental well-being.
- Non-indigenous health professionals need training in cross-cultural care before they can work effectively with Aboriginal and Torres Strait Islander peoples.
- It is imperative that nurses value the wisdom and spiritual powers of traditional healers, and collaborate with them.
- Mental health services with Aboriginal clients must become more culturally responsive.

# DISCUSSION QUESTIONS

1. If Aboriginality is not in itself a cause of mental illness, how do you explain the disproportionate number of Aboriginal people with serious mental health problems?

2. What cultural values are taken for granted in the way clients of mental health services are assessed, treated and discharged? What effect are these processes likely to have on indigenous clients?

3. How could you prepare yourself to provide culturally safe care for Aboriginal clients and their families?

4. What nursing interventions could you use to reinforce the cultural identity of (a) a young Aboriginal man who is an inpatient in a psychiatric unit in a general hospital, and (b) a middle-aged Aboriginal woman living in an urban area?

# EXERCISES

1. Ask your lecturer to arrange a clinical placement in an Aboriginal community for a group of students in your course. Keep a journal on your experiences and thoughts during the placement and discuss your reflections with your tutorial group when you return. What do you now understand about your own cultural values and cultural identity?

2. Contact the unit that has responsibility for supporting Aboriginal and Torres Strait Islander students in your university and find out how it sets about reinforcing their cultural identity. How could similar principles be applied in mental health services?

3. Apply the principles of the primary health care model outlined in Chapter 16 to Aboriginal mental health.

4. Debate the probability that non-indigenous nurses can be effective in reinforcing the cultural identity of Aboriginal and Torres Strait Islander people.

5. Find out if there is an Aboriginal Health Unit in your area. Invite an Aboriginal health worker to speak to your group. Find out what services and resources they provide in the area of mental health. Is there any information they can give you about Aboriginal and Islander communities in your area?

# FURTHER READING

- Eckerman, A., Dowd, T., Martin, M., Nixon, L., Gray, R. & Chong, E. (1992) *Binangoonj. Bridging Cultures in Aboriginal Health*, Armidale: University of New England Press. This book is a manual of cultural issues in Aboriginal health care. It was produced in conjunction with the Council of Remote Area Nurses of Australia and provides an excellent analysis of the issues concerning Aboriginal health, with useful guidelines for practitioners to follow.

- Edwards, C. & Read, P. (1989) *The Lost Children*, Sydney: Doubleday. This book tells the stories of thirteen families of stolen children and their efforts to return to their families and communities.
- Human Rights and Equal Opportunities Commission (1993) *Human Rights and Mental Illness*, Vols 1 & 2. Canberra: AGPS. The section on Aboriginal mental health presents an overview of the issues surrounding mental health for Aboriginal and Torres Strait Islander peoples.

# REFERENCES

Eckerman, A., Dowd, T., Martin, M., Nixon, L., Gray, R. & Chong, E. (1992) *Binangoonj. Bridging Cultures in Aboriginal Health*. Armidale: University of New England Press.

Edwards, C. & Read, P. (1989) *The Lost Children*, Sydney: Doubleday.

Holland, R. (1995) personal communication.

Human Rights and Equal Opportunities Commission (1993) *Human Rights and Mental Illness*, Vols 1 & 2. Canberra: AGPS.

McKendrick, J., Thorpe, G., Austin, G. & Roberts, W. (1992) *Victorian Aboriginal Mental Health Network*. Discussion Paper.

McCloud, N. (1993) 'Early intervention in East Arnhemland rural mental health', *Mental Health in Australia* 5(2), pp.76–81.

Menere, R. (1992) *Remote Area Nursing Manual*, Lismore: University of New England.

National Aboriginal Health Strategy Working Party (1989) *National Aboriginal Health Strategy*, Canberra: AGPS.

Ramsden, I. (1990) 'Cultural safety', *New Zealand Nursing Journal* 83(11), pp.18–19.

Reid, J. & Trompf, P. (1991) *The Health of Aboriginal Australia*, Sydney: Harcourt Brace Jovanovich.

Richards, J., Shields, R. & Holland, R. (1993) *Building Bridges and the Big Picture. Primary Community Mental Health Development*, National Aboriginal Mental Health Conference, Sydney University, November 1993.

Royal Commission on Aboriginal Deaths in Custody (1991) *Final Report and Recommendations*, Canberra: AGPS.

Swan, P. (1991) '22 years of unfinished business', *The Lamp* 48(11), pp.40–3.

# Dance

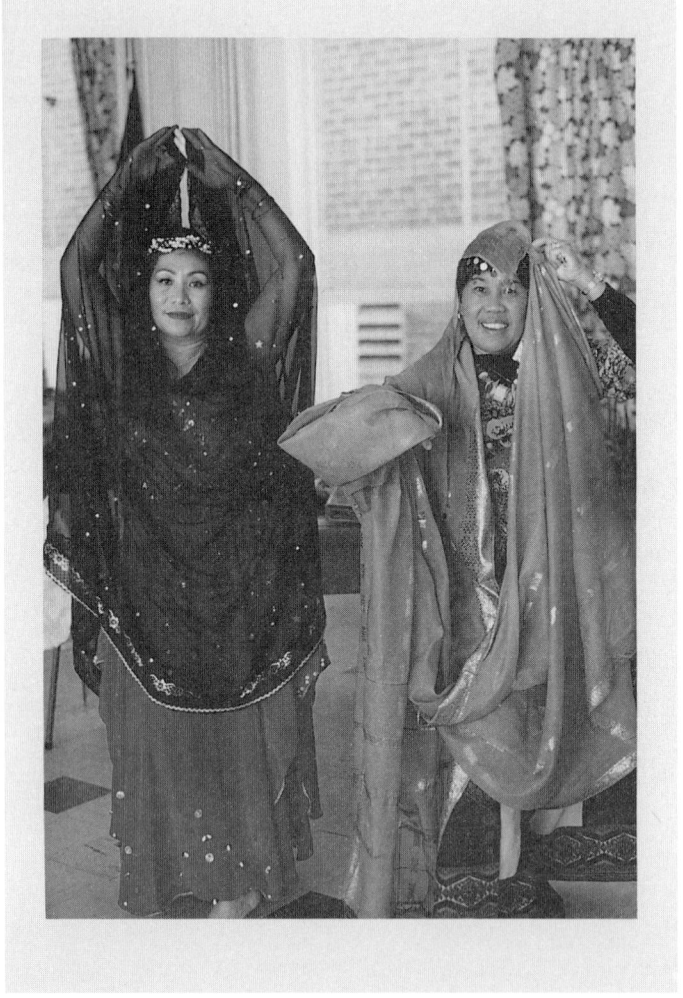

ROBERTA JULIAN

Dance can provide a means for maintaining physical
and mental health among the ethnic elderly.

Alicia Young and Ludivina Cooley perform multicultural dances
at a regular meeting of elderly migrants in Hobart.

## CHAPTER 7

# MENTAL HEALTH AND ETHNICITY

Gary Easthope and Roberta Julian

## CONTENTS

# LEARNING OBJECTIVES

This chapter will assist the reader to:

- develop an understanding of the relationships between mental health and ethnicity;
- appreciate the wide variation among ethnic groups in their understanding of mental illness and ways of dealing with it;
- understand that it may be more important to learn individuals' migration experiences, whether as refugees or voluntary migrants, than to know the ethnic group to which they belong;
- recognise that patients' social location is often more important than ethnicity in understanding their mental health.
- be aware that the point in a person's life course at which migration occurs may be central to understanding his or her mental health.

# INTRODUCTION

Let us start by admitting ignorance. Current knowledge of the incidence of mental illness among Australian migrant groups is sketchy at best. Three types of studies have been conducted which provide epidemiological data (National Health Strategy 1993, pp.46–8; Wooden et al. 1994, pp.176–80):

1. Hospital admission studies. This work found increased levels of **depression** among migrants, and increased rates of **schizophrenia** among migrants from non-English speaking backgrounds (**NESB**) from southern and eastern Europe.
2. Community surveys. A survey based on self-reported incidence in a general population found NESB migrants more likely to report mental ill-health.
3. Ethnic community surveys. These report lower figures than the previous two methods but still report a higher rate among NESB migrants. They have also found that the prevalence of mental illness is high among socioeconomically disadvantaged ethnic communities.

We have not provided any figures from these surveys as a range of methodological problems makes the interpretation of the data problematic. In addition, we believe that to present such figures is to suggest that ethnicity is a stable category with explanatory power. Rather we are concerned with migration as a process which is, in part, affected by ethnicity. Nonetheless, the figures from the Australian epidemiological and community studies do provide weak evidence of higher rates of mental illness among NESB migrants when compared to people born in Australia. The meaning that can be placed on these findings is discussed in the next section.

# *T*HE RELATIONSHIP BETWEEN ETHNIC IDENTITY AND MENTAL ILLNESS: EXPLANATIONS

There are four arguments that try to explain the broad findings noted above. The first argument considers whether ethnic identity causes mental illness. Does being Polish or Vietnamese predispose a person to mental illness or to specific mental illnesses? Despite cultural stereotypes of the depressed Slav and the excitable Latin American, it is extremely unlikely that ethnic identity in itself causes mental illness. Such a conception of ethnicity is racist (Ahmad 1993, p.19; Sashidharan & Francis 1993).

The second argument suggests that variation in mental illness is a function of cultural misunderstandings and treatment opportunities. Cultural differences have been found to affect both diagnosis and treatment (Wooden et al. 1994; Jayasuriya, Sang & Fielding 1992; Sashidharan & Francis 1993). Instruments designed to assess psychiatric disorder lack accuracy in cross-cultural situations even when questionnaires are stringently translated (Minas 1990). Studies have also demonstrated that the language of interview has a strong effect on self-assessments of mental health (Angel & Guarnaccia 1989). Communication difficulties clearly contribute to the problems of overdiagnosis, underdiagnosis and incorrect diagnosis (Minas 1990). They may also affect the treatment provided—for example, patients diagnosed with schizophrenia were more likely to receive electroconvulsive therapy if they came from a non-English speaking background (Minas 1990). Further, the type of treatment opportunity offered may affect presentation for treatment (see discussion of Vietnamese below).

The third explanation suggests that it is not ethnicity but the process of immigration that can cause mental illness. Immigration, particularly as a refugee, is stressful and can precipitate mental illness. Immigration challenges taken-for-granted assumptions and ways of behaving. For some, such challenges affect their adaptive functioning and cause mental illness. This argument is supported by research findings, but not in a simple manner. A study of Vietnamese **refugees** in the United States five years after arrival (Chung & Kagawa-Singer 1993) found that the number of traumatic events experienced prior to migration, the length of time in refugee camps, low income and poor proficiency in English were predictors of mental ill-health, particularly for women and older people. A Norwegian study seven years after arrival (Hauff & Vaglum 1993) found, on the contrary, that the refugee camp experience did not predict mental health problems and only war traumas were important predictors. The only longitudinal Australian study (Krupinski & Burrows 1986) found that on arrival the refugees showed more mental health symptoms than native-born Australians, but had lower rates than the native-born two years after arrival.

The fourth argument suggests that the apparently higher rate of mental illness among immigrants is a function of their social location. Many migrants, particularly those with limited English skills, are forced to take jobs that are stressful and exhausting. Such jobs can create mental and physical ill-health, especially if the migrants formerly had high-status positions in their country of origin, Furthermore, a lack of facility in English makes it more difficult for such migrants to access support services, both medical and welfare, which may help to prevent the development of mental illness (Easthope 1989, revised edition in press).

In considering these arguments we conclude that ethnicity in itself is not a significant factor in mental health. We argue that immigration is a long-term process of adaptation involving a complex interplay between culture, social location, stage of life and biographical experiences. Thus, any individual has a lifestyle (culture), a set of life chances (based on social location), has reached a certain point in the life cycle, and undergone certain life experiences. This formulation enables us to talk about people of the same culture without falling into the trap of presuming that all those with the same lifestyle are the same; in short, it stops us reifying ethnicity and culture as simple explanatory variables.

We are thus able to discuss the adaptation made by a young, single (life cycle) Italian (lifestyle) arriving from industrial Milan (life experience) who gains a job immediately (life chance), and compare it with the adaptation made by an elderly (life cycle) Italian peasant woman (life experiences) arriving under family reunion provisions who has no marketable skills and no English (life chances). She may have more in common, in terms of her adaptation, with an elderly Vietnamese woman arriving to join her family than with the young Italian.

In more formal terms, any understanding of migrant adaptation must take into account class, gender and biographical experience, as well as ethnicity, if a full understanding of mental health is to be achieved.

# IMMIGRANT ADAPTATION

While stressing the need to examine the biographical experiences of immigrants rather than assuming the significance of cultural factors, it is important that we do not replace a simplistic 'cultural effect' argument with an equally simplistic 'migration effect' argument. Immigration *per se* does not cause mental health problems. Nevertheless, immigration may be stressful at the premigration, migration or postmigration stages, thus contributing to the development of mental illness.

For example, settlement may be **stressful**. The major settlement stressors are employment and accommodation difficulties, downward social mobility, separation from family and social networks, and communication problems as a result of language differences (NHS 1993). Racism and discrimination are additional structural factors that contribute to mental illness (Jayasuriya et al. 1992). To reiterate earlier arguments, while migrants of similar ethnic origin and cultural backgrounds often have similar immigration and settlement experiences, this does not mean that ethnicity and/or culture is the most important factor in their mental health. For example, migrants with qualifications not recognised in Australia are likely to be in lower-status occupations than those held in the society of origin. Such experience of downward mobility may contribute to the development of mental disorders which have little to do with cultural factors.

Immigration may thus precipitate mental health problems (Cox 1989). Some experiences, including nostalgia and culture shock, can be considered 'normal' characteristics of the dislocation of migration. Nevertheless, immigrants experiencing such problems do present with symptoms of mental illness. European studies (e.g. Zwingman 1973, cited in Cox 1989, p.33) identify the symptoms of nostalgia as decrease in efficiency, idealisation of the past, lowered capacity for empathy, guilt feelings over family members back home, fatigue and loss of vitality, sensitivity with paranoid tendencies, accident proneness, decreased frustration tolerance and feelings of hostility.

It is important for those working with migrants to be aware that these symptoms may be part of a nostalgic reaction to migration. Informing immigrants about nostalgia can help them to develop coping strategies so that they do not develop more serious mental health problems (Cox 1989). Such symptoms should not be treated simply as medical conditions but rather viewed as behavioural patterns consistent with a particular stage of settlement. Health workers can then reduce the symptoms of nostalgia by assisting migrants in the settlement process; for example, by acquainting them with their new social environment and by helping them to develop meaningful social contacts, in order to maximise their participation in society.

## M IGRANTS AT RISK

A number of factors contribute to the development of mental illness among Australia's multi-ethnic population. Some are ethnic and/or cultural while others have more to do with migration and settlement experiences. The latter are more clearly located within a 'life stressor' framework. The interplay of various factors enables the identification of the populations most at risk: refugees, women, children and adolescents, and the aged.

### Refugees

When working with refugees it is important to be aware that symptoms of mental ill-health are likely to be associated with premigration traumatic experiences such as war, imprisonment, sexual assault and torture. The 'causes' of mental health problems among refugees settling in Australia may therefore be different from those of other migrants. It is for this reason that Jupp (1994) and others have called for refugees to be distinguished from other migrants, particularly in the provision of health and welfare services. He notes that the lack of appropriate specialised services for refugees may be due to the limited knowledge among Australians (including the medical, nursing and psychology professions) of the nature and extent of the atrocities experienced by some refugees:

> It is almost incomprehensible to many mainstream service deliverers that such viciousness can be routinely exercised by states against their citizens. They often lack knowledge of the social and political situations which make torture almost 'normal' in some particularly disturbed societies, and tend to dismiss accounts as exaggerated. It should be an essential part of any cross-cultural sensitisation program for service deliverers and medical or paramedical professionals that some attempt be made to include an understanding of this phenomenon. (Jupp 1994, pp.61–2)

Differences among refugees have been identified on the basis of age and gender as well as stage of the life cycle. The study by Krupinski and Burrows (1986) of young Indo-Chinese refugees found that, among young adults, over one-third had been diagnosed as having a psychiatric disorder. However, they also found differences between age groups: specifically, that stressful premigration experiences were not related to the frequency of disorders among adolescents or young adults, but that a relationship did exist for those in the 10–14 year old age group. They argue this was because 'these children experienced a number of severe stresses at critical periods in their psychological development' (Krupinski & Burrows 1986, pp.208–9). Interestingly the key determinant was found to be whether the individual interpreted those experiences as stressful rather than the actual experiences.

There is contradictory research evidence regarding the chronicity of mental illness in refugee immigrants. Research suggests that the trauma of refugee migration is overcome within a few years—the frequency of psychiatric symptomatology was found to be at a very low level within 24 months after arrival in Australia (Krupinski & Burrows 1986). Studies of postwar displaced people, on the other hand, argue that refugees are likely to have chronic mental health problems (e.g. Krupinski, Stoller & Wallace 1973). This is supported by the fact that the centres for the survivors of trauma and torture, recently established in most Australian capital cities primarily to meet the needs of recent refugees, are finding that now-elderly postwar displaced persons comprise a significant proportion of their clientele. Recent studies in Australia, based on psychiatric casework (e.g. Silove et al. 1991), also demonstrate the chronicity of post-traumatic stress symptoms. This indicates the need for health workers to be aware of the importance of the premigration experiences of refugees, even among long-term residents, so that they do not automatically, and inappropriately, medicalise mental health problems.

## Women

Studies of postwar immigrants emphasised the prevalence of psychiatric disorders among single male immigrants (e.g. Martin 1965). Studies of recent migrants, however, emphasise that women comprise a key at-risk category. For example, Krupinski and Burrows (1986) found that females were diagnosed with twice as many psychiatric disorders as males at first interview. While the significance of the role played by women in the settlement process is often acknowledged, very little research has been conducted on the effects of this role on women's mental health.

The life experience of a migrant woman is stressful in that it involves changing role expectations. A number of factors contribute to this stress: for example, not being involved in the decision-making process leading to migration and being expected to manage the emotional life of the family in an unfamiliar context without the resources on which she would normally rely. Separation from social support networks in the country of origin is a particularly important life stressor for migrant women.

Psychiatric illness among immigrant women is often attributed to high levels of isolation from the receiving society (Cox 1989). This is true for women in the paid workforce and for those who are not. Employed migrant women are likely to be 'tracked' into industries such as clothing (Yeatman 1992) regardless of skill level. Here they work with other NESB women, thus contributing to their level of isolation from the receiving society. In this way, their experiences of isolation are similar to NESB women who are isolated within the home.

In analysing mental illness among migrant women, we need to consider the cultural construction of gender as well as the cultural expectations of appropriate roles within the family. It has been argued, for example, that the 'typical' situation of migrant women in the 1960s produced a particular pattern of psychiatric illness:

> ... this late (7 to 14 years after arrival) mental breakdown in married, non-assimilated female migrants could be due among other things to the end of the mother's usefulness in a grown-up, now assimilated family, which has left her behind. This would inevitably result in frustration and hence a greater likelihood to develop mental disorder. (Reeves 1973, cited in Cox 1989, p.84)

However, cultural expectations in relation to gender and familial roles change over time, across generations and in different sociohistorical contexts. While the above account may have been characteristic of migrant women in the 1960s, it is important to recognise that gender expectations have been changing in the countries of origin, just as they have been changing in Australia. Furthermore, there has been a significant shift in source countries since the 1950s (ABS 1994, p.xvii). As a consequence, we may expect that this pattern of mental illness will not continue.

If we examine more recent migrant women, we find an increased proportion with high levels of education and an increased proportion of refugees. This variation in migrant intake is likely to alter the profile of mental illness. In particular, the experiences of refugee women are markedly different from those of voluntary migrants (Pittaway 1991). The onset of mental illness among these refugees may be earlier than that for other migrant women, and the need for different treatment strategies is clear.

When examining refugees and mental health, some argue that the effect of gender is greater than that of ethnicity in the management of stress. This may be due, in large part, to the similarity of premigration experiences. It is estimated that over 60% of refugee women in Australia have suffered from torture, sexual assault and rape (Pittaway 1991). As with many sexual assault survivors, it is not uncommon for the invasive techniques associated with childbirth in hospital settings to trigger psychological responses which relate to premigration experiences. Some knowledge of the experiences of refugee women is therefore important for nursing staff working in obstetrics.

## The aged

The ethnic aged include aged arrivals under the Family Reunion Program as well as those migrants who have grown old in Australia. Research (Ames 1991) has found that the ethnic aged experience a number of life stressors that make them vulnerable to psychological distress and depression. These include low incomes, social isolation and language problems. For example, Thomas and Balnaves (1993) found high levels of psychological stress among aged Vietnamese and argue that this was predominantly due to financial stress and isolation from kin. The tendency for the ethnic aged to revert to their first language has been well documented, although the extent to which this depends on age-related psychosis is debated (Rowland 1991, pp.40–1).

There is clearly a need for innovative programs to cater for the diverse needs of the ethnic elderly, who differ in terms of cultural background, socioeconomic status, access to family and ethnic support networks, age at migration and English language proficiency. A wide range of programs is evident throughout Australia's capital cities, including ethnic nursing homes, ethnic respite care and the concentration of the ethnic elderly in particular wards within geriatric hospitals.

While many of these measures are successful, additional programs of an innovative nature have also been canvassed. As an example, Bottomley (1992) describes the success of dance as a positive expression of ageing among elderly Greek-Australians. She notes that, given the significance of dance in traditional Greek culture (and thus in the villages from which many Greek migrants come), dance can have cathartic effects. It helps to dissolve some of the tensions and contradictions that arise from the migration experience by stimulating memory and reactivating earlier bases of identity formation. Thus dance can provide an affirmation of the sociocultural identity formed prior to migration but affected by the experience of migration and minority status (Bottomley 1992, pp.139–43). In short, she argues that dance as a 'kind of embodiment of memory can work powerfully against the silencing that marks both migration and ageing'.

## TREATMENT: PREVENTION AND INTERVENTION

The **prevention** of mental illness among Australia's immigrant populations depends on our ability to identify the life stressors associated with immigration and settlement. Prevention strategies will only be successful if they occur at the right time and place (see Chapter 5). Thus we need to know whether the major life stressor occurred prior to migration (e.g. trauma or torture in the country of origin) or if it was associated with settlement experiences in the receiving society (e.g. unemployment, non-recognition of qualifications). These will vary for different at-risk populations.

For example, among refugees, reactions to premigration experiences may be triggered by current situations—clinical settings may create panic attacks among those tortured in medical settings. Knowledge of this can (a) assist in the prevention of symptoms of mental disorder by providing more sympathetic environments during therapy, and (b) help nurses in a hospital setting to understand why they may find themselves listening to refugees' self-disclosures.

If settlement experiences are a major precipitator of mental health problems, then prevention requires an understanding of settlement conditions. In particular, the nature of the ethnic community and the migrant's level of involvement in it are significant. Since the Galbally Report (1978) there has been an assumption that ethnic communities will play a large part in managing migrant welfare. This argument does not take into account the fact that most ethnic communities (particularly among recently arrived immigrants) have very limited financial and human capital resources (Jupp, McRobbie & York 1991). Furthermore, since the prevalence of mental disorders is higher among socioeconomically disadvantaged ethnic groups than among the socioeconomically advantaged (Minas 1990), prevention strategies must also address social class factors affecting access to services.

## Intervention

While we argue that ethnicity or culture does not explain the differential incidence of mental health problems among different ethnic categories, cultural factors may well affect the presentation of symptoms. It should be clear that cultural considerations are extremely important in the *treatment* of health problems (see Julian & Easthope, in press), especially mental health problems. There are three main reasons for the significance of cultural factors.

1. Mental health has different 'meanings' in different cultures and these will affect (a) the identification and definition of the behaviour as 'a problem', and therefore the likelihood of seeking treatment, (b) whether treatment will be sought within the family and/or community or within the public sector, and (c) the nature of the treatment sought (e.g. physical or psychological).

2. The treatment of mental health is highly language-intensive. Whether the language used is the patient's preferred language or not is thus likely to have a significant effect on the success of intervention. Research has also shown that the language used tends to alter the nature of the intervention prescribed (Cox 1975, cited in Wooden et al. 1994, p.23).

3. Cultural understandings of mental health and illness, the nature of the ethnic community, and the level of resources available in it are all factors affecting the migrant's perception of, and access to, available treatment options.

# VIETNAMESE UNDERSTANDINGS OF MENTAL HEALTH

Insight can be gained into the divergent cultural understandings of mental health by considering Vietnamese ideas on mental health. According to traditional Vietnamese cultural beliefs there are several possible causes of mental illness. First, it can be caused by possession by ancestral spirits who have been offended and become angry. **Psychosis** can be caused by having a black magic spell cast upon the victim by a malevolent person, a magician or a sorcerer (Lien 1992, p.97).

Second, mental illness can be caused by being born at a bad astrological time, or by the house being built facing the wrong direction or on a bad piece of land. Traditional Vietnamese believe that such events influence a person's fortune and misfortune, including illness (Lien 1992, pp.97–8; Lien & Rice 1992).

Third, 'weak nerves' may cause mental illness. Since the nervous system is believed to be the source of all activities, a change in mental activity is perceived as being caused by a disturbance in the nerves. Mental illness is thus viewed as hereditary, making marriage impossible if it is known that there is a history of psychiatric illness in the family. Stress can affect the nerves and so mental illness can be caused by working too hard, thinking too much or worrying too much (Lien 1992, p.98).

Finally, the Vietnamese believe that good health is the product of a balance between two opposite forces: *am* and *duong* (similar to *yin* and *yang*). Physical and emotional illness is caused by an imbalance in these elements. Similarly, the element of 'wind' (as in breeze) can cause physical and emotional illness. Illnesses are also understood to be caused by unbalanced diets, and dietary treatments can prove effective in these cases.

Vietnamese understandings of mental health and illness have significant implications for the use of mental health services. This is because there is a strong **stigma** attached to psychiatric illness and admitting to such an illness brings shame on patients' ancestors, extended family and nuclear family (Lien 1992). There are also other consequences, since such patients and their siblings will not be able to marry. As a consequence of these cultural beliefs, the Vietnamese are likely to conceal mental illness rather than seek professional help (Lien 1992; Lien & Rice 1992).

Seeking treatment is likely to be a last resort, occurring when an acute illness is particularly severe or a chronic illness has become intolerable. It is also likely that a range of alternative therapists has already been approached, including traditional healers, Chinese herbalists, parish priests and others. Therapy often takes place without the knowledge of family, friends or neighbours (Lien 1992;

Lien & Rice 1992). **Somatisation,** the expression of mental illness through physical symptoms, is a cultural response to mental illness among the Vietnamese.

Somatisation has been identified among the working class in western societies (Davidson 1981) and may also be class-related among the Vietnamese (see Kleinman 1980, 1988). Vietnamese immigrants do not feel comfortable discussing personal feelings and interpersonal conflicts, but will readily discuss somatic problems. When combined with communication problems because of language differences, this often leads to misdiagnosis, as general practitioners without knowledge of Vietnamese culture are unlikely to recognise somatic problems as indicative of mental illness. Clearly, while it is not possible for health professionals to be familiar with all cultures, this does highlight the need for awareness of the importance of cultural factors in illness (Tham, Climidis & Minas 1991). It also emphasises the advantages of using trained interpreters to overcome the problems associated with cross-cultural communication, particularly in such important interactions as those between doctor or nurse and patient (Minas 1990, p.279).

Knowledge of Vietnamese cultural understandings of mental illness, and of the experiences of refugees and survivors of torture, has implications for the development of appropriate treatment of mental disorders among Vietnamese refugees. The psychotherapeutic counselling model, which focuses on self-disclosure, is based on a western scientific view of mental illness and carries with it western values, such as individualism, which may not be shared by other cultures. Family counselling and community-based therapies may therefore be more appropriate than individual counselling—for example, in addressing problems of **domestic violence** in Vietnamese families.

Furthermore, the delivery of health services to torture survivors needs to take account of their experiences. Among those who have experienced extreme physical torture it has been found that the use of physiotherapy and massage may be a more effective method of therapy than self-disclosure to a counsellor (McGorry 1991). As McGorry notes, '[t]orture represents a perversion of the healing relationship ... [so that] ... [t]he power relationship between client and professional must be very sensitively handled' (1991, p.168). Also, since torturers are sometimes assisted by medical practitioners (Silove et al. 1991), community-based therapy outside the clinical setting may be most effective. In short, rather than counselling Vietnamese refugees as individuals in a clinic, it may be more effective to consider community-based physical therapies involving therapists who have a knowledge and understanding of Vietnamese language and culture. Such culturally sensitive therapies, which also take into account the experiences of refugees, are more likely to achieve the goal of providing a sense of self-mastery and thus enabling them to 'regain a sense of empowerment in their struggle for survival as refugees' (Silove et al. 1991, p.173).

Minas, Silove & Kunst (1993) and others (e.g. Jayasuriya et al. 1992; HREOC 1993) have argued that the current structure of mental health services is inadequate. One measure of this is the very low rate of utilisation by NESB Australians. In particular, mainstream services are not meeting the needs of women, the elderly (Minas et al. 1993, p.20) or refugees (Jupp 1994).

There is a need for therapists with knowledge of the patient's language, cultural understandings of mental health and illness, and perceptions of culturally appropriate treatment (Minas 1990, p.279). It has been argued that a relationship of trust which enables self-disclosure is often more likely when the counsellor shares the same cultural traditions and biographical experiences as the client (Lien 1992; Rice & Lien 1992). Furthermore, misdiagnoses occur at a high rate when mental health professionals of the same ethnic background are not present at assessment (NHS 1993, p.47).

However, it is important not to replace traditional western psychotherapy entirely with culturally specific therapies. Cultures change in the context of new social conditions so that, as migrants and refugees adapt to new social experiences, they may also become more receptive to 'western' therapeutic methods. Those working in the field have therefore argued for the advantages of adopting multi-modal therapies that are multidisciplinary. Such approaches take account of the criticisms of clinical psychiatry that come from sociology and medical anthropology (e.g. Littlewood 1991) but do not 'throw out the baby with the bath water'. A number of very successful programs which adopt this approach (NHS 1993, p.111) have been established in Australia. These include the New South Wales Service for the Treatment and Rehabilitation of Torture and Trauma Survivors (STARTTS) (Reid, Silove & Tarn 1990) and those provided by Western Australia's Multicultural Psychiatric Centre and the Victorian Transcultural Psychiatry Unit in Melbourne.

It is important that mental health nurses are aware of the complexity of the relationship between ethnicity, immigration and mental illness, so that they do not make inadequate and inappropriate assumptions about cultural factors as causes of mental illness (see also Manderson & Reid 1994). It is also important that simplistic 'cultural' explanations are not replaced by equally simplistic 'immigrant' explanations. While the processes of immigration and settlement place immigrants in stressful situations, this does not mean that all will experience mental illness. Clearly, treating patients as either 'ethnic' or 'immigrant', and assuming that their ethnicity or their immigrant status is the major causal factor in their mental illness, does not take into account the variety of life experiences among ethnic Australians. It would be the same as employing the category 'woman' as a way of explaining an individual's behaviour. It is essential that such simplistic arguments, which reinforce essentialist notions of ethnicity and contribute to the stereotyping of immigrants as 'people with problems', be removed from current health care frameworks.

The life stressor framework adopted in this book highlights the need for the mental health nurse to be aware of the complex interplay between ethnicity, culture and immigration in the development and treatment of mental illness. Recognition that the process of immigration is potentially stressful should alert the mental health nurse to the advantages of exploring the immigrant's perceptions of the migration and settlement experience. For different types of migrants there will be particular life stages at which they are most at risk of mental disorder. Knowledge of these stressful life stages, and a sensitivity to the cultural factors affecting perceptions of mental illness, will enable the mental health nurse to play a vital role in the prevention of mental illness among Australia's ethnic minorities.

## SUMMARY

- Neither culture nor ethnicity causes mental illness, although cultural factors clearly play a part in definitions of mental health and illness, as well as in the choice of appropriate strategies for prevention and intervention.
- Migration and settlement do not cause mental illness. Nevertheless, some categories of migrants can be described as at-risk populations in that they are more likely than others to experience migration and settlement as stressful.
- Severity, chronicity and types of mental illness vary across at-risk categories.

## DISCUSSION QUESTIONS

1. How important is it that cross-cultural training is included in nursing education in Australia? What forms should this take? Should it be included in other health care training? For which health workers?

2. Discuss the kind of patients likely to have mental health problems as a consequence of migration. Which migrants are least likely to have mental health problems? What factors might produce exceptions to these generalisations?

3. To what extent is it possible to prevent mental illness among Australia's immigrants and ethnic minorities?

4. Identify ways in which the health care system creates barriers to the delivery of mental health care to Australians of non-Anglo Celtic and immigrant backgrounds. How could the system be changed? What can nurses do to assist the delivery of mental health care to NESB migrants?

5. A refugee who is a patient in a general hospital establishes a cathartic relationship with you, the nurse, and begins to disclose experiences of torture. What would you do?

# EXERCISES

1. Read the case study material in *one* of the following articles and answer the question: To what extent should the problem be treated as 'cultural' or as a consequence of immigration?

    (a) Holloway, G. (1994) 'Susto and the career path of the victim of an industrial accident: a sociological case study', *Social Science and Medicine* 38, (7), 989–97.

    (b) Lien, O. (1992) Case Vignette in 'The experience of working with Vietnamese patients attending a psychiatric service', *Journal of Vietnamese Studies* No.5, pp.102–3.

    (c) Minas, I. H. (1990) The case of Mehmet Yenisey in 'Mental health in a culturally diverse society' in J. Reid & P. Trompf (eds) *The Health of Immigrant Australia: A Social Perspective* Sydney: Harcourt Brace Jovanovich, p.251, p.265 & p.271.

2. Interview family, friends or peers and obtain four or five migration stories. Discuss these stories in small groups and delineate the mental health stressors experienced as a consequence of the migration experience. What factors influenced whether people had a positive or negative experience?

3. Perform a role play where a person is suffering from a mental illness and is being interviewed by a nurse through an interpreter. Try it with a telephone interpretor and/or a child interpretor. Discuss the difficulties involved.

# FURTHER READING

- Julian, R. & Easthope, G. (forthcoming) 'Ethnicity and Health' in C. Gerbich (ed.) *Sociology of Health and Illness*, Prentice Hall Australia. A summary of the findings on migration and health in Australia and the implications of those findings for nursing practice. Particular reference is made to the Hmong community in Hobart.

- National Health Strategy (1993) *Removing Cultural and Language Barriers to Health*, Issues Paper no. 6. Canberra: AGPS. Section 1 provides a useful summary of the ethnic composition of the population, ethnic health status and health service use. Section 2 looks at the response of the health system to the ethnic population.

- Krupinski, J. and Burrows, G. (eds) (1986) *The Price of Freedom: Young Indochinese Refugees in Australia*, Sydney: Pergamon Press. The only longitudinal study of the health of migrants in Australia. The section on mental health is particularly interesting. However, it should be read with caution as it takes mental health to be an unproblematic medical category.

- Cox, David R. (1989) *Welfare Practice in a Multicultural Society*. Sydney: Prentice Hall Australia. A practical approach to the problems experienced by those responsible for the welfare of immigrants in Australian society. Written for social workers and welfare practitioners, its case study approach makes it a useful text for nurses.

- Jayasuriya, L., Sang, D. & Fielding, A. (1992) *Ethnicity, Immigration and Mental Illness: A Critical Review of Australian Research*, Canberra: AGPS. An accessible research-based report on the mental health of immigrants and ethnic minorities in Australia.

- Minas, I. H. (ed.) (1991) *Cultural Diversity and Mental Health*, Melbourne: RANZCP-VTPU. An edited collection of papers covering a wide range of theoretical and practical issues. The papers are based on research conducted in Australia and provide a degree of depth and detail not available in texts with a broader health focus. An excellent selection of readings for nurses and others working within the Australian health care system.

- Cunningham, M., Becker, R. & Aroche, J. *STARTTS Eye of the Needle Trainers' Kit*. Produced with the assistance of the NSW Education and Training Foundation, Eastway Communication and the Department of Health. A 40-minute video and teaching package which provides excellent training material for counsellors and others working with refugees in Australia. A highly recommended resource package.

# REFERENCES

Ahmad, W.I.U. (1993) *'Race' and Health in Contemporary Britain*, Buckingham: Open University Press.

Ames, D. (1991) 'Geriatric psychiatry in a culturally diverse society' in I.H. Minas (ed.) *Cultural Diversity and Mental Health*, Melbourne: Royal Australian and New Zealand College of Psychiatrists–Victorian Transcultural Psychiatry Unit (RANZCP-VTPU), pp.115–24.

Angel, R. & Guarnaccia, P.J. (1989) 'Mind, body, and culture: somatization among hispanics', *Social Science and Medicine* 28 (12), pp.1229–38.

Australian Bureau of Statistics, Queensland (1994) *The Social Characteristics of Immigrants in Australia*, Canberra: AGPS.

Bottomley, G. (1992) *From another Place: Migration and the Politics of Culture*, Cambridge: Cambridge University Press.

Chung, R.C. & Kagawa-Singer, M. (1993) 'Predictors of psychological distress among southeast Asian refugees', *Social Science and Medicine* 36 (5), pp.631–9.

Cox, David R. (1989) *Welfare Practice in a Multicultural Society*, Sydney: Prentice Hall Australia.

Davidson, K.R. (1981) 'Conceptions of illness and health practices in a Nova Scotia community' in D. Coburn, C. D'Arcy, P. New and G. Torrence, pp.80–95 *Health and Canadian Society*, Toronto: Fitzhenry and Whiteside.

Easthope, G. (1989) 'Ethnicity and health' in G.M. Lupton and J.M. Najman (eds) *Sociology of Health and Illness: Australian Readings*, South Melbourne: Macmillan (revised chapter in press).

Fincher, R., Foster, L. & Wilmot, R. (1994) *Gender Equity and Australian Immigration Policy*, Canberra: AGPS.

Galbally, F. (1978) (Chairperson) *Migrant Services and Programs: Report of the Review of Post-arrival Programs and Services for Migrants* (Galbally Report), Canberra: AGPS.

Hauff, E. & Vaglum, P. (1993) 'Vietnamese boat refugees: the influence of war and flight traumatization on mental health on arrival in the country of resettlement', *Acta Psychiatrica Scandinavica* 88, pp.162–8.

Human Rights and Equal Opportunities Commission (1993) *Human Rights and Mental Illness*, Canberra: AGPS.

Jayasuriya, L., Sang, D. & Fielding, A. (1992) *Ethnicity, Immigration and Mental Illness: A Critical Review of Australian Research*, Canberra: AGPS.

Julian, R. & Easthope, G. (forthcoming) 'Ethnicity and Health' in C. Gerbich (ed.) *Sociology of Health and Illness*, Ringwood: Prentice Hall Australia.

Jupp, J. (1994) *Exile or Refuge? The Settlement of Refugee, Humanitarian and Displaced Immigrants*, Canberra: AGPS.

Jupp, J., McRobbie, A. & York, B. (1991) *Settlement Needs of Small Newly Arrived Ethnic Groups*, Canberra: AGPS.

Kleinman, A. (1980) *Patients and Healers in the Context of Culture*, Berkeley: University of California Press.

Kleinman, A. (1988) *The Illness Narratives: Suffering, Healing and the Human Condition*, New York: Basic Books.

Krupinski, J. & Burrows, G. (eds) (1986) *The Price of Freedom: Young Indochinese Refugees in Australia*, Sydney: Pergamon Press.

Krupinski, J., Stoller, A. & Wallace, L. (1973) 'Psychiatric disorders in east European refugees now in Australia', *Social Science and Medicine* 7, pp.31–49.

Lien, O. (1992) 'The experience of working with Vietnamese patients attending a psychiatric service', *Journal of Vietnamese Studies* no.5, pp.95–105.

Lien, O. & Rice, P. (1992) 'Concepts of mental illness of Vietnamese and the attitude toward psychiatric services', *Tap San Y Si* (Medical Journal of the Vietnamese Medical Association, Canada) vol.115, April, pp.69–77.

Littlewood, R. (1991) 'Anthropology and psychiatry' in I.H. Minas (ed.) *Cultural Diversity and Mental Health*, Melbourne: RANZCP-VTPU, pp.5–18.

McGorry, P. (1991) 'The significance of torture: theoretical and therapeutic aspects' in I.H. Minas (ed.) (1991) *Cultural Diversity and Mental Health*, Melbourne: RANZCP-VTPU, pp.165–70.

Manderson, L. & Reid, J.C. (1994) 'What's culture got to do with it?' in C. Waddell & A.R. Petersen (eds) *Just Health: Inequality in Illness, Care and Prevention*, Melbourne: Churchill Livingstone, pp.7–25.

Martin, J. (1965) *Refugee Settlers*, Canberra: ANU Press.

Minas, I.H. (1990) 'Mental health in a culturally diverse society' in J. Reid & P.Trompf (eds) *The Health of Immigrant Australia: A Social Perspective*, Sydney:

Harcourt Brace Jovanovich.

Minas, I.H., Silove, D. & Kunst, J.P. (1993) *Mental Health for a Multicultural Australia: A National Strategy.* Report of a consultancy to the Commonwealth Department of Human Services and Health, December 1993. The Victorian Transcultural Psychiatry Unit, St Vincent's Hospital, Melbourne.

National Health Strategy (1993) *Removing Cultural and Language Barriers to Health,* Issues Paper no. 6. Canberra: AGPS.

Pittaway, E. (1991) *Refugee Women—Still at Risk in Australia,* Canberra: AGPS.

Reid, J., Silove, D. & Tarn, R. (1990) 'The development of the New South Wales Service for the treatment and rehabilitation of torture and trauma survivors (STARTTS): the first year', *Australian and New Zealand Journal of Psychiatry* 24, pp.486–95.

Rowland, D.T. (1991) *Pioneers Again: Immigrants and Ageing in Australia,* Canberra: AGPS.

Sashidharan, S.P. & Francis, E. (1993) 'Epidemiology, ethnicity and schizophrenia' in W. I. U. Ahmad *'Race' and Health in Contemporary Britain,* Buckingham: Open University Press.

Silove, D., Tarn, R., Bowles, R. & Reid, J. (1991) 'Psychotherapy for survivors of torture' in I.H. Minas (ed.) *Cultural Diversity and Mental Health,* Melbourne: RANZCP-VTPU, pp.171–93.

Tham, G., Klimidis, S. & Minas, I.H. (1991) 'Psychiatric nurses: their awareness of cultural factors in patient management' in I.H. Minas (ed.) *Cultural Diversity and Mental Health,* Melbourne: RANZCP-VTPU, pp.195–209.

Thomas, T. & Balnaves, M. (1993) *New Land, Last Home: The Vietnamese Elderly and the Family Reunion Program,* Canberra: AGPS.

Wooden, M., Holton, R., Hugo, G. & Sloan J. (1994) *Australian Immigation: A Survey of the Issues,* Canberra: AGPS.

Yeatman, A. (1992) *NESB Migrant Women and Award Restructuring,* Canberra: AGPS.

# $S$*tructure*

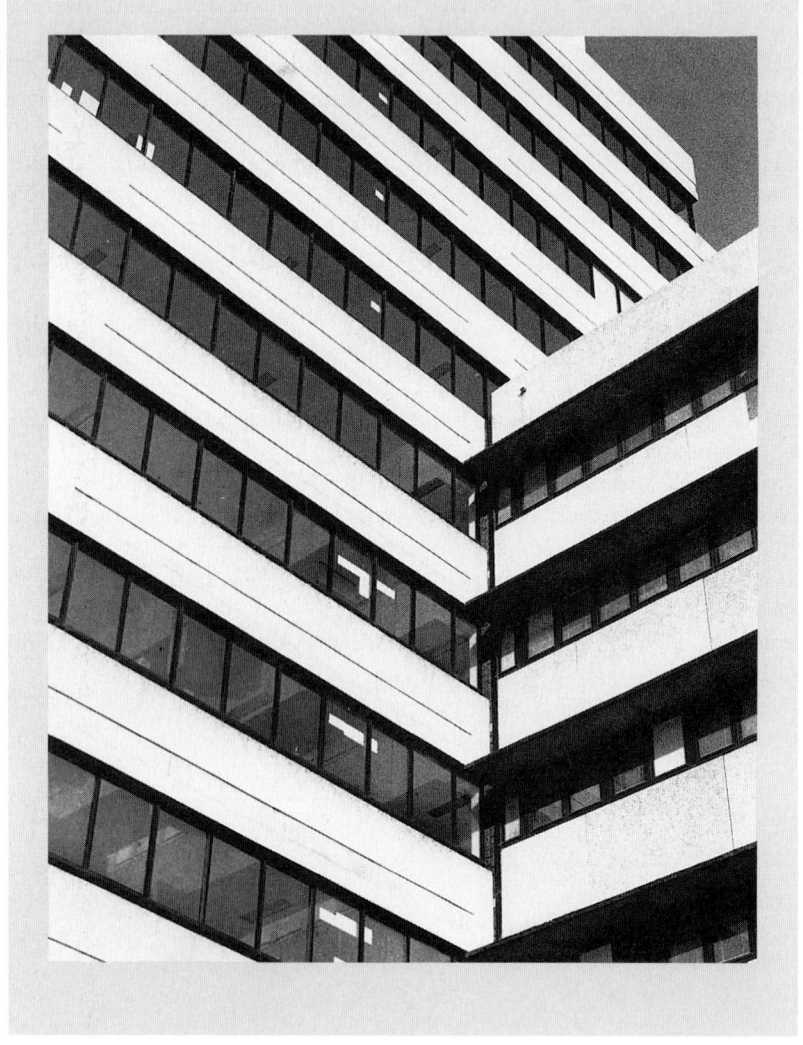

TIM OWEN

The mental health system creates and limits opportunities for mental health.

## CHAPTER 8

# MENTAL HEALTH CARE SERVICES

Michael Clinton and Sioban Nelson

## CONTENTS

## LEARNING OBJECTIVES

This chapter will assist the reader to:

- compare the structures, components and costings of the Australian and New Zealand health care systems;
- discuss the provision of mental health care;
- examine the role of non-government organisations (NGOs) in supporting people with a mental illness;
- argue a case for greater intersectoral collaboration in mental health care;
- examine the role of private hospitals;
- discuss the impact of deinstitutionalisation on the development of community services.

## INTRODUCTION

This chapter examines structural aspects of mental health care in Australia and New Zealand. The discussion commences with an outline of the components and costings of the Australian and New Zealand health care systems. Institutional and community service provision, the public and private sectors, and the structural reform of both systems are examined. The discussion then moves to an analysis of aspects of service provision that extend beyond health care systems *per se*. Here, issues such as housing, income protection, social support, employment, and **intersectoral** links in the provision of services for those suffering from mental illness are examined.

## HEALTH CARE

The promotion of health and the provision of health care, programs to improve the mental health of the population, to treat mental illnesses, and to manage the care of people with chronic debilitating conditions such as **schizophrenia** or major **depression**, are the tasks of the health care system. Knowledge of this system is therefore important in understanding the delivery of mental health care.

### Australia

The Australian health care system is pluralistic and complex. Federal, State and local governments, institutions and individual providers, private and public interests are all involved in the delivery of health care. The delineation of responsibilities and authority through Federal, State and local government agencies is not static; it is frequently negotiated between the Commonwealth and States, and between local governments and States, and is therefore subject to change. Consequently, although the Commonwealth is responsible for

*T*ABLE 8.1: Who pays for what in Australia's specialised mental health service network?

| STATE AND TERRITORY GOVERNMENTS | COMMONWEALTH GOVERNMENT | PRIVATE HEALTH INSURANCE FUNDS | COMMUNITY, INCLUDING NON-GOVERNMENT ORGANISATIONS |
|---|---|---|---|
| • Specialist psychiatric hospitals | • Medical benefits for services by private psychiatrists | • Private hospitals | • Accommodation<br>• Psychosocial rehabilitation<br>• Social and personal support<br>• Advocacy<br>• Information services<br>• Recreation<br>• Respite care |
| • Public acute hospitals | • Public acute hospitals (via Medicare agreement) | • Day patient care | |
| • Community mental health services | • Department of Veterans Affairs: services to war veterans | • Gap insurance for inpatient care by psychiatrists | |
| • Specialist nursing homes and hostels | • Specialised disability support services funded via CSDA, including NGOs | • Clinical psychologists' rebates | |
| • Specialised disability support services, including non-government organisations (NGOs), funded through the Commonwealth State Disability Agreement or other channels | • National mental health plan funding | | |
| | *plus significant contributions by:*<br>• General medical practice/ primary care<br>• Pharmaceutical Benefits Scheme | | |

funding health care (directly and indirectly) and the States for administering those funds—a state of affairs that has existed since Federation in 1901—there have been many changes to this arrangement over that time. The components of the current arrangements are shown in Table 8.1.

## New Zealand

The New Zealand health care system is nationally organised and coordinated. However, four regional health authorities (RHAs) have autonomy within program guidelines, while the central government has responsibility for planning, finance and policy direction. The New Zealand health care system has recently undergone major reform. The RHAs have been established to manage the purchasing of, and contracting for, health services throughout New Zealand. The RHAs have responsibility for funding primary care provided by general practitioners and others in the community, and for hospital care. Unlike the area health boards they replaced, the RHAs have no obligation to concentrate funding on their own services. They are free to purchase services from the public, private or voluntary sectors.

Large public hospitals have been established as Crown Health Enterprises (CHEs) with appointed boards of directors. The CHEs operate along business lines, and a Minister of Crown Health Enterprises has been appointed to represent the interests of the Crown, as the owner of public hospitals and associated services. Over time, communities are to be given the opportunity to take over their local hospitals and run them as community trusts. The interrelationships between sections of the New Zealand health care system are shown in Figure 8.1.

## Service provision

In Australia, national, State and regional lines of responsibility and funding structures, institutional and community provision of care, and private and public sectors of the economy combine to form an industry that employs 600 000 people, or 7.6% of the entire employed Australian workforce (Grant & Lapsley 1993). Health care is the second largest item of government expenditure, and accounts for approximately 8.5% of Gross Domestic Product (GDP) or $34.39 billion in Australia (AIHW 1994). In New Zealand the total cost of health care is $5.8 billion, or 7.57% of GDP (McKendry & Mathumala 1994). Clearly, the health care system in developed countries such as Australia and New Zealand comprises a significant sector of the economy.

## FUNDING HEALTH CARE: AUSTRALIA AND NEW ZEALAND

Health care in the two countries is funded quite differently. State versus Commonwealth pressures characterise the Australian system, whereas a national reform process dominates the New Zealand scene.

FIGURE 8.1: *The New Zealand health care system*

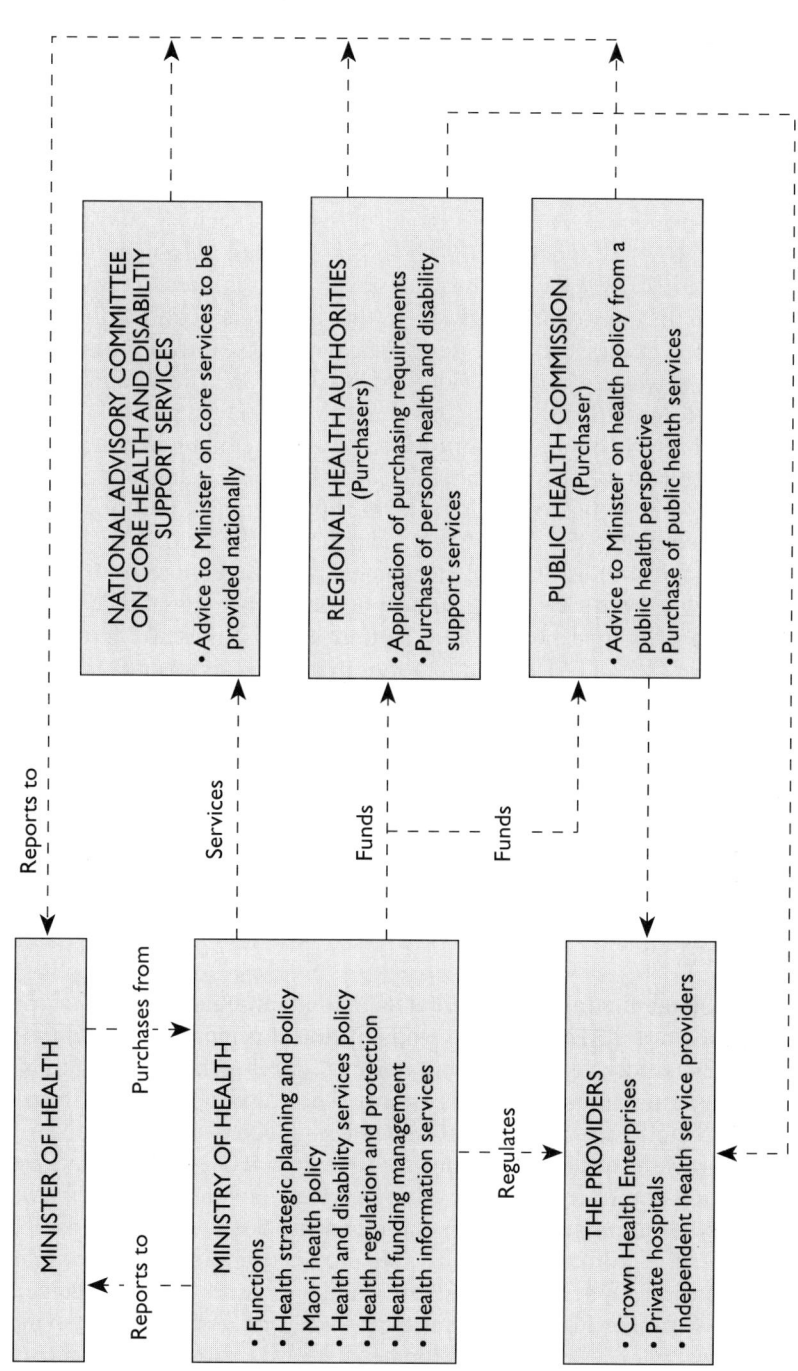

## Australia

In Australia the imperative to provide a consistent high-quality service to all Australians, and the need for the integration of health with other Commonwealth programs such as social security, housing or even research funding, has led to far less autonomy for State and local agencies. By tying funds to specific programs the Commonwealth has been able to develop national health programs and services. Through conditional grants to the States, the Commonwealth has implemented programs involving the administration, funding and regulation of a wide range of services such as nursing homes, pharmaceuticals, and medical and hospital services. Through the *Health Insurance Act (1973)* the Commonwealth government is directly responsible for the regulation and payment of private health providers. The Medicare rebate system largely bypasses the State level of government and negotiations take place directly between service provider organisations and the Commonwealth.

The Commonwealth also has an important role to play in public health issues in that it decides the national priorities for health, including health promotion activities. Commonwealth agencies decide whether a campaign should be conducted at a national or a State level. For example, the Better Health Commission conducts the HIV/AIDS campaign and the Campaign Against Drug Abuse (CADA) as national campaigns, because a strategic, coordinated approach is considered vital to the success of these programs (AIHW 1992).

In the area of mental health the adoption of the National Mental Health Policy and Plan (1992) has led to alterations in funding arrangements governing mental health services between the Commonwealth and the States. Since 1 July 1993, public psychiatric hospitals have been covered under the Medicare Agreement between the States and the Commonwealth (Whiteford, MacLeod & Leitch 1993). The terms of this agreement outline reforms to improve patient access to services, and the planning and integration of health services to improve efficiency and quality of services (Department of Health, Housing, Local Government and Community Services 1993).

## New Zealand

In New Zealand funding has been a perennial problem for mental health services. Abbott and Kemp (1993) comment that the appropriation of funds by annual parliamentary vote has been a source of funding insecurity. Funding in the past has gone to area health boards, with no specifically targeted or 'ringmarked' funds for mental health services. Elected board members have determined mental health allocations for their regions against the background of competition for resources with other services. An uneven distribution of health resources to mental health is the result and is evident across the board. For example, the Ministry of Health has provided grants to assist workforce development and support research into workforce issues. Expenditure in this area was $5.4 million in 1988–89, yet only 4.4%, or $240 000, went to mental health. Furthermore, service development loans contributed $2.3 million

(11.9%) to the development of mental health services in 1988–89 from a budget of $19.3 million. In 1991 an additional $25 million was allocated to area health boards for service development. In the same year, 8% of an estimated $2267.2 million funding to area health boards, or $181.4 million, was allocated to psychiatric services. Area health boards spent about 20% of health dollars on mental health, although mental health accounts for 42% of patient bed days in hospital (Abbott & Kemp 1993). Yet despite the level of activity in the mental health sector, most area health boards have not kept accurate figures on expenditure in mental health.

In comparison with other OECD countries, Australia and New Zealand rate well. Notwithstanding the difficulties in making comparisons across countries with different health care systems and different methods of costing those systems, Australia and New Zealand compare favourably, consistently spending proportionally more than the UK and Japan, but less than the United States. Australia's spending was proportionally equivalent to that of Canada in 1980, although in 1990 Canadian spending exceeded that of Australia, increasing to approximately 9% of GDP (AIHW 1994).

These comparisons across countries need to be adjusted for demographic characteristics. For example, age composition of a particular population is a significant determinant of a country's health costs (see Chapter 5). As New Zealand and Australia have similar age structures, a comparison is possible. From 1970 to 1993 Australia has consistently spent more than New Zealand on health care. Current data indicates a full percentage point difference in spending, with New Zealand spending 7.5% in 1992–93 (McKendry & Mathumala 1994) and Australia 8.5% in 1992–93 (AIHW 1994).

## Where the dollars go ...

The institutional sector is by far the most expensive part of the health care system. In Australia in 1989–90 the hospital system accounted for expenditure of over $10 billion, funding 3.7 million admissions and extensive non-inpatient services (National Health Strategy 1991). In both Australia and New Zealand, 1993 figures reveal that the institutional sector accounts for over half the total spending on health (McKendry & Mathumala 1994; AIHW 1993).

## The non-institutional sector

While the institutional sector of health care accounts for most of the costs, the area of substantial growth has been the community sector. Throughout the health care system there has been a demonstrable shift in recent years from institutional care to community-based care. In acute services, three measures have led to a dramatic reduction in the average length of hospital stay:

- the increase in day surgery (AIHW 1992);
- the extension of domiciliary nursing to accommodate early discharge patients under the Medicare Incentives Scheme (Blue Nursing Service, Brisbane 1994); and

- the increase in home-based palliative care treatment funded under HAAC or Medicare Incentives (Blue Nursing Services, Brisbane 1994; Queensland Health 1993).

In Australia in 1991–92, the mean duration of an inpatient stay was 5.0 days, for private hospitals it was 4.2 days, and for public hospitals 5.3 days. This is a marked reduction from the 1985–86 mean level of 6.5 days, a private hospital level of 5.5 days, and 6.9 days for public hospitals (AIHW 1994).

## Deinstitutionalisation

In mental health too there is now the belief that institutional care is not the preferred system of care, and the community sector has become the sector of growth in psychiatric care. **Deinstitutionalisation** is the term used to designate this policy shift that has occurred in the provision of care for people with mental illness over the last twenty years.

> Deinstitutionalisation has two facets. First, the discharge of existing patients into the community, and secondly a policy of reducing new admissions and treating people outside specialised psychiatric institutions... In Australia the population of the psychiatric hospitals declined from 29 500 in the early 1960s, when Australia's population was 10.5 million (281 beds per 100 000) to 6750 inpatients for a population of 17 million today (40 beds per 100 000). (National Health Strategy 1993, p.20)

It is not only the number of beds that has declined—public psychiatric hospitals have also witnessed a decline in average length of inpatient stay. In the past, the length of stay for patients with mental illness was measured in years. Now it is considered uncommon for residents to stay in psychiatric units for more than three months (Ministry of Health 1994).

## Mainstreaming

The institutional sector of mental health services is undergoing further restructuring with the move to mainstream services. This means that the services of health professionals are now to be provided in a range of settings as part of general health service provision. This shift to a model of integrated services is occurring in Australia in line with the implementation of the National Mental Health Policy (1992). Under mainstreamed services, the care of those experiencing an acute episode of mental illness occurs in designated psychiatric beds in general hospitals. Ongoing support for recovering patients and people with chronic illness is to be given in the community (Whiteford, MacLeod & Leitch 1993; National Mental Health Policy 1992).

The mainstreaming of psychiatric services puts mental health into the main arena, subject to the same policy developments, quality assurance procedures, and outcome evaluation as the rest of the health sector. It is thought that many of the inequities in mental health care—the poor services, under-resourced staff,

**stigma**, and infringements of patient rights—will be improved through the integration of psychiatric services with mainstream health services (Whiteford, MacLeod & Leitch 1993). The concern with mainstreamed services is that the specific needs of the mentally ill may be overlooked when funds are allocated. To protect against this possibility it has been argued that monies should be 'ringmarked' as mental health funds, so that the mental health budget will not be vulnerable to competing interests (National Health Strategy 1993).

## PRIVATE HOSPITALS

In Australia, private hospitals form an increasingly important part of the institutional sector of the health care industry. Not only is there marked growth in the number of private hospitals, and in employment in the private sector, the private sector is now poised to assume a role in the provision of services in the public sector. The New South Wales privately run public hospital of Port Macquarie is a significant development in the Australian health care industry (NSW Health 1993; Mayne Nickless 1993).

There are clear differences between the provision of private psychiatric services in New Zealand and Australia. In both countries public sector psychiatric services provide four psychiatrists per 100 000 population (Andrews 1989). In both countries one-third of all patients are seen in hospital; this group is likely to be suffering from **psychosis** and is unlikely to be in the workforce. However, in 1989, the year of Andrews' survey, Australia had twice the psychiatrists and half the psychiatric beds of New Zealand in 1989 (Andrews 1989). Furthermore, in Australia, 77% of patients were seen privately whereas the corresponding figure for New Zealand was 15%. Interestingly, 55% of Australia's private sector patients suffered from neuroses or personality disorders, and only 26% suffered from psychoses. However, in New Zealand, half suffered from psychoses and only one-third from neuroses or personality disorder. Nonetheless, due to the large number of patients seeing private psychiatrists in Australia, more patients with psychoses were seen in the private than in the public sector (Andrews 1989).

The private sector is increasingly providing an extensive range of health services in Australia. The 1986 census reveals that 47.5% of health industry employment was in the private sector; by 1991 this had risen to 51.9%. This increase is substantial in that it absorbs a 2.1% fall in government sector employment and a 16.9% increase in private sector employment (AIHW 1994). In Australia, 25 private hospitals provide a total of 1370 licensed private psychiatric beds (ABS 1993). The Private Hospital Survey, conducted by ABS, provided data on the extent of the utilisation of these beds. Of the 76.6% of hospitals that responded to this particular question, the primary diagnosis of 'mental disorder' accounted for 34 686 separations (deaths and discharges) (ABS 1993). However, unlike the State system, which provides for an extremely high proportion of people with chronic mental illness, the private sector caters largely for the better off and less severely ill client. In fact, the use of private psychiatrists has been demonstrated to be correlated with higher socioeconomic status (Jorm, Rosenman & Jacomb 1993). Thus, in Australia, the private sector to a great extent treats the less ill, less impaired patient (Andrews 1989).

This problem does not apply exclusively to psychiatrists. In a recent UK study it was found that mental health nurses who had undertaken additional training as counsellors or therapists, and who were attached to general practices, provided virtually no care at all to people with serious mental illness (Gournay & Brooking 1993). This is not to say that the provision of care to those with less serious mental health problems is unimportant. The point is that there is a service gap between those with less serious mental health problems and those suffering from severe mental illness, and the provision of care to those in greatest need is not a commercial imperative for the private sector.

One imperative that does exist for the private sector is that, in addition to State licensing arrangements, a private hospital must meet the requirements of insurance funds so that patients are eligible for cost reimbursement. The private health insurance funds require hospitals to demonstrate that they provide structured programs for mental health problems. Examination of these programs by officers of the larger insurance companies is required before the programs are eligible for insurance rebate. The programs tend to be organised on a modular basis and individual treatment prescribed from a set format. Commonly, these include programs for eating disorders, drug and alcohol problems, anxiety disorders, depression, and acute programs. As the insurance rebate is higher for a psychiatric bed than a general medical bed or rehabilitation bed, the payment rate alters with length of stay. For example, the Medical Benefits Fund recognises various categories of care depending on length of stay; with Medibank Private the rebate is evaluated on a program-only basis (MBF QLD, personal communication, January 1994; Health Insurance Commission, personal communication, January 1994). Given the importance for hospitals to conform with insurance requirements, it is inevitable that to some extent the structure of the private mental health care provided is determined by these funding criteria.

## Community care

Most mental health care is provided in the community by general practitioners. Along with other types of health services, the GP is the gatekeeper of mental health services. In the Christchurch psychiatric epidemiology study, it was shown that not only do most people in New Zealand go to the GP with mental health problems, but most people who suffer from pre-existing mental illnesses also go to GPs. People with pre-existing psychiatric conditions are only marginally more likely to visit a psychiatrist than the rest of the population (Hornblow et al. 1990). In fact less than 7% of those with a psychiatric disorder in the previous six months had received specialist treatment (Hornblow et al. 1990). These findings support earlier work by Goldberg and Huxley (1980) who argue that 'it is quite clear that even in the developed countries of the world, most mentally disordered patients are not being treated by psychiatric services'.

Furthermore, community studies conducted in Christchurch and Dunedin demonstrate that about one-third of adults and nearly a quarter of adolescents have, at some stage, met DSM-IIIR criteria for at least one of the main psychiatric disorders (Public Health Commission 1993). Such studies show that mental illness is common in the community and that there is an unmet need for appropriate help, whether from counsellors, general practitioners, psychiatrists, or other service providers. The fact that the majority of those with a disorder have not received help for their disorder, let alone help from mental health specialists, is of serious concern.

In New Zealand, as part of the process of deinstitutionalisation and the expansion of the community sector, two hospitals, Carrington Hospital in Auckland and Cherry Farm Hospital in Dunedin, were closed in 1992. The replacement services in Auckland and Dunedin provide examples of two models for community care. The Auckland model has one management structure, with few hospital beds and all other services based in the community in a more extended approach to community treatment. The Dunedin model is based on three separate management structures with largely hospital-based services.

The Controller and Auditor General of New Zealand undertook an audit of the efficiency and effectiveness of the community care services in the two areas previously served by the hospitals (Controller and Auditor General 1993). The audit team found that three of the four crisis teams operating in central Auckland were responding to the same group of people, that 61% of community care staff had only minor involvement in rehabilitation, and that crisis intervention was the dominant activity of community care staff. The prominence of **crisis intervention** work was found to limit the ability of staff to concentrate on their 'key worker' role, to the detriment of ongoing support for clients and the coordination of services. The Dunedin audit found that there was a need for closer liaison between hospital and community care staff. Another finding was that there was inadequate follow-up of clients in the community after they were discharged.

This relationship between hospitals and community centres has been found to be a significant issue of mental health care. In some areas the separate development and organisation of community centres has led to competition between institutional and community services for resources and power, and to the provision of fragmented and ill-coordinated services (National Health Strategy 1993).

The community:hospital resource ratio has been found to be an important determinant of the success of mental health programs. It is argued that the better services, both overseas and in Australia, 'consistently spend a higher proportion of the mental health budget on community services'. The current ratio for Australian community:hospital spending is 24:76; in Queensland it is 12:88. A model program in New Hampshire, US, has a spending ratio of 65:35 (National Health Strategy 1993).

An important point to note is that quality community care is not necessarily cheaper to provide than institutional care. The wide range of allied health services, and medical and nursing services required, and the provision of extended hours care and the emergency care essential to the successful management of clients in the community, comes at substantial cost. Evidence indicates that demand for this range of services does not in fact decline. On the contrary, the successful maintenance of clients in the community is actually reliant on the continuation of intensive support (Dermer & Landeen 1991).

## WIDER SERVICE PROVISION: INTERSECTORAL LINKS

The intensive support of clients in the community can be provided by a wide range of organisations and people in the community. General practitioners, hospital medical specialists, nurses and other service providers are central to the delivery of health care. However, the boundaries of the health care system are somewhat arbitrary. In this chapter the boundaries of the health care system are defined by considering typical mental health needs and the ways in which these are met by different service providers, agencies, community groups and government programs. Once these needs are considered, it becomes clear that a wide range of health and other support services is required to promote mental health and to meet the needs of people with a mental illness.

Mental health services can be divided into those provided by specialist mental health workers (psychiatrists, clinical psychologists, psychotherapists, mental health nurses) and those provided by individuals and organisations outside the specialist mental health services (general practitioners, generic family support services, housing programs, non-government organisations). The focus of this chapter is specialist and non-specialist mental health services. However, the distinction between specialist and non-specialist is not completely satisfactory because some community organisations, particularly **self-help groups**, specialise in their activities despite not being part of a specialist treatment service. For example, Alcoholics Anonymous provides specialised support to people with drinking problems, but is not regarded as specialised in the sense of a professional specialisation. Service components available to most sufferers of mental illness include specialised psychiatric services, psychological services, inpatient and outpatient facilities, physiotherapy and occupational therapy services, and community care programs. Specialist psychiatrists are available in services for children and parents, adolescents, the elderly mentally ill and people with disturbed and law-breaking behaviours (Puckett 1993).

Services typically provided outside specialist mental health services include:

- *Income*: Income security, Disability Services Program, emergency relief, consumer-managed businesses, employment programs, skills training.
- *Health*: General practitioner care, outpatients clinics, medical benefits, pharmaceutical benefits, nursing home benefits, sessions between primary care personnel and specialist psychiatric teams.

- *Social services:* Telephone hot-lines, drop-in centres, HAAC services, respite care, community development services.
- *Accommodation:* Access to public housing, special needs housing schemes, consumer managed housing schemes, crisis housing.
- *Community services:* Self-help groups for consumers and carers, advocacy to governments and service providers, information and advisory services, consumer-run social centres and 'clubhouses'.

People with chronic mental illness have 'the right equal to other citizens to health care, income maintenance, education, employment, housing, transport, legal services, equitable health, and other insurance and leisure appropriate to one's age' (Mental Health Consumer Outcomes Task Force 1991). However, people with mental illness in Australia encounter barriers to mainstream health, social and disability services, although some of these barriers have been addressed by recent positive initiatives. It is a relatively recent development that long-term patients in mental hospitals have been eligible for income security. Previously the Commonwealth had assumed that their needs for health, welfare, housing, disability support and income support were being met by the States. Older people with mental illness and a history of hospitalisation were ineligible, prior to 1990, for Commonwealth-supported aged care services. It was only after significant community pressure that the *Commonwealth Disability Services Act* (1986) recognised psychiatric **disability,** but recognition in legislation is not matched with funding or access to generic disability services.

Following the trend towards community care, State mental health authorities have begun to fund non-governmental organisations for support services, but the level of funding is low. This is due partly to a lag in the transfer of hospital expenditure to community services as deinstitutionalisation has progressed, and partly to the traditionally low expenditure on mental health services. The outcome is a confusion of services provided by different agencies. Therefore, people with chronic mental illness have difficulty accessing the mental health, general health, and social and disability services they need (National Health Strategy 1993).

## Housing

Access to housing is a key issue for people with mental illness. In a Western Australian study that surveyed patients with schizophrenia about to be discharged from hospital, and a second group who attended a community centre, it was found that housing was the primary concern of clients (Harries et al. 1991). Too often, deinstitutionalisation has led to people with chronic mental illnesses having to depend on underfinanced, fragmented and often inaccessible services, with those lost to the mental health system commonly found in shelters, in jail, or on the streets (see Chapter 17). The difficulty of providing services to this group is compounded where there is abuse of alcohol or drugs, homelessness or poor continuity of care (Mechanic & Aiken 1987). The serious problem of people with frank mental illness surviving on the streets of the major cities throughout the western world has led to a call by many for a moratorium on deinstitutionalisation, and the reminder that 'asylum' means protection (Bacharach 1984; Lamb 1992) (see Chapter 1).

In Australia, housing options are required for people with mental illness that allow for personal choice and flexibility. Unfortunately, people with chronic mental illness have been excluded from mainstream housing and support services. There has been a marked failure to link housing with community support services, and matters are made worse by the scarcity of low-cost accommodation (National Health Strategy 1993). Recent public housing policy reforms have improved access to housing services for people with psychiatric disabilities, through programs for single and young people (National Housing Strategy 1992). Yet in most States private boarding houses and hostels remain the main option. People living in boarding houses and hostels receive support from mental health workers. However, those with mental health problems have wider support needs, which may include meals, cleaning, washing and assistance with personal hygiene (National Health Strategy 1993). The need for these services inhibits people with chronic mental illness from moving to independent housing where this level of support is not provided. These accommodation problems are exacerbated by widely varying standards in boarding house and hostel accommodation.

In New Zealand, funding is provided directly to people with psychiatric disability (and intellectual handicaps) by the Housing Corporation, through the rental housing program. People with mental illness can also receive indirect support for accommodation through the program, and supported accommodation is available in some areas. In 1988 $2.3 million was allocated to 22 special tenancies, $5 million was loaned to community agencies for supported housing, and 100 houses were allocated to people discharged from psychiatric hospitals (Abbott & Kemp 1993).

In other countries, notably the United States, a range of accommodation options has been developed, from regular apartments supported by key workers to consumer apartments with live-in caretakers, often former **consumers**, to group homes with on-call staff. The trend is to more consumer-owned and -staffed facilities. A positive aspect of this trend is to provide consumers with tapering levels of support as they gain in independence; staff gradually withdraw their involvement and leave consumers in familiar surroundings to which they have adapted, rather than transfer them to new accommodation as their confidence and independence improves. Staff move, rather than consumers (Kirkpatrick 1994). However, businesses providing 24-hour support for these consumers have no incentive to improve the functioning of individual residents (Hallwright 1993).

## Psychiatric disability: service delivery and income protection

In general, people with psychiatric disabilities in Australia have not had access to personal and respite care services funded under the Home and Community Care Program (HACC). Therefore, there has been limited access to home help and home maintenance services, delivered meals, home respite care and transport services for people with chronic mental illness. Substantial additional funding for HACC would be required if these anomalies were addressed. No programs have been developed for people with mental illness who require intensive personal care similar to that provided by attendant carers, such as help with showering, shaving, dressing and housework. Reforms are required to housing support services and respite care programs if people with chronic mental illness are to enjoy better access to services.

The need for such a multifaceted, multidisciplinary approach to service delivery and analysis has been reiterated in the National Mental Health Policy (1992), which emphasises the importance of linking mental health and other services. The objectives of the 'intersectoral links' policy are:

- to eliminate barriers to services that are based on discrimination against people with chronic mental illness;
- to formalise policy and planning arrangements at all levels of government and administration;
- to ensure that all relevant programs meet the needs of clients adequately; and
- to encourage linkages between agencies to ensure access to services that meet clients' needs.

## Social support

An important model in community support systems for people with chronic mental illness is the Clubhouse model. Established in New York in 1948, this model has been replicated successfully at Bromham Place in Melbourne, and a second Australian Clubhouse has been established by the Schizophrenia Fellowship in Queensland with funding from Queensland Health and the Silvia and Charles Viertel Foundation. A Clubhouse is a club run for and by its members. The members are typically people with chronic mental illness. Although the general focus of Clubhouse activities is vocational, the Clubhouse is not an education or training centre. The Clubhouse provides daytime support that includes food for members, shelter, occupation, social contacts, structure and guidance. In the Clubhouse model the trend is towards greater participation of consumers. The Clubhouse philosophy centres activities on each person's strengths, and stresses that people with chronic mental illness can look forward to the future with optimism because they have opportunities to use their knowledge and skills in the restorative environment of the Clubhouse (see Chapter 1).

The Clubhouse model demonstrates the contribution of voluntary organisations to the support of people with mental illness in the community. In addition, other **non-governmental organisations**, including the Association of Relatives and Friends of the Mentally Ill, GROW, Step Out of the Shadows, and State mental health associations, are playing an increasingly important role in supporting people with mental illness and psychiatric disabilities in the community.

In New Zealand, a similar range of services exists and people with chronic mental illness face similar problems and barriers to services as those in Australia. People with psychiatric disability are often unemployed and on low incomes, but may only qualify for limited employment benefit entitlements. The Department of Social Welfare provides funds through the income maintenance system under the *Disabled Persons Community Welfare Act (1975)*. The income supports used by people with psychiatric disabilities include Sickness Benefits, Invalid Benefits, Special Benefits, Accommodation Benefits, Disability Allowance and Residual Care Supplement. About 20% of Invalid Benefits go to people with mental illness. Seventeen per cent of Sickness Benefits, plus a significant proportion of benefits going to ill-defined conditions, probably go to people with mental illness (Abbott & Kemp 1993).

## Employment

In employment programs the trend is towards increased consumer-based skill development schemes and away from specialised units and personnel, which are considered less effective. Specialised workshops have become less popular because of the difficulties found when trying to transfer skills from the workshop to the regular workplace. A benefit of the new approach is that specialised mental health workers form relationships with employers that actively facilitate new employment opportunities for consumers (Hallwright 1993). A number of new model employment schemes are listed below.

- Contracts are given to consumer cooperatives for cleaning mental health service premises, either on a preferential basis or through open tender.
- Supported work schemes help consumers to obtain work skills, often with the assistance of a personal coach, usually a former consumer.
- In transitional employment schemes, mental health services contract with employers to identify positions for consumers and to ensure their jobs are well done. The service guarantees to protect employers from absenteeism and recruitment and training costs.
- Job sharing allocates the benefits of the scheme among consumers, allowing each to contribute at an optimum level, while maintaining a reasonable level of work output for the employer.

Refinements to such schemes include mental health workers substituting for consumers if required, and job rotations to ensure that skills are transferred among consumers.

Several model employment and training programs for people with chronic mental illness have been established in Australia. In Newcastle, NSW, is a tripartite DEET-funded program which specifically targets people with psychiatric disabilities; the Ground Work Program in Victoria offers a support program of up to two years for people with chronic mental illness who get a job; and the ACT Mental Health Service Pre-vocational Training

Program, based in Canberra, provides training in employment skills and paid work experiences (National Health Strategy 1993).

The care of those with serious mental illness necessarily involves far more than the health care system. The collaborative model requires that a wide range of government services, such as housing, social security, disability services, and employment and training, integrates with health services. At the same time, the primary role of non-government organisations and the informal care of families and friends must be acknowledged, so that services can begin to develop the types of programs that consumers need, and that consumers want.

# FUTURE TRENDS

Mental health service provision must be seen to extend beyond the parameters of the health care system and to encompass issues of housing, employment and income security. The role of the nurse has made that extension too. As nurses have followed patients out of the large psychiatric hospitals, the care of patients has extended to a broader definition of 'needs': people need housing, people need income, people need employment, people need to be part of a social network.

The Australian and New Zealand health care systems have taken similar but distinctive paths in developing their models of service provision. In both countries at least 80% of expenditure on mental health goes to 20% of the clients (Hallwright 1993); in both countries the institutional sectors account for over half the total health expenditure (McKendry & Mathumala 1994; AIHW 1994); in both countries idealistic models of care struggle against economic rationalism to provide care that is, at times, innovative and full of promise, and at other times underresourced and indefensible. It is likely that the successful innovations from around the world, such as the Clubhouse model and consumer-managed accommodation and businesses, will prove to be the growing trends in Australia and New Zealand.

For nurses, the continuing requirement will be to function well in a multidisciplinary health care environment while supporting growing specialisation in new approaches to long-term care. The needs of the small number of long-term patients who remain in hospital will pose an enormous challenge to future practice, as will the need to define and establish the role that nurses have in the delivery of mental health care in this climate of change and innovation.

# SUMMARY

- Mental health care systems in New Zealand and Australia have undergone significant reform. Worldwide trends such as deinstitutionalisation, the development of community care, and the adoption of intersectoral approaches to service provision are the dominant trends.

- Non-government organisations are playing an increasing role in the provision of services for the seriously mentally ill, with consumer-run advocacy and support services providing exciting innovations in community care.
- The provision of quality mental health care must encompass intersectoral services, including income support and employment, health care, social services, housing and community support services.
- Mental health nurses will increasingly provide care for those with serious mental illness as part of multidisciplinary teams.

## DISCUSSION QUESTIONS

1. What are the structural differences between the Australian and New Zealand health care systems?
2. How are mental health services in Australia and New Zealand funded?
3. What recent structural reforms have been made in mental health services in Australia and New Zealand, and why have they been introduced?
4. Why is it necessary for service initiatives for people with mental illness to extend beyond the health care sector?
5. What is meant by *intersectoral collaboration* in mental health care? Illustrate your answer with three examples.
6. What have NGOs contributed to the deinstitutionalisation of people with mental illnesses?

## EXERCISES

1. Compare and contrast the assumptions implicit in the arrangements for funding mental health services in Australia and New Zealand.
2. Write a short case study on any major reform in mental health care introduced in Australia or New Zealand in the past five years (1000 words).
3. Map out the services that a person with mental illness would ideally expect to receive. As examples, (a) use a client who has never required admission, and (b) one who has required repeated admissions and extensive rehabilitation.
4. List the factors that promote and impede intersectoral collaboration in mental health care.
5. Prepare a submission arguing that access to mental health services should be more equitable (1000 words).
6. Select a mental health service in your area and evaluate its integration into the general health care sector.

# FURTHER READING

- National Health Strategy (1993) *Help Where Help is Needed: Continuity of Care for People with Chronic Mental Illness*, National Health Strategy, Issues Paper no. 5, Melbourne. This publication outlines the problems in the delivery of services to the severely mentally ill. It argues for a multidisciplinary and intersectoral approach to the problem and outlines a number of model programs.
- Abbott, M. & Kemp, D.R. (1993). 'New Zealand' in D. Kemp (ed.) *International Handbook on Mental Health Policy*, New Zealand: Greenwood Press. This chapter discusses the history of mental health care in New Zealand and analyses the current challenges faced in the delivery of mental health care.

# REFERENCES

Abbott, M. & Kemp, D.R. (1993) 'New Zealand' in D. Kemp (ed.) *International Handbook on Mental Health Policy*, New Zealand: Greenwood Press.

Andrews, G. (1989) 'Public and private psychiatry: a comparison of two health care systems', *American Journal of Psychiatry* 146(7), pp.881–6.

Australian Bureau of Statistics (1993) *Private Hospitals in Australia, 1991–92*. Cat.no. 4390.0.

Australian Institute of Health and Welfare (1992) *Australia's Health, 1992*. Canberra: AGPS.

Australian Institute of Health and Welfare (1994) *Australia's Health, 1994*. Canberra: AGPS.

Australian Institute of Health and Welfare (1993) *Health Expenditure Bulletin. Number 8*.

Bacharach, L.L. (1984) 'Asylum and chronically ill psychiatric patients', *American Journal of Psychiatry* 14(8), pp.957–78.

Blue Nursing Service Brisbane (1994) Unpublished data.

Controller and Auditor General (1993) *Report of the Controller and Auditor General on Community Care for People with Mental Illness*, December. Wellington, New Zealand.

Department of Health, Housing, Local Government and Community Services (Aus) (1993) *Annual Report*, Canberra: AGPS.

Department of Human Services and Health (1994) *First National Mental Health Annual Report 1993*, Canberra: AGPS.

Dermer, S.W. & Landeen, J.L. (1991) 'Establishing a model for care in schizophrenia: one program's experience', *Canadian Journal of Psychiatry* 36, pp.588–93.

Goldberg, D. & Huxley, P. (1980) *Mental Illness in the Community*, London: Tavistock.

Gournay, K. & Brooking, J. (1993) *A structure, process and outcome study of community psychiatric nursing in primary health care*. Unpublished report to the

Department of Health and Social Security, UK.

Grant, C. & Lapsley, H.M. (1993) *The Australian Health Care System*. Australian Studies in Health Service Administration no. 75. Sydney: University of NSW.

Hallwright, S. (1993) *Report on Best Practices Study of the US*. Ministry of Health, Wellington.

Harries, M., Jayasuriya, L., Wearne, A. & Dickinson, J. (1991) *Schizophrenia and Social Needs*, Department of Social Work and Social Administration, University of Western Australia.

Hornblow, A.R., Bushell, J.A., Wells, J.E., Joyce, P.R. & Oakley-Browne M.A. (1990) 'Christchurch psychiatric epidemiology study: the use of mental health services', *New Zealand Medical Journal* 103(897), pp.415–17.

Jorm, A.F., Rosenman, S.J. & Jacomb, P.H. (1993) 'Inequalities in the regional distribution of private psychiatric services provided under Medicare', *Australian and New Zealand Journal of Psychiatry* 27, pp.630–7.

Kirkpatrick, H. (1994) 'Transforming a long-stay unit to a psychosocial rehabilitation program'. Presented at the Provincial Implementation Forum, Mental Health Reform. Sponsored by the Ontario Ministry of Health, Toronto.

Lamb, R.H. (1992) 'Is it time for a moratorium on deinstitutionalisation?' (editorial) *Hospital and Community Psychiatry* 43(7), p.669.

McKendry, C.G. & Mathumala, D. (1994) *Health Expenditure Trends in New Zealand: Update to 1993*, Wellington: New Zealand Ministry of Health.

Mayne Nickless (1993) *Annual Report*.

Mechanic, D. & Aiken, L.H.(1987) 'Improving the care of patients with chronic mental illness', *New England Journal of Medicine* 317(26), pp.1634–8.

Mental Health Consumer Outcomes Task Force (1991) *Mental Health: Statement of Rights and Responsibilities*. Report of the Mental Health Consumer Outcomes Task Force, Canberra: AGPS.

Ministry of Health (NZ) (1994) *Mental Health Data*, unpublished.

National Health Strategy (1991) *Hospital Services in Australia—Accessing and Financing*, Issues Paper no. 2, Melbourne.

National Health Strategy (1993) *Help Where Help is Needed: Continuity of Care for People with Chronic Mental Illness* National Health Strategy, Issues Paper no. 5, Melbourne.

National Housing Strategy (1992) *Housing Choice: Reducing the Barriers*. Issues Paper no. 1, National Housing Strategy, Melbourne.

National Mental Health Policy (1992) Canberra: AGPS.

New South Wales Health (1993) *Annual Report 1992–1993*, Sydney: State Health Publication.

New Zealand Public Health Commission (1993) *Our Health Our Future. Hauora Pakari, Koiora Roa*. Wellington: Public Health Commission.

Puckett, A. (1993) *Community Mental Health*, Sydney: Harcourt Brace & Co.

Queensland Health (1993) *Review of Medicare Incentives Scheme*. Internal report.

Whiteford, H., MacLeod, B. & Leitch, E. (1993) 'The National Mental Health Policy: implications for public psychiatric services in Australia (1992)', *Australian and New Zealand Journal of Psychiatry* 27, pp.186–91.

# CLINICAL FOCUS

PART IV PROVIDES AN OVERVIEW of aspects of mental health nursing knowledge and practice. The material presented has been organised around the theme 'clinical focus', to draw attention to the way mental health nursing is shaped by clinical assumptions. The view of mental health nursing that emerges is one dominated by assessment and diagnosis, physical and structured psychiatric and psychologically oriented treatment options, and related interventions. This approach is not intended to be comprehensive. Rather, the opportunity has been taken to stress the importance of the biological and psychological components of the biopsychosocial model of mental illness. The three chapters taken together show how nursing interventions are related to treatment options derived from careful assessment and accurate diagnosis.

Psychopharmacologic options and their rationale have been stressed because they play a central role in the management of mental disorder. The modes of action of the therapeutic compounds discussed have been described because undergraduate students of nursing often have difficulty accessing this information at the right depth in a form that is readily understood by those with no previous knowledge of neurophysiology.

Chapter 9 comments on how notions of mental disorder have changed and introduces the biopsychosocial model that informs mental health nursing practice. The need for rigour in the classification of mental disorders and in clinical assessment is emphasised. Consideration of taxonomies relevant to mental health nursing practice leads on to detailed advice on how to conduct a mental status examination.

Chapter 10 describes the clinical features of the serious mental disorders found in Australia and New Zealand. Chapter 11 completes the section by discussing selected treatment options and nursing interventions.

# Classification

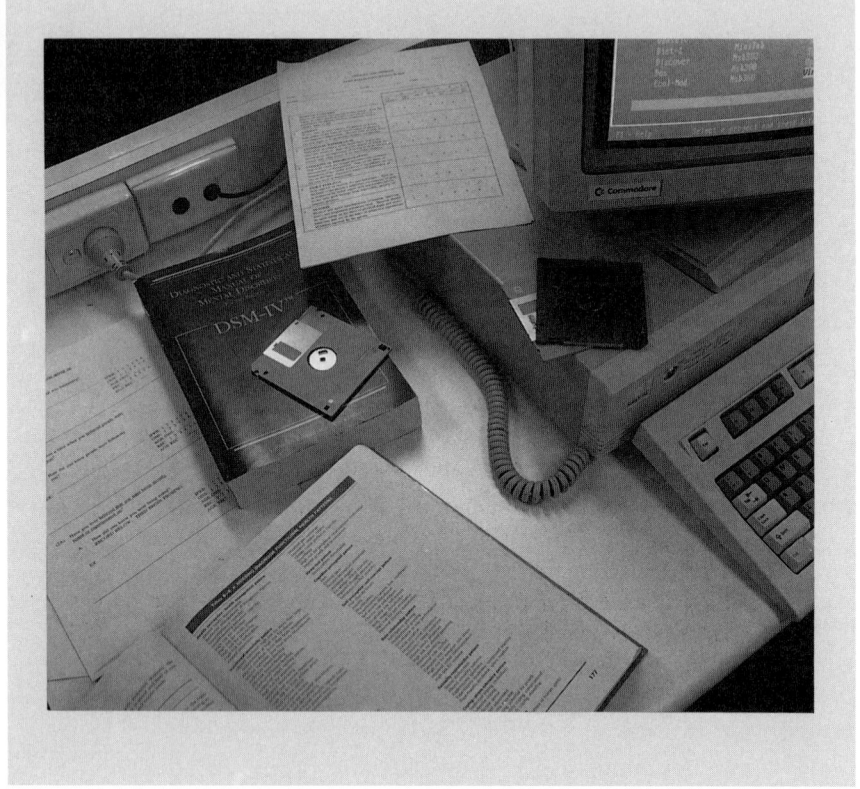

All taxonomies are a way of making sense of complexity

## CHAPTER 9

# MENTAL DISORDER: CONCEPTUAL FRAMEWORK, CLASSIFICATION AND ASSESSMENT

Derek Weir and Tian Oei

## *C*ONTENTS

# LEARNING OBJECTIVES

This chapter will assist the reader to:

- understand the emergence of modern concepts of mental disorder;
- appreciate the need for rigour in the clinical assessment and classification of mental disorder;
- identify appropriate nursing, medical and interdisciplinary taxonomies of mental disorder;
- conduct a mental status assessment.

# INTRODUCTION

At the end of the twentieth century, our understanding of mental illness has come a long way from early explanations dependent on ethereal beliefs (alien forces, evil spirits, sin or transgressions) to the current view of mental disorder as a complex interaction of biochemical, psychological, socio-cultural and environmental influences. It can also be assumed that the advances in scientific methods and techniques that have underpinned the dramatic increase in research, as well as increased public concern, will continue to improve the understanding and treatment of mental disorder. It is now obvious that some of the conditions recognised as mental disorders have well-established aetiology or pathophysiology, and these give rise to different treatment options. For most mental disorders, however, the causes are still unclear or unknown. There are many theories that attempt to explain how these disorders arise and substantial evidence to support them. Some evidence confirms theories of biological aetiology, some findings support psychological theories, and some evidence implicates interaction between biological, psychological and social factors in the causation of mental disorders.

# THE BIOPSYCHOSOCIAL MODEL

Expanding knowledge of neuroendocrinology, immunology and the effects of stress on biological systems further supports the importance of considering the interaction of biological, psychological and social factors in the causation of mental disorders. An approach that integrates these perspectives is justified, as it combines the benefits of biological psychiatry with knowledge drawn from psychosocial research. This composite view is referred to as the **biopsychosocial model** (Amchin 1991) and provides a more comprehensive conceptual framework for assessing and treating mental illness.

According to the biopsychosocial model, the clinician's approach to the client focuses on three integrating dimensions of the client's functioning: biological (physical or organic processes), psychological (aspects of mental functioning, including thought, emotion and behaviour); and social (interactions with others, including family, friends, colleagues at work, professionals and others important to the client) (Amchin 1991). Reflecting this philosophy, psychiatric abnormalities are becoming increasingly designated as 'disorders' rather than diseases. However, it may not always be necessary or practical to pursue all three aspects of the biopsychosocial model fully with each client. Therefore, the mental health worker should retain the biopsychosocial perspective and, if possible, individualise diagnostic assessment and intervention. For example, if a client's problems clearly reflect a primary biological process, it is appropriate to focus on the biological dimension in assessment and treatment.

The integration of behavioural and biomedical ideologies has provided direction to treatment. The appropriate approach is one that combines the study of the human brain and its connections to the body, with investigation of the problems of developing interpersonal bonds, the effect of social organisation and the disorders of communication. Practice in mental health has been medically derived and there is a need to retain a balance between scientific and compassionate concerns for the person. Nurses need to be at ease in understanding the brain, the complexity of neural pathways and neurotransmitters, and the drugs that act on them. However, they must also be sensitive to the uniqueness of each client's personality, with its specific mix of cognitive and emotional styles, patterns of adaptation and defence, and internal conflicts and fantasies.

Models of mental disorder, like other theoretical models, are limited in what they can explain. They can also limit mental health practitioners in their work if too much value is attached to one model at the expense of others. For example, if genes turned out to have something to do with deviant behaviour, it would not mean that knowledge about the psychodynamics of behaviour should be abandoned. It is equally true that someone who has a problem with an organic basis can be helped by 'talking' therapies. There are many studies which show that behavioural and psychodynamic therapy are effective in decreasing symptoms in **depression**, senile **dementia** and **schizophrenia** (Lazarus 1973; Simpson & May 1982; Wetzel 1984; Free & Oei 1989; Robinson, Berman & Heimayer 1990), despite the fact that the biological model has been the most avidly accepted explanation for these disorders.

The use of models provides the essential framework for understanding and conceptually organising the client's specific psychiatric symptomatology, for hypothesising about the underlying aetiology, and for developing treatment plans. The biological, psychological and social perspectives all need attention in arriving at a psychiatric diagnosis.

# CLASSIFICATION OF MENTAL DISORDER

In introducing the concept of classification, it helps to reflect on the labels often applied to clients. Labels such as 'non-compliant', 'refusers' and 'dropouts' are indicative of the perspective of the labeller (see Chapter 1). It is common for medical labels to be readily applied to people suffering from distressing social problems (i.e. they are 'anxious', 'depressed', 'confused', 'distraught', 'agitated', 'suicidal'). While some of these labels may be appropriately used, it is worth remembering that many people display disabilities and handicaps similar to those associated with mental disorder, such as interpersonal difficulties, poor social skills, inefficient problem solving, antisocial behaviour, lack of motivation, or poor vocational achievement. Sometimes the behaviour of distressed people may be more a reflection of past experiences, or of having received inadequate help in the past, than an indicator of some intrinsic attribute. Many of the psychosocial interventions that are effective in treating these psychosocial problems are also effective in the management of mental disorders. Without the application of clear definitions of mental disorders, abuse of these labels is frequent.

Research has led to the development of sophisticated methods of classifying mental disorders. High levels of agreement between clinicians can be attained when standardised diagnostic interviews and classification systems are used (DSM-IV 1994). The increasing complexity of the assessment criteria required to differentiate known and recognisable clinical entities makes it essential that nurses have a fundamental grasp of current diagnostic terminology. Such knowledge enables nurses to communicate effectively and professionally with other disciplines, to participate collaboratively in patient care management, to contribute to clinical research, and to organise and use data in clinical problem solving and choice of effective nursing interventions. In addition, the knowledge and use of a classification system presumes a systematic and logical procedure for intervention. Such knowledge increases the nurse's efficacy in providing professional assistance to the client. An awareness of the objective data, as distinct from the subjective interpretation that stems from a particular theoretical orientation and conceptual framework, allows nurses to make maximum use of their creativity and uniqueness in clinical practice.

As with concepts of physical disorder and mental health, no single definition adequately specifies the precise boundaries for mental disorder. The term 'mental disorder', by implication, suggests conditions which are separate from physical disorders as if there were no interaction between the two. This is problematic, because such separation is not the case (DSM-IV 1994). The term 'mental disorder' persists, however, and in the absence of any more satisfactory terminology it remains in current use. The APA describes mental disorders as those conditions that can be:

> ...conceptualised as a clinically significant behavioural or psychological syndrome or pattern that occurs in an individual and that is associated with present distress (a painful symptom) or disability (impairment in one or more important areas of functioning) or with a significantly increased risk of suffering death, pain, disability, or an important loss of freedom ... [which is not] merely an expectable response to a particular event (for example the death of a loved one). (DSM-IV, p.xxii)

Whatever its original cause, the mental disorder must be considered a manifestation of a behavioural, psychological or biological dysfunction in the person. But DSM-IV warns that neither behaviour which deviates from established political, religious or sexual norms, nor conflicts that are primarily between one person and society are mental disorders, unless the deviance or conflict is a symptom of a dysfunction as described.

It is also important to recognise that any one mental disorder is not a discrete entity with sharp boundaries that separate it from any other mental disorder or, in fact, the absence of a mental disorder. Many people who experience the clinically significant disruption that justifies the label 'mental disorder' may manifest symptoms that are common to several disorders, but have a predominance of those symptoms that are essential defining features of a particular disorder. Similarly, not every person who meets the defining criteria for a particular disorder will present exactly the same features—he or she may well differ in important ways that may have effects on clinical management and outcomes.

According to DSM-IV, a common misconception is that a classification of mental disorders classifies *people*, when what are actually being classified are the *disorders* that people have. For this reason, the text of DSM-IV avoids the use of such expressions as 'a schizophrenic' or 'an alcoholic' and instead uses the more accurate, but admittedly more cumbersome, 'an individual with schizophrenia' or 'an individual with alcohol dependence'. This approach is used throughout this book.

# NURSING DIAGNOSTIC SYSTEMS FOR MENTAL HEALTH AND MENTAL DISORDER

A nursing diagnosis for a person with a **mental disorder** is a way of conceptualising the human response from a nursing perspective—a way of making sense of the data collected during assessment. The diagnosis reflects judgments and decisions about the pattern of interactions between client and environment, from which goals and interventions can be logically derived and evaluated (Varcarolis 1994). Nursing as a profession has not yet adopted a standard diagnostic format. Several possibilities that link assessment data, dictate logical outcome and evaluation criteria and suggest appropriate nursing interventions are being considered. In general terms, nursing diagnoses for people with mental disorders address broad categories of actual or potential health problems. These broad categories reflect:

- limitations of self-care and impaired functioning;
- emotional stress;
- changes in self-concept and life processes;
- alterations in cognitive abilities;

- physical symptoms accompanying altered psychological functioning; and
- behavioural risks to self or others.

The diagnosis is made through an assessment process carried out by the nurse and validated with the client. In clinical settings, there is a wide range of nursing diagnostic systems, and readers are encouraged to refer to specific diagnostic texts for further details and guides to using these systems. While recognising that nursing diagnostic systems have the potential to provide a common frame of reference for nurses, it is important to remember that they are still undergoing refinement and standardisation, and are not widely understood by other health disciplines.

# INTERDISCIPLINARY DIAGNOSTIC SYSTEMS FOR MENTAL DISORDER

Classification systems that are widely used in interdisciplinary mental health care settings are required, in order to provide a functional, standardised and validated system of classification that can be used by appropriately trained mental health professionals. These systems need to reflect the breadth of available evidence and opinion. One such system, based on medical concepts, has become widely used. The American Psychiatric Association's *Diagnostic and Statistical Manual of Mental Disorders*, 4th edn (DSM-IV), was released in 1994 as a classification of mental disorders that was developed for use in clinical, educational and research settings. It is intended to provide a clear description of the diagnostic categories to enable diagnosis, communication about, study of and interventions for people with various mental disorders. This extensive list of descriptive terms and symptoms covers almost all kinds of unusual or deviant behaviour. DSM-IV describes the major disorders that are thought to be consistent across varying cultures and throughout history.

## Issues in classification

Legitimate interdisciplinary and nursing diagnoses can only be made when a complete assessment of a client has been carried out. Nursing diagnoses are meant to illustrate a broad range of possibilities that might eventuate for a client with a particular medical psychiatric diagnosis. Any taxonomy attempting to classify disruptions as mental disorders has some limitations:

- the system must be properly used and may require specialised training;
- the system may not be complete; and
- cultural and ethnic differences in language, values, behavioural norms and the manner in which distress is expressed, may be unaccounted for by the chosen taxonomy (see Chapters 6 and 7).

The realities presented by the interdisciplinary nature of mental health services mean that those professionals who work in these settings must be familiar with diagnostic systems that enable accurate, comprehensive and appropriately focused diagnosis and clinical decision making. Since theories of the aetiology of mental disorders are subject to refinement and some controversy, a descriptive, objective approach that is neutral with respect to theory or aetiology may provide a more useful system of clinical classification.

# THE EVALUATION OF MENTAL STATUS

How, then, do nurses initiate the nursing process with a client, and how do they obtain the information about the client's thoughts, feelings and behaviours that is needed to assess psychopathology? When should they stop collecting information? How and when should they develop a treatment plan? How do they follow up (evaluate) a client's progress?

There is an art to eliciting clinical information. Empathy, common sense and intuition are necessary to develop trust and rapport, and to encourage disclosure of the necessary information. The emotional fragility of clients, regardless of how disorganised they appear, must also be considered. When the initial assessment is conducted during a crisis, or when the client is emotionally distraught, the evaluation must be brief as well as accurate in order to avoid adding to the client's stress; it must also be accompanied by whatever acute interventions the situation demands. As the initial assessment marks the beginning of a therapeutic relationship, it should help clients feel that their concerns are understood and regarded as primary, even when the nurse feels there are more important things to explore. It helps to have a logical framework to follow when collecting this information, but sound clinical judgment in how far or how relentlessly to pursue the various criteria is also needed.

Assessing the mental status of a client typically involves a semi-structured interview and a formalised mental status examination (MSE) that deals with the client's thoughts, feelings and behaviour at a particular time point. While the MSE entails a systematic collection of relevant data about the client's level of functioning, it is only part of the evaluation. The semi-structured interview provides a framework for the total assessment—it functions to establish rapport, gain knowledge of characteristic patterns of living and coping behaviours, elicit the past history of the client, and form an assessment of cognitive functioning. Throughout the interview, data is obtained both by communication with and observation of the client. There is no single best way to perform such a psychiatric interview and so the approach and line of enquiry should vary, depending on the nature of the presenting problem and the individual client being assessed.

## The semi-structured interview

In this interview, use open-ended questions. Ask the specific questions later in the formal part of the assessment. Unless clients are extremely uncooperative or incapable of free expression, encourage them to tell their story with little interruption during the first 5 to 15 minutes. An open-ended question such as 'What is the problem that brings you here?' or 'How can we help you?' will suffice. (Clients are often tense early in the interview and this tension may stimulate the information flow.) A client who has a formal thought disorder (where the thoughts do not connect coherently) will quickly reveal this. Much of the information needed for the diagnosis can be provided in the first few minutes if the client proceeds without interruption. Remember that being too prescriptive in your questioning at this point may cause you to miss important material. On the other hand, if a client is particularly tense, more structure at the beginning may lead to easier communication—sometimes clients need to be guided into channels that provide the information required for a diagnosis. With a client who is very tense, the interviewer can ask specific questions that are emotionally neutral—about background, growing up, school, marital status, job history.

### Establish the chronology of the illness

The course of a mental disorder is as important as the symptoms. When did the symptoms begin? What was going on in the client's life at the time? (Look for evidence of other stress/trauma.) Was the client ever free of symptoms? When? (Age of onset is important for diagnostic purposes.) Has the illness been continuous, always present with fluctuations, or episodic in the sense that symptoms sometimes go away entirely? How rapid was the onset? (This factor is often relevant to prognosis.) Have professional interventions (medication, other treatment) altered the course of the illness? Look for evidence of past psychiatric history. Has the client tended to improve or to get worse?

## Client's perception of problem

Having got a clear account of the presenting problem, it is important to determine how the client perceives the problem. For example, is it something they think they can change? Something someone else is responsible for? Something no one can control? This should move you towards the mental status examination itself—the more formal part of the total evaluation. While you are obtaining information about the presenting problem and taking the history, you are also informally and indirectly accumulating information about the client's mental state. However, you still need to ask questions to complete an accurate and comprehensive mental status examination. Often there may be little time to conduct the evaluation, but, for the evaluation to be complete, it should include attention to mental status. The purpose of the mental status format is to help the interviewer organise and communicate observations about a client. Some framework is necessary to facilitate thinking and communication. The format presented here is commonly used.

# Mental status examination

The purpose of the formal mental status examination is to determine objectively the observable aspects of the client's psychological functioning. This contrasts with taking the client's history, which is based not on observable behaviour but on the client's recollections. The performance and recording of a mental status examination has several major functions:

- it is an agreed-on method of organising clinical observations;
- it provides a clinical baseline for the client's psychological state; and
- it provides specific information that assists in establishing certain diagnoses.

Record verbatim examples of speech as these help to present a precise picture. Mental status examinations generally include investigation of the following areas.

- *General observation,* which includes specific details of those characteristics that appear outstanding to the interviewer, such as appearance and motor behaviour.

- *Sensorium and intelligence,* which describes, first, the client's state of consciousness and ability to perceive the environment accurately. Second, the client's orientation, memory, intellectual function, judgment and comprehension are assessed. Impairment in more than one area may point to a diagnosis of an organic mental disorder. Since the disorder can vary from mild, transient disruptions to permanent alteration of all areas, it is important to document each area carefully.

- *Thought processes,* which alert clinicians to the content and form of thinking, the patterns of verbalisation and the content of speech.

- *Affect and mood* which are the subjective and objective manifestations of the emotional state, and provide clues to the appropriateness of that state.

- *Insight,* which is the understanding clients have about the nature of their problem and how it affects their feelings, thoughts, behaviours, judgment and attitudes. Insight also includes clients' current understanding of the situation in which they find themselves, and possible solutions to it. Those with insight will know whether they are (or were) psychiatrically ill. If a man, for example, says that his voices are 'real', he lacks insight. If he says it was simply his imagination playing tricks on him, he has insight. Psychosis and organic brain disorders are both associated with lack of insight; so-called neurotic disorders are usually accompanied by insight.

A simple acronym will help you to recall the main areas for mental state assessment: OSITAMI for Observation, Sensorium, Intelligence, Thought (content and form), Affect, Mood and Insight.

## General observation

Under this heading you assess appearance and motor behaviour.

1. *Appearance.* Specific aspects of the client's appearance that appear out-standing to the interviewer are often relevant to the diagnosis. The appearance of a person with a schizophrenic disorder (e.g. poor grooming and poor personal hygiene) may reflect underlying cognitive disorganisation. Someone with a depressive disorder may also lack the motivation to pay attention to clothing and personal hygiene. A person in the manic phase of a bipolar disorder may wear bizarre combinations of clothes, and may change them several times in the course of an hour, in keeping with the distractability and overactivity that accompanies the disorder.

   When describing appearance, do so in terms of its consistency with age and station in life. Focus on the manner of dress (conservative, meticulous, inappropriate, extreme, bizarre, seasonal appropriateness) and on facial expressions (impassive, expressionless, vacant, sad, bewildered, excited, alert, angry, hostile, degree of eye contact).

2. *Motor behaviour.* Assessment is for consistency of behaviour and should include any overt motor behaviour, such as finger tapping, hand-wringing, hair twirling, pacing, posturing, or bizarre movements, that may indicate changed mental functioning.

   In addition to assessing posture and gait, the *speed* at which tics, posturing, grimacing and other abnormal body movements occur is important. Is there a general slowness of movement? Is much effort expended just to talk, walk or gesture? Or do the movements appear to be intense and rapid?

   There are several abnormal motor behaviours that frequently relate to specific mental disorders, but it is important to note that some drugs used in the treatment of mental disorders may also produce motor abnormalities. Box 9.1 describes some examples of abnormal motor behaviour. There are others.

B O X   9 . 1 : *Examples of abnormal motor behaviours associated with certain mental disorders*

- **Echopraxia:** pathological repetition by imitation of the movements of another person.

- **Cerea flexibilitas (waxy flexibility):** holding the arms or legs in the same position for a long period of time.

   Both echopraxia and cerea flexibilitas may be seen in catatonic schizophrenia.

- **Catalepsy:** a generalised condition of diminished responsiveness, often characterised by trance-like states and immobility; can occur in organic and psychological disorders.

*continued …*

- **Cataplexy:** temporary loss of muscle tone; may be precipitated by surprise, laughter or anger, and is seen in schizophrenia.

- **Compulsion:** an insistent, repetitive, intrusive and unwanted urge to act in a way designed to reduce overwhelming anxiety (often accompanies intrusive and unwanted obsessional thoughts); present in subtypes of anxiety disorders.

- **Akathisia:** a restlessness produced by neuroleptic drugs—the client cannot sit still and feels compelled to walk. Neuroleptics may also produce **parkinson-like** symptoms, including tremor, 'pill rolling', dyskinesias (abnormal muscle movements, especially of the mouth) and sometimes extremely severe, frightening and painful torticollis reactions (eyes evert and neck becomes dorsiflexed).

## Sensorium and intelligence

Under this heading you assess level of consciousness, orientation, memory, intellectual functioning, judgment and comprehension.

1. *Level of consciousness.* A variety of terms can be used to describe the current level of consciousness, such as 'alert', 'awake', 'stuporous' and 'sleepy'. Is the client easily distracted or hyperalert? Can attention be sustained to both external and internal stimuli? A clouded state of consciousness is an essential feature in **delirium**, and it is therefore essential for accurate diagnosis and treatment to assess the level of consciousness.

2. *Orientation.* Clients are questioned about orientation to time, place and person. Do they know who they are, where they are, how they got there, the people around them, the date? To be disoriented for time means being more than one day off the correct day of the week, and more than four or five days off the current date. Misidentifying people (e.g. thinking the clinician is a relative when this is not so) is a clear case of disorientation, as is giving the wrong year, or the wrong city or hospital.

    Clients with organic disruptions may give grossly inaccurate answers, especially for time relationships. In contrast, in schizophrenic disorders, clients may be appropriately oriented to place, but not to person—believing, for example, that they are someone else.

3. *Memory.* Memory impairment can be a prominent behaviour that can range from forgetfulness to total lack of understanding of significant people and events in the individual's life. There are three areas to be tested in memory—immediate recall, recent memory and remote memory.

    Immediate recall involves attention and concentration as well as an ability to retain material just learned. One test of immediate recall is the 'digit span test', which requires the client to repeat digits either forwards or backwards within a 10-second interval. The interviewer recites a series of randomly selected digits, beginning with three digits and increasing the number until it is clear that the client is unable to repeat the digits in proper sequence. The same procedure is repeated, but the client is asked to reverse the order of the numbers. An example is given so that the procedure is understood. It would be reasonable to expect someone with unimpeded function to recall between seven and nine digits correctly. Remember that high levels of anxiety may interfere with a client's ability to concentrate, and this should be taken into consideration if the performance is poor.

Recent memory can be tested by asking clients when they came to hospital, and to recall the events of the past 24 hours. A reliable informant may be needed to verify this statement. Another test of recent memory is to ask clients to remember three words (e.g. an object, a colour and a suburb) and have them repeat the words back during the interview 15 minutes later.

The ability to give a consistent account of past history requires an intact remote memory. Available records or reliable informants are needed to verify information such as date of birth, age, when started and finished school, date of marriage, birth dates of children, and other significant life events.

4. *Intellectual function.* This has to be assessed relative to the educational, occupational and attainment levels that each individual has achieved. Testing the client's vocabulary, counting and calculating ability, ability to extract meaning from events (referred to as abstraction) and fund of general knowledge provides some information about intelligence. Vocabulary can be assessed by asking for word definitions or synonyms. Counting and calculating involve doing simple arithmetic problems (e.g. $9 \times 6$; $21 + 7$) and performing a serial subtraction of 7 from 100. If this is too difficult, subtract 3 from 20 serially. This task also involves attention and concentration.

The ability to conceptualise and abstract can be tested by explanation of a series of proverbs. Give an example of a proverb and its interpretation, then have the client explain what several proverbs mean. Frequently used proverbs are: 'When it rains, it pours'; 'A stitch in time saves nine'; 'A rolling stone gathers no moss'; 'The proof of the pudding is in the eating'. Most adults are able to interpret proverbs as a representation or symbolisation of human behaviour or events. Cultural background is a factor that should be considered when the client is unable to complete the task.

If the educational level is relatively low, asking clients to list similarities between a series of paired objects (e.g. bicycle and bus; apple and pear; television and newspaper) is one means of assessing their ability to abstract. A good reply would be in terms of the items' function, whereas an answer in terms of their physical structure may indicate a tendency towards concrete thinking. To determine general knowledge, clients could be asked to name the last three prime ministers, the mayor of a large city, five large cities, the capital of Australia or New Zealand, or similar questions suited to their educational background. A client who does not read or work may not be able to state recent events or local news, but could relate the plots of television shows.

5. *Judgment.* Judgment involves the ability to understand facts and draw conclusions from relationships between events. You might inquire about past decisions and how these were reached. In discussion of recent events, does the client appear to exhibit sound judgment? It is useful to determine if the judgments were deliberate, impulsive or inappropriate. Several hypothetical situations can be presented to the client to evaluate: 'What would you do if you found a stamped addressed envelope lying on the ground?' 'How would you find the way out of a forest in the daytime?' 'What would you do if you entered your home and smelled gas/smoke?'.

6. *Comprehension.* Throughout the interview, assess clients' ability to understand the meaning of questions, as well as their ability to comprehend incidents in the environment, such as local, political and personal events that affect them and the community. Does the client understand the client role, and, if hospitalised, the hospital routine?

The assessment data obtained in the area of sensorium and intelligence is of particular importance in determining disorders classified as organic mental disorders. The acute picture presented to the clinician is often easy to identify, whereas the more subtle changes that can occur as a result of a degenerative disease or brain tissue lesion require attentive observation and careful documentation of behaviours.

## Thought processes

Under this heading you assess both the form and the content of thought.

1. *Form of thought* refers to intelligibility as it relates to associations. Through the client's speech, it is possible to make observations about thought processes. The patterns, or forms, of verbalisation, rather than the content of speech, are assessed here. What is the rate, or flow? Is it overly fast or retarded? Does the speech progress in a clear, logical, goal-directed manner? As clients talk, you can note whether they can express themselves in an understandable manner, or if the ideas are vague, leaving you uncertain about their meanings. Is the client able to move freely from one topic to another?

   There are several characteristics to consider when assessing thought processes:

   - Is there continuity of thought, or are the associations between thoughts disconnected or haphazard (referred to as *loose*)?
   - Are thoughts constantly and rapidly changing from one topic to another (*flight of ideas*)?
   - Are comments wide of the point of conversation (*tangential*)?
   - Are answers full of unnecessary detail and explanation (*circumstantial*)?
   - Is speech interrupted suddenly (*blocked*)?

- Is there repetition of exactly the same response to different questions (*perseveration*)?
- Are the words used by one person repeated pathologically (*echolalia*)?
- Is speech distorted and bizarre, as when new words are made up to express ideas symbolically (*neologisms*)? or rapid and unstoppable (*pressure of speech*)?

Note though that elderly respondents are often circumstantial. People with schizophrenic disorders often have marked tangentiality, while the speech of those with mood disorders (particularly mania) and those with schizophrenic disorders is often marked by pressure of speech and flight of ideas. The difference between pressure of speech and tangentiality is that in pressured speech there is a connection between the thoughts.

2. *Content of thought*. Content encompasses perceptual disturbances. Recurring patterns of content, such as delusions, hallucinations or illusions (see Box 9.2) may be observed, reflecting a disruption to perception. Misperceptions include a variety of thoughts, feelings or fears the client may have that interfere in some way with reality testing.

## Box 9.2: *Misperceptions in mental disorders*

**Hallucinations** refer to sensory perceptions for which there are no external stimuli. Sometimes, client behaviour will indicate that they are hallucinating: they may adopt a listening attitude, mumble, pick at unseen objects, or stop suddenly as if guarding themselves. Asking clients if they have heard noises or voices when no one was around, or have had any unusual experiences will provide an opportunity for them to describe such experiences to you. Characteristics such as the source, manner of reception, content and time of the experience should be described.

Hallucinations can have different origins, such as psychosis, brain tumour, drug reaction toxicity or withdrawal, sleep deprivation and hepatic failure. They may be vague sounds, flashes of light, or recognisable voices, faces, insects or odours. They may affect any of the senses—most common are auditory; others are visual, olfactory, tactile (touch), gustatory (taste) or visceral (sensation). More unusual hallucinations are extracampine—that is, sufferers see objects outside the sensory field, usually behind their head.

**Delusions** are recurring false beliefs that are not congruent with the clients' culture or background, and from which no logic or experience can dissuade them. There are five types of delusion:

- those relating to the belief that there is an organised conspiracy to hurt or harm the person in some way (*persecutory*);

*continued ...*

- those which convince the person that his body is deteriorating from within or that someone is in his brain (*somatic*);
- those which convince the person she is famous or important, or has some special status above others (*grandeur*);
- belief that a person's 'bad' thoughts have the power to affect or influence others (*guilt*); and
- the belief that a person is being controlled by external objects or individuals (*influence*).

Tactful questioning will help clients to focus on delusional material. Do they misinterpret what is happening to them, giving it special or false meaning? Do they feel they are being singled out or watched? Do they think their thoughts or actions are being controlled by an external force?

**Illusions** are misinterpretations of actual sensory stimuli. Seeing shadows of a tree branch on a wall and thinking they are insects crawling on the wall, or hearing a door or window bang in the wind and misinterpeting this as voices, are examples of illusions.

## Affect and mood

Under this heading you assess the client's mood and emotions.

1. The term **affect** refers to what the individual is expressing emotionally, and specifically to the outward appearance, which may or may not be appropriate to the client's reported mood and content of thought. For example, if a woman smiles happily while telling of people 'trying to poison her', the affect would be described as inappropriate. Several areas can be noted when assessing affect:

   - *range*—the variety of emotions expressed in the course of the interview (may be described as limited, narrow or blunted);
   - *intensity*—the quality of emotion expressed when referring to significant life events (may appear 'flat', meaning that the usual fine modulation of facial expression is absent; or 'exaggerated', with great energy);
   - *type*—the different categories of emotion, described as sad, happy, fearful, angry, elated, etc;
   - *lability*—the rapidity of shift from one emotional state to another; and
   - *appropriateness*—does the affect expressed fit the content expressed?

   People with schizophrenic disorders often demonstrate flat affect, but so do those taking neuroleptic drugs; and a depressed client may show little change of expression while speaking.

2. **Mood** refers to the subjective description of feeling—what clients say about their internal emotional state. 'I am happy/sad/angry' are statements describing mood. The questions facing you, the interviewer, are: What is the dominant, pervasive, enduring mood during the interview? Does the client's appearance reflect that mood? Does the client look 'down in the dumps'? How does the client describe his or her mood? Does it remain the same or change throughout the day, or from day to day? Are these changes rapid, cyclic or situational? Asking clients to rate their mood on a scale of 1 to 10 can be useful to determine changes over time. When the clinical picture is highlighted by a continuous intensification or change in the client's mood, a mood disorder is suspected.

When eliciting client's feelings, if a potential for suicide is perceived, attempt to bring out the client's thoughts about self-destruction. Information about suicidal or homicidal thoughts should be directly addressed. Has there been any desire to self-harm or harm someone else? Have any suicide attempts been made and, if so, what events surrounded those attempts?

To make a judgment about the degree of suicidal or homicidal risk present, the nurse must assess details of plans, ability to carry these out, plans for implementation (availability of weapons, etc.), client's attitudes to death, and the support systems available to them.

## Insight

The degree of **insight** that clients have about the nature of their problem, and how it affects their feelings, thoughts and behaviour, may be assessed informally as they talk about their problems. It is important to determine whether clients see the problem as something brought on by external factors or arising from within themselves. Whether clients see treatment needs realistically will affect the treatment plan and the setting of mutual goals to meet these needs. Several questions may be helpful to ascertain the degree of insight:

- 'What do you think about all you have told me?'
- 'What do you want to do about it?'
- 'What do you think that others and you can do about it?'

How long should the mental status examination take? Time is never wasted in collecting data because the process of assessment is, in itself, therapeutic. The relief associated with the feeling that someone is trying to understand and wants to help has enormous benefits to the client. It is rare that data collection ever stops. Since mental status is variable over time, assessment is a continuous process which, in itself, has therapeutic value in enabling feedback to the client, evaluation of the interventions, and approriate modification of interventions. Just as the emotional fragility of the client determines how rigorously to pursue the interview, it is useful to remember that the context in which the mental status examination is conducted influences the information obtained. In professional relationships, information is gained under conditions of privilege and, thus, appropriate attention to privacy and confidentiality is essential.

# SUMMARY

- Explanations of mental disorder have shifted from those that have stressed ethereal explanations to those that recognise the complex interaction among biochemical, psychological, sociocultural and environmental influences. Advances in scientific methods and techniques as well as increasing public concern have resulted in a dramatic increase in research, and research will continue to shape how mental disorders are understood and how they are treated.

- The biopsychosocial model is now dominant among explanations of mental disorder. Expanding knowledge of neuroendocrinology, immunology, and the effects of stress on biological systems supports the importance of considering the interaction of biological, psychological and social factors in the causation of mental disorders. An approach that integrates these perspectives is justified, as it combines the benefits of the biological treatment of mental disorder with those of knowledge drawn from research into psychosocial aspects of mental health.

- Nurses need to be at ease in understanding the brain, the complexity of neural pathways and neurotransmitters, and the drugs that act on them. However, they must also be sensitive to the uniqueness of each client's personality, with its specific mix of cognitive and emotional styles, patterns of adaptation and defence, and internal conflicts and fantasies.

- Sophisticated methods of classifying mental disorders and of conducting clinical assessments using these taxonomies have been developed. The American Psychiatric Association's Diagnostic and Statistical Manual of Mental Disorders, fourth edition (DSM-IV) and the North American Nursing Diagnosis Association's (NANDA 1994) approach to nursing diagnosis are two approaches with which mental health nurses should be familiar, although further work is required to modify the NANDA approach for use in Australia and New Zealand.

- A mental status examination is the first step in initiating the nursing process. Conducting the structured assessment enables the nurse to assess the client's needs, to communicate effectively with members of other mental health professions, and to devise a plan of care in collaboration with the client.

# DISCUSSION QUESTIONS

1. The biopsychosocial approach to mental disorder provides an interactive model of functioning. Discuss.

2. Discuss the benefits professionals and clients gain from using standardised systems of classifying mental disorders. Are there any limitations to the use of these systems?

3. Define the term 'mental disorder'.

4. Outline the essential components of a mental status examination, and provide examples of normal and abnormal findings in each category of assessment.

5. Consider the problems associated with conducting a mental status examination on a client of Aboriginal, Maori or non-English speaking background. Refer to Chapters 6 and 7.

# EXERCISES

1. Next time you undertake learning experiences in a psychiatric setting, note any informal labels that are used to refer to clients and compare them with the terminology nurses use when undertaking nursing assessments. Account for any tendency for nurses to apply labels to clients in an unreflective way and assess the impact of these labels on clients.

2. With the permission of the client, observe how an experienced mental health professional conducts a mental status examination.

3. Conduct a mental status examination on a friend, and then have the same friend conduct one on you. Discuss your conclusions. Compare notes on how it feels to be the assessor and the person being assessed. Discuss how the process can be made as non-judgmental as possible.

4. With the informed consent of the client, arrange to carry out a mental status examination under the supervision of your clinical facilitator or a registered nurse. Compare your conclusions with those of the clinical facilitator or registered nurse. Rewrite your conclusions, using NANDA terminology.

# FURTHER READING

- Varcarolis, E.M. (1994) *Foundations of Psychiatric-Mental Health Nursing*, 2nd edn, W.B. Saunders, Philadelphia. Outlines the process of examination of a client, and refers to the conceptual frameworks for classification and assessment. Varcarolis provides excellent examples of nursing approaches to client care.

- Arthur, D., Dowling, J. & Sharkey, R. (1992) *Mental Health Nursing. Strategies for Working with the Difficult Client*, Sydney: W.B. Saunders/ Balliere Tindal. See Appendix 2 for a discussion of NANDA and related nursing diagnoses. The authors provide a summary of the diagnoses of relevance to mental health nursing.

# REFERENCES

Amchin, J.K. (1991) *Psychiatric Diagnosis: A Biopsychosocial Approach using DSM-III-R*, Washington DC: American Psychiatric Press.

*Diagnostic and Statistical Manual of Mental Disorders*, 4th edn (1994), Washington DC: American Psychiatric Press.

Free, M.L. & Oei, T.P.S. (1989) 'Biological and psychological processes in the treatment and maintenance of depression', *Clinical Psychology Review* 9, pp.653–88.

Lazarus, A.A. (1973) 'Multimodal behaviour therapy: treating the "Basic ID"', *Journal of Nervous and Mental Disease* 156(6), pp.404–11.

North American Nursing Diagnosis Association (1994) *NANDA Nursing Diagnosis: Definitions and Classification* 1995–1996, St Louis, NANDA.

Robinson, L., Berman, J. & Heimayer, R. (1990) 'Psychotherapy for treatment of depression: a comprehensive review of controlled outcome studies', *Psychological Bulletin* 108, pp.30–48.

Simpson, G.M. & May, P.R. (1982) 'Schizophrenic disorders' in J.H. Greist, J.W. Jefferson & R.L. Spitzer (eds) *Treatment of Mental Disorders*, Oxford University Press, Oxford pp.143–76.

Varcarolis, E.M. (1994) *Foundations of Psychiatric-Mental Health Nursing* (2nd edn), Philadelphia: W.B. Saunders.

Wetzel, J.W. (1984) *Clinical Handbook of Depression*, New York: Gardner Press.

# Fear

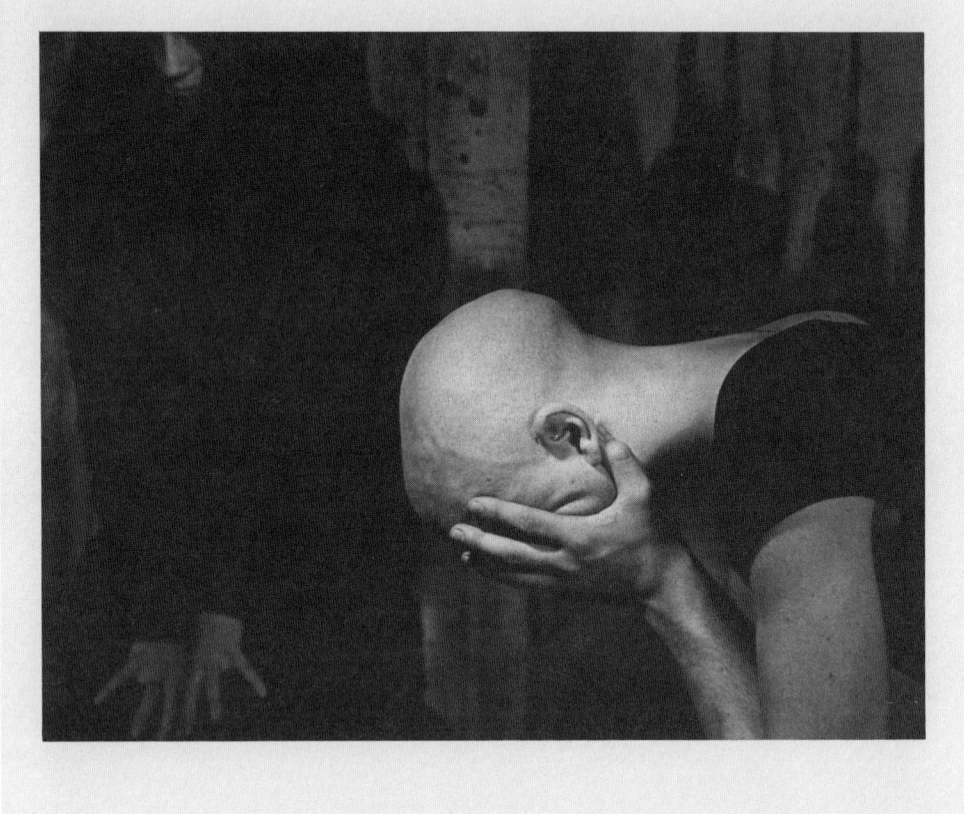

GRAHAM BURSTOW

Some people fear the mad, others the terror of their own thoughts.

## CHAPTER 10

# SERIOUS MENTAL DISORDERS

Derek Weir and Tian Oei

## CONTENTS

# LEARNING OBJECTIVES

This chapter will assist the reader to:

- discuss serious mental disorders found in Australia and New Zealand;
- identify relevant clinical indicators for serious mental disorders, associated aetiological factors and the psychosocial impact of the disorders;
- review options for the clinical management of these disorders, based on the framework presented in Chapter 9;
- identify essential elements in initiating the nursing process with clients experiencing serious mental disorders.

# INTRODUCTION

The incidence of mental disorder in Australia and New Zealand is difficult to determine because of the absence of national databases and few epidemiological studies (see Chapter 5). In addition, unlike sufferers of physical disorders, people with serious mental disorders often do not seek help from medical services (Goldberg & Huxley 1980). One recent study also indicates that a substantial portion of patients who present to general practitioners are not recognised as suffering from mental disorder (Human Rights and Equal Opportunities Commission 1993). Some of these patients would undoubtedly involve complex presentations requiring sophisticated assessment techniques to diagnose their disorder (Goldberg & Bridges 1987). Even patients who are detected as having a mental disorder by their GP may not receive a referral to specialised services, or attend those services. This 'hidden morbidity' presents a considerable problem for epidemiological studies on mental disorders (see Chapter 5).

Identifying the prevalence of mental disorders is not just an academic exercise. There is a potent argument that resources allocated to the provision of mental health services ought to reflect the incidence of mental disorders (Ellard 1994). This view is countered by an equally persuasive argument that the disorders that have the most significant impact on both the individual and the community deserve a proportionally greater share of services, as the people affected are likely to be vulnerable when it comes to accessing appropriate treatment. The allocation of funds to the provision of services and treatment for mental disorders is critical because of the impact which mental health problems can have on national productivity (see Chapter 8).

In order to make an appropriate contribution to the services necessary for the care of those suffering from mental disorders, it is imperative that mental health nurses understand the impact these disorders may have on the people who suffer from them. Mental disorders are not selective of social class. People who suffer from these disorders and those who care for them (often their immediate families) have for years experienced poor care and social ostracism, due to widespread ignorance and stereotyping of mental disorders. It is only necessary to seek out the reports of several recent Commissions of Inquiry in Australia to confirm this view. The greatest impact of mental disorder relates to the stigmatisation and marginalisation which accompanies the diagnosis and also, until comparatively recently, the treatment provided. These negative perspectives carry over into health care settings and are found among health care workers, sufferers themselves, family members, peers, social contacts, work environments, and the community to which the sufferer belongs.

This chapter discusses several of the most commonly encountered serious mental disorders. It is not a comprehensive list of all disorders—a cursory perusal of the DSM-IV (1994) will reveal a vast listing of mental disorders and conditions, ranging from those which are first evident in childhood to those afflicting the elderly. The intention of the discussion here is to promote an awareness of the characteristic features of some of the most debilitating mental disorders.

The definition of serious mental illness, adopted by the medical workforce commissioned as part of the National Mental Health Policy reform process in Australia, describes serious mental illness as a group of specific disorders which, although varying in cause, course and treatment, share the common characteristics of being long-lasting and/or producing significant levels of impairment:

> Severe mental illness is defined through diagnosis, disability and duration and includes disorders with psychotic symptoms such as schizophrenia ... as well as severe forms of other disorders such as depression, panic disorder and obsessive compulsive disorder. (Department of Human Services and Health 1994)

The National Mental Health Policy presents an abbreviated list of serious mental disorders, which forms the basis of the discussion in this chapter.

## SCHIZOPHRENIC DISORDERS

Schizophrenia represents a group of reactions whose chief characteristics appear to be an inability to form relationships, disturbances in the boundaries of self-image, and distortions in the affective and cognitive domains. These disorders are collectively referred to as 'psychotic' disorders. Schizophrenia is not, as commonly misconstrued, a split personality.

The term 'psychotic' has historically received a number of different definitions, none of which has achieved universal acceptance. In schizophrenia, schizophreniform disorder, schizoaffective disorder and brief psychotic disorder, the term 'psychotic' refers to delusions, any prominent hallucinations, disorganised speech, or disorganised or catatonic behaviour. Schizophrenia is 'arguably the worst disease affecting mankind' (*Nature* 1988). Due to its early onset and chronic nature, this mental disorder is probably the most prevalent of the psychotic disorders treated in hospital settings.

Schizophrenia is a disturbance that lasts for at least six months and includes at least one month of active-phase symptoms—that is, two (or more) of the following: delusions, hallucinations, disorganised speech, grossly disorganised or catatonic behaviour, negative symptoms (DSM-IV 1994). There are several subtypes of schizophrenia—paranoid, disorganised, catatonic, undifferentiated, and residual (the reader is advised to refer to psychiatric texts for a description of these).

The course of schizophrenia often begins with prodromal symptoms (markedly peculiar behaviour, abnormal affect, unusual speech, bizarre ideas and strange perceptual experiences); the onset of more pronounced symptoms may be acute (over just a few days) or gradual (a few months). Schizophrenia often begins during adolescence and there may be a demonstrable precipitating event, such as moving away to college, experience with a hallucinogenic drug, or the death of a relative. The prodromal symptoms may be present for a year before a diagnosis is made, making diagnosis and acceptance of treatment often a difficult process. The classic course of schizophrenia is one of exacerbations and remissions, and the individual's life is frequently characterised by aimlessness, inactivity, frequent hospitalisations, homelessness and poverty. During the acute illness phases (referred to as the 'florid' stages), patterns of thinking, feeling and acting become grossly disorganised and distorted. Frequently, these exaggerated and disturbed manifestations are not only frightening to the sufferers of schizophrenia, but also to those they come into contact with.

Although schizophrenia is discussed as if it were a single disease, it probably includes a variety of disorders that present with similar behavioural symptoms, and patients whose clinical presentations, treatment responses and course of illness are varied. Currently, no laboratory diagnostic test for identifying schizophrenia is available, so its diagnosis depends exclusively on the psychiatric history *and* mental status examination. Epidemiological studies of schizophrenia indicate an incidence of 1:1000 of the population, with approximately 2 million new cases worldwide each year (Kaplan & Sadock 1988). There is variability in the reported prevalence of schizophrenia because different studies have varied in study population and clinical definition. Estimates of prevalence have ranged from 0.2% to 2.0% across many large studies. Prevalence rates are similar throughout the world, but pockets of high prevalence have been reported in some specific areas. Overall, the lifetime prevalence of schizophrenia is usually estimated to be between 0.5% and 1% (DSM-IV 1994) (see Chap. 5).

## Aetiology of schizophrenia

Over the decades, diverse theoretical views have been proposed to explain the aetiology of schizophrenia. These theories mostly reflect the different approaches in treatment that have been developed, including biological (usually biochemical and/or neural structural alterations), genetic, psychological and familial. However, no single causative factor has been isolated in the condition. The most likely theory is that of multiple causation, taking into account such factors as the individual's vulnerability and sensitivity to stress, the type of premorbid personality, the specific modes of adaptation used by the individual in response to stress, the type of sociocultural and economic background that influenced development, the biophysiological and chemical makeup, and familial hereditary factors.

Biological alterations do seem to occur and the symptoms associated with schizophrenia, such as delusions or hallucinations, are found in people who are not suffering from a mental disorder only when they are in a state of metabolic imbalance or suffering from organic diseases. The symptoms are believed to result from overactivity of the dopaminergic system. Many of the neuroleptic agents used in the treatment of schizophrenic disorders block dopamine (DA) receptor activity, and this is thought to account for the consequent reduction in disorganised activity. Alternatively, psychological theories of schizophrenia encompass problems in information processing, attention and arousal, and family communication. (These only manifest as the disorder when a genetic vulnerability also exists.)

## Diagnostic criteria for schizophrenia

The schizophrenic disorders are characterised by a range of cognitive and emotional dysfunctions affecting perception, inferential thinking, language and communication, behavioural monitoring, affect, fluency and productivity of thought, speech, hedonic capacity, volition, drive and attention.

As no single symptom is solely associated with schizophrenia, the diagnosis involves the recognition of the constellation of signs and symptoms associated with impaired occupational or social functioning (DSM-IV 1994). Characteristic symptoms fall into two broad categories—'positive' and 'negative', reflecting the exaggeration or reduction of normal functioning. The **positive symptoms** include distortions or exaggerations of inferential thinking (delusions), perception (hallucinations), language and communication (disorganised speech) and behavioural monitoring (grossly disorganised or catatonic behaviour). **Negative symptoms** include restricted range and intensity of emotional expression (flattened affect), restricted clarity in thought and speech (alogia) and limitations in the initiation of goal-directed behaviour (avolition).

### Postive symptoms

*Delusions* are erroneous beliefs that usually involve a misinterpretation of perceptions or experiences. These may include a variety of themes (e.g. persecutory, referential, somatic, religious, or grandiose). More concisely, **delusions** are a disorder in the content of thought. Persecutory delusions are most common: sufferers believe they are being tormented, followed, tricked, spied on, or subjected to ridicule. Referential delusions are also common; patients believe that certain gestures, comments, passages from books or newspapers, song lyrics or other environmental cues are specifically directed at them (DSM-IV 1994).

*Perceptual changes*, which may occur in all senses (not just one or two), may include not only distortions in sensory reception and interpretation, but the presence of the phenomena known as illusions and hallucinations. **Hallucinations** are perceptions occurring in any sensory modality (auditory, visual, smell, taste and touch) in the absence of external stimuli. Auditory hallucinations are by far the most common and are usually experienced as voices, whether familiar or unfamiliar, that are perceived as distinct from the person's own thoughts. The content may be variable, although highly critical or threatening voices are especially common. Illusions are misinterpretations of sensory stimuli (such as misinterpreting sounds of the wind in trees as voices).

*Changes in communication* methods are frequent, and people with schizophrenia have difficulty responding appropriately to events and people they encounter. These difficulties arise because of their distorted perceptions, the interpretation of those perceptions and problems in communicating responses clearly. The degree of clarity of communication displayed by the sufferer may reflect the degree of thought disorganisation.

*Disturbances in thought processes* are characteristic of schizophrenia. Thinking is often muddled or unclear, with disjointed thoughts and looseness of associations—revealed by the content of speech in which the person may 'slip off track' from one topic to another. Responses may be simply inappropriate to the situation or conversation. There may be evidence of thought blocking, circumstantial communication, or tangentiality, in which answers to questions may be obliquely related or completely unrelated. Rarely, speech may be so severely disorganised that it is nearly incomprehensible and resembles receptive aphasia in its linguistic disorganisation ('incoherence' or 'word salad') (DSM-IV 1994).

## Negative symptoms

*Disruptions in emotional responses* are commonly presented by patients with schizophrenia, with either restricted or inappropriate expression of emotions. Behaviour may appear at best aimless and disruptive or, at worst, grossly disorganised. The range of disorganised behaviour includes childlike activity, unpredictable agitation, impoverished goal-directed behaviour so that activities of daily living are severely impeded, lack of care for personal attention and in hygiene the person appears dishevelled and may dress in an unusual manner—such as wearing many jumpers or coats on a hot day—or clearly inappropriate sexual behaviour and unpredictable agitation (such as shouting and swearing).

The symptoms within an individual change with time and may remit or worsen. There is *almost* always a characteristic deterioration from a previous (premorbid) level of functioning (family and friends often observe that the person is 'not the same'). A variety of factors are associated with good and poor prognosis. For instance, late onset, obvious precipitating factors, acute onset and variability in course tend towards a good prognosis, whereas factors opposite to these tend towards a poor prognosis. The range of recovery rates in the literature is 10–60% and a reasonable estimate is that 20–30% are able to lead somewhat normal lives. About 20–30% continue to experience moderate symptoms, while around 40–60% remain significantly impaired by the illness for their entire lives.

The emotional and behavioural responses to the apparently disordered world in which a person with florid schizophrenia exists can be both unpredictable and impulsive. The condition can thus be extremely frightening to the sufferers, and to their family and friends. Partly due to the nature of the condition and partly to others' reactions to their symptoms, people with schizophrenia experience withdrawal and isolation from their environment. This widening social distance from the activities and lives of others may sadly progress to a pathological state of loneliness. Nursing interventions for schizophrenic patients focus on changing patterns of activity, cognition, emotion, interpersonal processes and perception.

# MOOD DISORDERS

Most people have felt 'depressed', have expressed feelings of 'depression' or have been described by others as being 'depressed' at some time in their lives. The words 'depressed' and 'depression' are common expressions in everyday conversation. People who experience *depressive symptoms* (as opposed to a depressive disorder) usually continue to function without much disruption to most aspects of their lives. The symptoms are usually short-lived and often spontaneously remit without treatment. So, the normal grief that accompanies the loss of a loved one is a depressive symptom that is not considered a disorder. The DSM-IV (1994) classification of mood disorder refers to a mental disorder exhibiting prominent and persistent mood and affect changes that are pathological. The most serious mood disorders are **depression** and **mania**. In an earlier version of the DSM-IV, depression and mania were called affective disorders, whereas now they are grouped together as mood disorders. Mood refers to the *internal* emotional state of an individual (i.e. a subjective experience described by the individual, such as 'I am happy', 'I am angry', 'I am sad'). Affect refers to the *external* expression of emotional content (i.e. objective, outward appearance and observable behaviours, such as facial expression or posture indicating feelings of sadness or anger).

## Aetiology of mood disorders

Theories of mood disorders encompass biological (including genetic), psychosocial (environmental) and psychological hypotheses. Considerable research has been conducted over the past twenty years to determine the physiological correlates of bipolar disorder. Two of the neurotransmitters—the biogenic amines norepinephrine (NE) and serotonin (5HT)—are most commonly implicated in mood disorders, with reported fluctuations in both mania and depression. Low levels of 5HT may predispose people to mood disorders, and the actual increase or decrease of NE is deemed responsible for the direction of the mood alteration.

In the mood disorders, these biologic amine abnormalities probably have resultant effects on a number of other neuroendocrine functions (including cortisol—hypersecreted; thyroid stimulating hormone (TSH)—decreased; luteinising hormone (LH)—decreased; follicle stimulating hormone (FSH)—decreased; and decreased testosterone in males). Variations in brain calcium levels and electrical activity are also thought to contribute to mood disorders. Genetic factors have been implicated in the development of mood disorders with strong evidence that mood disorders can be inherited. About 50% of bipolar patients have at least one parent with a mood disorder, most often major depression. If one parent has bipolar disorder, there is about a 27% chance that the offspring will have a mood disorder; if both parents have bipolar disorder, the chance of mood disorder in the offspring rises to 50–75% (Kaplan & Sadock 1988). As in the twin studies of schizophrenia, the closer the genetic linkage to parents, the greater the likelihood of developing mood disorder.

Psychological theories of mood disorders focus on a personal history of deprivation, trauma or significant loss, financial problems, perceived or real failure, and life transition crises.

## Diagnostic criteria for mood disorders

The mood disorders are a group of psychiatric diagnoses characterised by disturbances in emotional and behavioural response patterns. These patterns range from extreme elation and agitation to extreme depression and a serious potential for suicide. Mood may be normal, elevated or depressed; a normal individual experiences a wide range of moods and has an equally large repertoire of affective expression, mostly feeling in control of both. The mood changes occurring in the mood disorders appear to be disproportionate to any cause and may continue over an extended period. Therefore, mood disorders are characterised by a disturbance of mood, a loss of that sense of control and a subjective experience of great distress.

Mood disorders are divided into two diagnostic categories—bipolar disorders and depressive disorders. **Bipolar disorders** are characterised by one or more periods of manic or hypomanic episodes (usually with a history of major depressive episodes). Someone who has only manic episodes is still classified as bipolar. The **depressive disorders** are characterised by one or more periods of depression, without a history of either manic or hypomanic episodes. Depression and mania, however, encompass a great variety of mood and symptom changes that vary in duration, frequency and intensity. The DSM-IV clarifies the definition of mood disorder by indicating that there are two bipolar disorders:

- bipolar disorder, in which there is one or more manic episodes (usually with one or more major depressive episodes); and

- cyclothymic disorders, in which there are numerous hypomanic episodes and numerous periods with depressive symptoms

Similarly, there are two depressive disorders:

- major depression, in which there is one or more major depressive episodes; and
- dysthymia, in which there is a history of a depressed mood on most days for at least two years and in which, during the first two years of the disturbance, the condition did not meet the criteria for a major depressive episode.

People with elevated mood show expansiveness, flight of ideas, decreased sleep, heightened self-esteem and grandiose ideas, and are referred to as manic. With the bipolar disorders, the episode that usually leads to first-time hospitalisation is a manic episode. Both manic and depressed episodes can occur, and often one type of episode under the bipolar category will be followed immediately by a short episode of the other kind. Thus, the person who experiences a manic disorder may appear to recover, only to develop symptoms of depression.

The depressive disorders are characterised by exaggerated and unwarranted feelings of sadness, melancholy, dejection, worthlessness, emptiness and hopelessness. People with depressed mood show loss of energy and interest, guilt feelings, difficulty in concentrating, loss of appetite, and thoughts of death or suicide. The fatigue reported in depression is chronic, with about 80% of depressed patients reporting fatigue, lethargy, an inability to motivate themselves, and an inability to perform usually expected activities. With regard to the suicidal preoccupation in depressed clients, about 66% contemplate suicide and 10–15% complete suicide (Kaplan & Sadock 1988). Other signs and symptoms of depression involve changes in activity level, cognitive abilities, speech and vegetative functions (e.g sleep, appetite, sexual activity and other biological rhythms).

The impact both of the present episode and of recurring mood fluctuations on the affected individual's life must be considered when conducting an assessment. When the impact of a depressed mood is great, the depressed person cannot function well because of disruptions to cognitive functioning; interpersonal relationships are likely to suffer due to difficulties with social interaction. With a manic individual, the dysfunction may be seen in failure to perform expected tasks, in risk taking or, due to the 'seductiveness' of the manic mood, in difficulties in setting personal limits. Certainly, recurring mood swings have a residual impact on the client's life, because feelings of embarrassment or guilt can prevail.

## Suicide

In both depressive and bipolar disorders, safety interventions are of primary importance. As mentioned earlier, suicide is one potential way for self-harm, and impoverished judgment produced by the condition itself may hasten a decision in this direction. Similarly, diminished concentration can lead to accidents. When clients with mood disorders demonstrate significant alterations in conduct, impulse control, motor behaviour, or self-care activities, they may need to be hospitalised for their own safety. Medication may be used to alter behaviour if it is severely manic or depressed. Clients who are actively suicidal must be protected in an environment that is free of all means of harm, and they may require constant observation. (See Chapters 13 and 16 for discussion of the assessment and nursing management of suicidal clients, and Chapters 5, 13 and 14 for a discussion of the gender and age risks associated with suicide.)

## Electroconvulsive therapy

Electroconvulsive therapy (ECT) is another effective somatic treatment used in the treatment of depression and, sometimes, in the treatment of other mental disorders. Compared with the use of TCAs, treatment for major depression by ECT is associated with shorter hospital stays and lower mortality rates after three years (Guttmacher 1988). Follow-up at six months has revealed fewer suicides and suicide attempts among patients treated with ECT than among those treated with antidepressants. Biologic signs and mood-congruent psychotic features are associated with better responses to ECT than to antidepressants or neuroleptics alone (Guttmacher 1988). That is, clients who experience significant weight loss, somatic symptoms and recurrent thoughts of death, including suicidal ideation, are likely to respond well to treatment with ECT. Clients treated with ECT require attentive nursing care. Readers are referred to any standard text on psychiatric nursing for further details.

## ANXIETY DISORDERS

**Anxiety** is a state everyone has experienced. Certain objects, people and situations provoke anxious feelings in us all. These feelings can, at different times, be minor irritations, cause better or worse performance, and prevent us from doing the things we want to do.

At low to moderate levels of anxiety, we experience a narrowing of perception—an optimal level for learning. We generally experience some increased muscle tension ('jitters'), our rate of speech increases, and we are likely to have feelings of challenge and a mixed sense of optimism, confidence and fear. Physiologically, anxiety activates the sympathetic nervous system, which increases blood pressure, heart rate and respiration and causes pupillary dilation and peripheral vascular constriction.

As anxiety levels increase to severe and extremely severe, the 'fight or flight' response signals a general sympathetic nervous system discharge, a stimulation of the adrenal medulla, an increase in circulating catecholamines, an increased heart rate and palpitations, increased muscle tension and rigidity, and hyperventilation (see Chapter 2). Our perceptual capacity becomes further restricted, problem solving becomes inefficient, and physical reactions become increasingly more agitated, random and disorganised, with pacing, wringing of hands, fidgeting and trembling. Speech is likely to contain stammering and become rapid and high-pitched, and eye contact is markedly impoverished. In some people, cardiovascular symptoms such as palpitation and sweating may occur, as well as gastrointestinal symptoms such as nausea, an empty feeling or butterflies in the pit of the stomach, and diarrhoea. In addition, some people experience urinary frequency, and some have respiratory symptoms such as shallow breathing and tightness in the chest. These are all visceral reactions.

In some people, muscle tension prevails and they experience muscle tightness, spasm, headache, neck tension and hypertension. Lightheadedness, dizziness, tingling in the extremities, restlessness and a desire to move around are also common. At panic levels of anxiety, the continued physical arousal is manifested in the inability to execute simple motor tasks, and in fumbling, gross motor agitation, withdrawal, mouth agape, rocking and accompanied feelings of impotence, helplessness, agony and desperation.

Anxiety is an alerting signal—it warns of impending danger and enables the person to take action to deal with the threat. We all attempt to cope with anxious feelings, and most of us are relatively adept at doing so. However, for about 8% of the population, the anxiety they experience makes them dysfunctional and seriously impedes daily life. Dysfunctional aspects of anxiety are marked by three major components: behavioural avoidance, catastrophic cognition and autonomic hyperarousal. This last condition produces neuroendocrine and physiological effects. None of these components, however, differentiates between 'normal' and 'pathological' anxiety—the only effective distinguishing criterion is interference in personal, occupational or social functioning.

## Aetiology of anxiety disorders

The biological view of anxiety disorders implies some sensitivity of the autonomic nervous system to arousal, thereby producing the cardiovascular, muscular, gastrointestinal and respiratory symptoms. Anxiety disorders are associated with changes in cerebral serotonin (5HT), and many of the anxiolytic agents specifically affect 5HT activity. Norepinephrine (NE) and gamma-aminobutyric acid (GABA) have also been implicated in the aetiology of anxiety disorders. There is also the theory that postulates a genetic basis to anxiety disorders by familial expression.

A major psychological theory of the aetiology of anxiety, which derives from behaviourism and learning, is that anxiety is a conditioned response to specific environmental stimuli. According to learning theory, anxiety is widespread because it has a biological survival value. All living things demonstrate specific responses to particular dangerous stimuli, and there is conclusive evidence that these responses are innate. In all animals, the fear response is remarkably consistent. In humans, the standard response is the 'fight or flight' mechanism and the autonomic consequences are the well-known tachycardia, increased blood pressure, sweating, and raised muscle tone and respiration rate. These are, of course, the effects that prepare us best for fighting or fleeing. It is the fight or flight response that causes us to tremble and feel faint when an anticipated threat fails to materialise. These responses probably have biological survival value in that they trigger behaviours which 'prepare' us for danger. Behaviourists claim that the anxiety response becomes learned and conditioned in the presence of high levels of anxiety, and the avoidance behaviour that results (termed 'escape training') serves as a powerful reinforcement for continuation of the behaviour.

A cognitive perspective broadens this view: behavioural, cognitive and autonomic systems are generally congruent with each other, in the sense that it is the negative cognitions about a particular situation that are accompanied by autonomic arousal and the behavioural response of avoidance. In some situations, this 'synchrony' breaks down—for example, the anxiolytic drugs have an effect on the physiological indices and the appraisal of threat, but not on the behavioural measure of approach and avoidance. The process of change during psychological treatment of phobic anxiety seems to involve an initial behavioural change that is followed by autonomic change (such as reduction in heart rate) and, finally, by attitudinal and other cognitive changes.

DSM-IV defines various types of anxiety disorders: panic disorders (with or without agoraphobia); phobic disorders (simple phobia and social phobia); obsessive-compulsive disorder; post-traumatic stress disorder; and generalised anxiety disorder. For brevity, only panic disorder, the phobic disorders and obsessive-compulsive disorder will be discussed. The reader is advised to refer to appropriate psychiatric texts for information on the other conditions.

## Panic disorder

Panic disorder is marked by spontaneous, episodic and intense periods of anxiety, usually lasting less than one hour. These panic attacks are discrete periods in which there is a sudden onset of intense apprehension, fearfulness or terror, with associated feelings of impending doom. During these attacks, symptoms such as shortness of breath, palpitations, chest pain or discomfort, choking or smothering sensations, and fear of 'going crazy' or 'losing control' are present. Attacks commonly occur several times each week, and sufferers may spend much of their waking time worrying about their recurrence. The first panic attack is usually spontaneous, although they can follow excitement, caffeine intoxication, physical exertion, sexual activity or moderate emotional trauma. Onset begins abruptly with about a 10-minute period of rapidly worsening symptoms. The psychological symptoms, in addition to extreme fear and a sense of impending doom, include a sense of being unreal or in a dream (derealisation and depersonalisation). The physical symptoms may include tachycardia, palpitations, dyspnoea, sweating and hyper-ventilation—this last symptom may produce respiratory alkalosis and further symptoms. During the panic, the immensely distressing nature of it usually motivates the person to flee the situation in order to seek help.

Panic attacks vary in length, but generally last only a few minutes (5–20 minutes). Typically, the person prone to panic attacks lives in fear of them and, between attacks, spends a great deal of time worrying about further attacks.

# Phobic disorders

Phobic disorders comprise an irrational fear resulting in conscious avoidance of a specific feared object, activity or situation. This reaction of an intense, recurrent, unreasonable fear attached to an object, event, activity or situation can be precipitated by exposure to that object. Unless there is intervention, phobic disorders are likely to become chronic. Examples of phobias are simple phobia, social phobia and agoraphobia.

## Simple phobia

Simple phobia is defined as the persistent, irrational fear and avoidance of a specific object or situation. The condition is relatively common, affecting about 15% of the general population. Simple phobias are so common that most people simply put up with them and never seek treatment. The irrational and overly intense fear of objects such as snakes, spiders, rodents and dogs is unlikely to interfere significantly with daily activities unless very intense. However, some simple phobias are more problematic—heights, enclosed spaces, crowds and fear of flying all involve a large amount of avoidance and can easily impair an individual's functioning in daily life.

Another common simple phobia which has an important clinical presentation is the fear of blood or injury. The physiological responses to this specific fear seem to distinguish it from other phobias. For example, someone with a phobia of injections will respond initially just like other phobics—with increased heart rate and blood pressure—but this is frequently followed by fainting. While other phobics fear fainting in anxiety-provoking situations, they rarely do so. An estimate of the prevalence of such fears, and the vagal response to them, is provided by the recorded incidence of fainting in blood donor clinics being as high as 17%. This, of course, excludes those who are so afraid of blood or injury that they avoid giving blood.

## Social phobia

Social phobia is characterised by an irrational fear of humiliation or embarrassment in public places, such as when eating or drinking in restaurants, urinating in public lavatories or public speaking. Episodes of social phobia are characterised by intense, prolonged, irrational and disabling fear, and behavioural avoidance of situations in which the individual might be scrutinised by others when expected to perform a particular social role or activity. Social phobia is less common than simple phobia (affecting about 3–5% of the population). The fear is often complicated by deficiencies in social skill performance, either because avoidance of contact with others has led to a lack of opportunity to acquire or rehearse these skills, or because the individual's anxiety is sufficiently high to have a detrimental effect on performance.

To some extent, everyone is socially anxious, in the sense that certain situations frighten the majority of us. Addressing a large group of prestigious strangers or being the centre of attention at formal social gatherings (such as weddings) are common experiences that evoke anxious feelings. For the socially phobic person, however, many everyday situations generate this degree of anxiety. Sometimes the fears are specific, such as writing, eating or drinking in front of others, because of a fear of possible tremor. More often, the fears tend to be diffuse and cause marked impairment in social functioning.

Onset seems to favour adolescents and is equally common in both sexes, although males more often tend to seek help (perhaps due to social role expectations). Social phobia is usually chronic, with a tendency for the cycle of anxiety to escalate to a level that produces avoidance and feelings of failure, thus creating greater impairment over time. Some people with social phobia complicate the problem by the use of self-medication, particularly alcohol, to combat their anxiety.

## Agoraphobia

**Agoraphobia** can occur with or without panic attacks, although the latter is not common. Most people with agoraphobia do experience panic attacks, which suggests that there is a close relationship between panic attacks and the development of agoraphobia. The main characteristic of agoraphobia is fear and avoidance of busy public places, particularly situations it would be difficult to get out of, or where help is unavailable 'should something go wrong'. Avoidance is pervasive and a variety of situations can be involved: being alone outside the home: being at home alone; being in a crowd of people; travelling in a car, bus or plane; being on a bridge or in a lift. Some people are able to expose themselves to the feared situations, but endure them with considerable dread. Other characteristics of those with agoraphobia include episodes of depersonalisation (body is unreal, floating or dead) or derealisation (perception that the environment is unreal), concern that some physical or social catastrophe will occur, mild depression, an emphasis on the physical manifestations of anxiety (giddiness, dyspnoea and cardiac phenomena) and the use of anxiolytics, sometimes to the point of physical dependence.

Epidemiological studies throughout the world consistently indicate the lifetime prevalence of panic disorder (with or without agoraphobia) to be between 1.5% and 3.5%. One-year prevalence rates are between 1% and 2%. Approximately one-third to one-half of individuals diagnosed with panic disorder in community samples also have agoraphobia, although a much higher rate of agoraphobia is encountered in clinical samples (DSM-IV 1994).

The onset of agoraphobia is typically in the early 20s, and women are marginally more likely than men to be affected. The course of agoraphobia is unpredictable—sometimes the handicap is minimal, at other times it is particularly severe. Frequently, the onset of agoraphobia is associated with the loss of a significant person, change in social circumstances or change in lifestyle. The phobic nature of the response is real to the individual, and avoidance patterns seem necessary to the person for survival. Agoraphobia is such a remarkably incapacitating disorder that it is not uncommon for sufferers to find themselves housebound (or town-bound) for many years, resulting in social and interpersonal impairment.

## Obsessive-compulsive disorders

Obsessive-compulsive disorders are probably the most notorious of the anxiety disorders and can be extremely debilitating. There are two essential features: obsessions and compulsions.

*Obsessions* are recurrent and intrusive mental events—thoughts, feelings, images, ideas or sensations—which feel alien to the person experiencing them, but cannot be attributed to any external source. These ideas or impulses have the capacity to intrude into conscious awareness and are experienced as unpleasant. The intrusive idea or impulse is recognised as irrational; the person feels a strong urge to resist, but usually does not. This is accompanied by feelings of anxious dread, which often lead the person to take some action to counter the ideas or impulses. The individual usually tries unsuccessfully to stop the obsessions. Examples of obsessions are preoccupation with cleanliness or safety, or morbid fear of contamination by 'germs'.

*Compulsions*, which are the second feature of the disorder, are conscious, standardised, recurrent behaviours, such as counting, checking or avoiding, that the individual feels compelled to undertake despite feeling that it is senseless. Such activities are stereotypes and, despite resistance to performing them, create high anxiety if unperformed. Excessive handwashing is an example.

For any of the anxiety disorders, it is important to remember that the person is experiencing real discomfort and distress, and that the overwhelming anxiety and associated fears are as significant as any physical pain or condition. The symptoms are consciously unwanted and viewed as undesirable—they produce irritation and distress, are felt to be strange and produce discontent with daily life. The clinical picture is not always clear-cut and more than one subtype can exist concurrently.

## CONCLUSION

For a significant portion of the general population, mental disorders can result in chronic disability and incapacitation. Current estimates indicate that the incidence of mental disorders is approximately one person in every four. The serious mental illnesses are problematic for a number of reasons: the nature of the condition; the impact the symptoms have on personal, social and occupational functioning; treatment availability and accessability; and attitudinal factors. The disorders presented in this chapter (schizophrenia, mood disorders and anxiety disorders) share the common characteristics of being long-lasting and/or of producing significant levels of impairment.

## SUMMARY

- It is important for mental health nurses to understand the impact of serious mental disorders on those who suffer from them, in order to make an appropriate contribution to the services necessary for these people.

- Schizophrenia represents a group of reactions whose chief characteristics are the inability to form relationships, disturbances in the boundaries of self-image, and distortions in the affective and cognitive domains. In schizophrenia, schizophreniform disorder, schizoaffective disorder and brief psychotic disorder, the term 'psychotic' refers to delusions, any prominent hallucinations, disorganised speech, and disorganised or catatonic behaviour.

- The most common mood disorders are depression and mania. There are two diagnostic groups—bipolar disorders and depressive disorders. Bipolar disorders are characterised by one or more episodes of mania or hypomania (usually with a history of major depressive episodes). Someone who has only manic episodes is still classified as bipolar. The depressive disorders are characterised by one or more periods of depression without a history of either manic or hypomanic episodes. However, depression and mania encompass a great variety of mood and symptom changes that vary in duration, frequency and intensity. Suicide is a risk in both depressive and bipolar disorders so safety interventions are of primary importance.

- Anxiety disorders are disabling. Their dysfunctional aspects are marked by three major components: behavioural avoidance; catastrophic cognition; and autonomic hyperarousal. None of these components differentiates between 'normal' and 'pathological' anxiety; the only effective criterion for making this distinction is interference in personal, occupational or social functioning.

- Panic disorder presents as spontaneous episodes of intense anxiety, usually lasting for less than an hour. These attacks are characterised by intense apprehension, terror and feelings of impending doom.

- Phobic disorders comprise irrational fears associated with continuous avoidance of the feared object, activity or situation.

- Obsessive-compulsive disorders are the most notorious of the anxiety disorders and can be extremely debilitating. They involve obsessions—recurrent and intrusive mental events which feel alien to the person experiencing them, but cannot be attributed to an external cause. Compulsions are the second feature of the disorder, characterised by conscious, standardised, recurrent behaviours (counting, checking, avoiding) that the person is compelled to undertake, despite feeling that the behaviour is senseless.

- For any of the anxiety disorders, it is important to remember that sufferers are experiencing profound discomfort and distress, and that their overwhelming anxiety and associated fears are as least as significant as any physical pain or condition.

# DISCUSSION QUESTIONS

1. Discuss the arguments for and against allocation of resources to provide services for people with mental disorders, based on the prevalence rates of the disorders.
2. 'The greatest impact of mental disorder relates to attitudes towards, and discrimination against, those diagnosed with a serious mental disorder.' Discuss this statement.
3. What constitutes a 'serious mental illness'?
4. Schizophrenia is characterised by periods of exacerbation and remission of symptoms. What symptoms would you expect to predominate during these phases?
5. Outline the clinical features displayed by a person with either major depression or bipolar disorder.
6. Anxiety disorders are categorised into a number of subtypes, including panic disorder, phobic disorders, and obsessive-compulsive disorder. What are the broad clinical features of each of these conditions?
7. Is mental illness hereditary? Justify your answer with reference to relevant research.

# EXERCISES

1. Consider two clients with the same diagnosis of a serious mental disorder. Identify the clinical features they share and those in which they differ. How do you account for these similarities and differences?
2. What advice would you give to an undergraduate student of nursing who cannot understand why people with obsessive-compulsive disorder cannot simply stop their senseless behaviour?
3. Refer to the NANDA taxonomy and identify the nursing diagnoses that may be associated with any three of the serious mental disorders described in this chapter.
4. Write a case study of a person with schizophrenia, identifying the clinical features of the illness that persist even when florid symptoms subside.
5. List the precautions that can be taken (a) in a client's home, and (b) in a psychiatric unit to reduce the risk of suicide in a person with either major depression or bipolar disorder.

6. Draw up a table showing the predisposing factors, age of onset, clinical features, and prognoses of the serious mental disorders discussed in this chapter.

# FURTHER READING

Consult any major psychiatry or mental health nursing text, such as the two listed below, for full information on the aetiology of mental disorders.

- Kaplan, H.I. & Sadock, B.J. (1988) *Synopsis of Psychiatry: Behavioural Sciences, Clinical Psychiatry* (5th edition), Baltimore: Williams & Wilkins.
- Varcarolis, E.M. (1994) *Foundations of Psychiatric-Mental Health Nursing* (2nd edition), Philadelphia: W.B. Saunders.

# REFERENCES

Department of Human Services and Health (1994) *First Mental Health Report 1993*, Canberra: AGPS.

*Diagnostic and Statistical Manual of Mental Disorders*, 4th edition (1994), Washington DC: American Psychiatric Press.

Ellard, J. (1994) 'Private psychiatry in a changing medical system', *Australasian Psychiatry* 2(1), pp.6–10.

Falloon, I.H.R. & Fadden, G. (1993) *Integrated Mental Health Care: A Comprehensive Community-based Approach*, Cambridge: Cambridge University Press.

Goldberg, D.P. & Bridges, K. (1987) 'Screening for psychiatric illness in general practice', *Journal of the Royal College of General Practitioners* 37, pp.15–19.

Goldberg, D.P. & Huxley, P. (1980) *Mental Illness in the Community*, London: Tavistock Press.

Guttmacher, L.B. (1988) *Concise Quide to Somatic Therapies in Psychiatry*, Washington: American Psychiatric Press.

Human Rights and Equal Opportunities Commission (1993) *Human Rights and Mental Illness* Vols 1 & 2. Canberra: Australian Government Publishing Service.

Kaplan, H.I. & Sadock, B.J. (1988) *Synopsis of Psychiatry: Behavioural Sciences, Clinical Psychiatry* (5th edition), Baltimore: Williams & Wilkins.

*Nature* (1988) editorial. 95 p.336.

# Listening

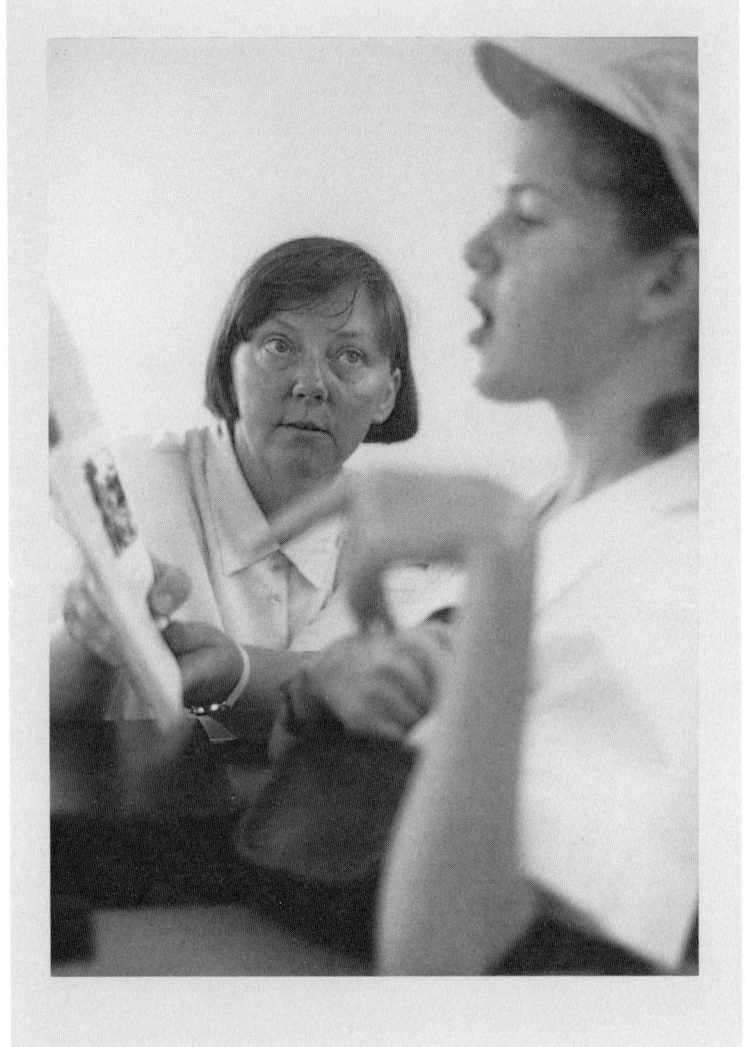

Remember that the listener creates the space for the other to speak.

## CHAPTER 11

# *T*REATMENT AND NURSING INTERVENTIONS

Derek Weir and Tian Oei

# *C*ONTENTS

## LEARNING OBJECTIVES

This chapter will assist the reader to:

- understand the basis of interventions that promote and restore mental health;
- identify measures to minimise maladaptive stress responses;
- consider options for the restoration of mental health;
- appreciate the rationale for intervention options in mental disorder.

## INTRODUCTION

People are not merely passive recipients of environmental events. They can (and do) make conscious choices to respond to the demands of the world. Many life events tend to be unpredictable and may have an impact for which people are unprepared. Despite the widely held lay view that **stress** is always a negative experience, some degree of stress is actually productive—it serves to keep people alert, safe and focused on the task at hand (see Chapter 2). When stress is experienced, it is better to accept that it is a 'manageable' rather than a 'controllable' phenomenon. To expect to be able to 'control' stress is not helpful. Stress is an inevitable by-product of daily life and we need to develop the capacity to occasionally tolerate quite high levels. Therefore, while the appropriate application of stress reduction strategies can reduce the unpleasant effects of stress to a level that is manageable, it would be fruitless to attempt to remove *all* experience of stress.

## MANAGEMENT OF STRESS

A key point for managing **stressors** is to be able to identify and use appropriate strategies, and also to recognise that sometimes the strategy selected may not work as efficiently as hoped and/or may not take effect immediately. At such times, flexibility in approach is needed. This raises an important point about stress management: personal expectations. It is quite common for people to set fairly unrealistic standards for themselves—and, for that matter, for others—standards which represent perfection (e.g. striving to attain 100%, or even 110%, all the time). When an individual is unwilling to compromise idealistic standards, disappointment and even maladaptation may result. In this case, the person will feel a failure, or attribute blame for the failure elsewhere. It is more productive to take a step back, to look a little more realistically at self-imposed standards and expectations, and to consider appropriate stress management options.

It is common for people to want immediate relief from their distressing symptoms. Sometimes, more or less immediate symptomatic relief is possible—for example, by the use of prescribed and non-prescribed drugs. However, it is useful to recognise that these remedies offer only temporary symptomatic relief, and the situations that generated the distress are unlikely to be affected by such action. This is an important point to consider in developing successful stress management strategies.

Management of stress is intended to enhance the capacity of individuals to cope with stressors. It involves the ability to assess current and potential stressors realistically, to gauge their likely effects, and to plan and execute effective strategies to deal with high stress levels before they threaten mental health status. Some interventions can be used successfully at the time the distress occurs, and many others can be rehearsed in advance of exposure to stressors.

Common stress management strategies can be classified into four categories: biological, psychological, environmental and psychosocial strategies. Some stress management techniques can be applied in two or more categories. Some of the strategies commonly associated with each of these categories, together with the relevant underlying mechanisms, are summarised in Boxes 11.1 to 11. 4.

## $B$ OX 11.1: *Common biological stress management strategies*

*Pharmacological means.* Caffeine, alcohol, prescribed and non-prescribed drugs, especially the antianxiety drugs (more properly called the **anxiolytics**). These are palliative rather than curative. All serve to decrease awareness of the environment and, thus, have no direct effects on stressors. These drugs have effects on the 'stress-related' hormones such as:

- adrenocorticotrophic hormone (ACTH)
- adrenaline, also known as epinephrine (E)
- norepinephrine (NE)
- dopamine (DA)
- 5 hydroxytryptamine (5HT)
- gamma-aminobutyric acid (GABA)
- prolactin (PRL)
- growth hormone (GH)

*Exercise.* Physical fitness is probably the most popular way to deal with stress. Even unintentional exercise such as slamming a door, throwing items or 'going for a walk around the block to cool off' serve to reduce tension. It is believed that regular exercise dissipates the build-up of stress-related hormones. The sense of well-being—the 'high'—that accompanies exercise is believed to be induced by release of brain peptides such as endorphins.

*continued ...*

*Muscle relaxation techniques.*    These typically use a modification of the original technique of Jacobsen (1938) and incorporate relaxing thoughts/images as well as tranquil breathing patterns in conjunction with systematic tension and relaxation of muscle groups. Some relaxation techniques incorporate autogenic training (an emphasis on sensations such as limb warmth or heaviness) to achieve this effect, or visual imagery in conjunction with physical relaxation. The goal of relaxation techniques is to provide deep muscular relaxation, based on the physiological responses of muscle cells, and to utilise the simple fact that muscle relaxation is the exact opposite of muscle tension.

*Meditative techniques.*    These may attempt to produce a 'relaxation response'. The techniques may use a repetitive deep breathing pattern and an associated focus on a word or a phrase with each expiration. This technique probably suppresses arousal responses and provides opposition to the 'fight or flight' response. Deep breathing, however, may alter blood gases in profound ways and these alterations may themselves produce unpleasant physical sensations (decreasing carbon dioxide ($CO_2$) can trigger a hyperventilation syndrome). Thus, such techniques are not always well tolerated.

*Biofeedback training.*    This enables individuals to learn to control a number of physiological activities previously thought to be involuntary. The most common training uses frontalis muscle tension (in the forehead), fingertip temperature or electrodermal response. The principle of biofeedback training is that, by receiving information on a continuing basis, the recipient can become aware of previously unknown bodily processes and can recognise stimuli or feelings that produce consistent changes in the required direction. Biofeedback training requires specialised equipment and, usually, individualised instruction.

B O X   *1 1 . 2 :  Common psychological stress management strategies*

**Behavioural strategies**
*Behavioural techniques* are based on the concepts of learning, conditioning and reinforcement. Outcomes, which depend on the selected behaviour, will reinforce the frequency (and likelihood) of that behaviour recurring. Some people engage in behavioural techniques that are not necessarily healthy: social isolation, 'throwing oneself into work', the use of non-prescribed drugs, smoking or overeating are sometimes used as stress reducers. These have obvious detrimental effects. Other techniques, such as jogging or breathing exercises, produce positive physiological effects that decrease the stress response.

*continued ...*

Improved behavioural skills such as improved communication, assertiveness training, hyperventilation control, exercise, time management and career development are useful psychological interventions for stress management. One of these techniques—hyperventilation control—has a biological basis but it also has the important psychological consequence of distraction. At times of high anxiety, breathing rates can change dramatically. This technique uses slowed inspiration and expiration cycles, typically of 5 seconds duration. Thus, one complete respiratory cycle will last 10 seconds, compared to a normal resting rate of about 5 seconds.

**Cognitive strategies**
*Cognitive techniques* aim at improving cognitive (or thinking) skills, and can provide stress reduction benefits. These techniques are based on the assumption that stress responses often result from an individual's past experiences in appraising threatening situations. These perceptions do not necessarily reflect the environment accurately. A person may externalise or internalise 'blame' for the events; engage in anxiety-producing thoughts (exaggerating, catastrophising, negativism) or develop unrealistic beliefs. Some examples of these techniques are:

- distraction
- thought stopping
- attention switching (from an internal to an external focus)
- exchanging negative catastrophic thoughts for neutral/positive ones; and
- covert rehearsal, in which the person learns to plan ahead. In each case, practise familiarises the routine for the person, and successful stress reduction provides the positive reinforcement needed to ensure that the desired changes are continued.

## BOX 11.3: *Environmental strategies*

Some physical structures of the environment, as well as the values attached to it, can be modified or manipulated, and thus decrease the advent of stressful stimuli. Making aspects of the environment more attractive usually makes people feel better about it and more inclined to tolerate day-to-day stressors.

Control or management of environmental stressors may require making some change, in which the focus may be shifted from individual to group responses. This change of emphasis capitalises on the buffering or supportive nature of group activities.

$B$*OX 11.4: Psychosocial strategies in stress management*

Psychosocial strategies incorporate personal management techniques that may improve the psychosocial settings in which people operate, and are thus of value in stress management. They include:

- social support;
- providing information about management of day-to-day problems;
- help with mental health awareness;
- flexibility in work hours, thus accommodating individual requirements for child care and other care services.

These approaches may focus on broader stressors, including those which may be generated outside one's environment (e.g. the workplace), but which transfer into it. The focus of these broader approaches can range from general counselling services to specific individualised programs (e.g. weight reduction, anti-smoking programs, and others aimed at reducing alcohol or other substance use and abuse).

The options shown in Box 11.1 are primarily biological in effect, and probably have the greatest utility when they assist an individual to manage unavoidable environmental demands. Psychological methods (see Box 11.2) are designed to improve *adaptive moderation* (whether behavioural or cognitive) of exaggerated or inappropriate psychological responses to stress. The environmental approach, shown in Box 11.3, deals with facets of the immediate environment that can be changed or modified to reduce high levels of stress. The thrust of the psychosocial approaches (see Box 11.4) is to provide a more supportive sociocultural group in which to function.

## *M*ANAGEMENT OF MENTAL DISORDERS

From time to time some people suffer from major problems that affect their mental health. However, in order to justify a clinical diagnosis of **mental disorder**, clearly defined criteria must be met. These criteria include a minimum time period for which the symptoms must be experienced (see Chapter 10). Fortunately, only a relatively small number of people meet these clinical criteria. Even the mental disorders that are most obviously connected to stress and coping (the anxiety disorders, particularly post-traumatic stress disorder) have explicit criteria that must be fulfilled for a specified time period.

Some of the conditions recognised as mental disorders have well established aetiologies or pathophysiology. For most, however, the causes remain unclear or unknown. There are many theories that attempt to explain how these disorders arise and substantial evidence is offered in support of them (see Chapter 10). Some evidence indicates biological aetiologies, some psychological, and some an interaction between biological, psychological and social factors (Free & Oei 1989). The recognition that psychological and social influences affect physical processes, and that all three dimensions interact, has been an important influence in treatment options. Interventions consist of a broad range of techniques that increase social abilities, self-sufficiency, practical skills and interpersonal communication, as well as pharmacotherapy, which is intended to reduce the disabling and distressing symptoms of the disorder.

The targets for intervention, as well as the intervention options, have to some extent been refocused. Since it is acknowledged that most mental disorders first manifest in the young adult population (18–24 years), the logical and imperative targets for these strategies must be young people (<18) (e.g. Oei & Baldwin 1992) (see also Chapter 5). In addition, there has been an increased awareness that people with mental disorders reside mostly in the community, not in hospital (Human Rights and Equal Opportunities Commission 1993).

In this chapter, major contemporary frameworks for intervening in mental disorders, together with some representative examples, are presented. The intention is to enable readers to make their own judgments and to identify which framework prevails in the health care settings they know best. Either explicitly or implicitly, clinicians (including nurses) choose one framework or a combination of frameworks to guide their interventions.

## Medical-biological interventions

The medical-biological model in psychiatry originated from the systematic observation, naming and classification of symptoms. According to this model, behavioural disruptions, including abnormal behaviour, are attributable to organic factors such as a disease process, probably originating in the central nervous system. Examples of organic factors are lesions, neuropathologic conditions, toxins introduced from outside the body, and biochemical abnormalities of neurotransmitters and enzymes. This indicates that, like any other disease, there is a process operating; the condition is likely to follow a predictable course and the prognosis can be estimated. If the causes can be identified and treated, the symptomatology will subside. Treatment depends on diagnosis and frequently includes somatic therapies in addition to interpersonal therapies. How much treatment is appropriate will depend on how the client's symptoms respond to intervention. There is a wide body of evidence for a biological basis for many mental disorders and this forms the core component of commonly prescribed somatic interventions.

Recent research provides an impressive body of scientific evidence suggesting that dysfunction in certain neurological pathways and/or disruptions to various neuroendocrine processes are associated with behavioural changes. In most cases, it is now recognised that there is no simple linear relationship between any one system (neurochemical, endocrine, immune) and behavioural change, but rather that complex relationships exist between a number of biochemical factors and how they are ultimately expressed.

Because the drugs used in the treatment of mental disorders have effects primarily at the neurochemical and molecular level, they will ultimately modify behaviour. The prescription of medication does not necessarily render the client symptomless. While there is a reduction in the obvious expression of clinical symptoms, aetiological factors may be unaltered by the medication. These pharmacological compounds are not always used alone but are often combined with other psychopharmacological agents, or used in conjunction with other therapies designed to promote insight into behavioural function. The compounds discussed here do not represent an exclusive list, but are representative of the general categories available and routinely used in Australia and New Zealand. There are several good basic texts on pharmacology, written for nurses, and many substantial texts written by pharmacologists for the wider health profession, which deal with this material at an advanced level. The reader is advised to refer to an appropriate text for a detailed outline of the basic pharmacology of the general categories of compounds, their clinical indications, contraindications, effects, common adverse effects, potential interactions and specific precautions (e.g. see Society of Hospital Pharmacists Australia 1985).

The compounds used to treat mental disorders are classified according to their effects on the CNS. They include the neuroleptics (sometimes inappropriately called 'antipsychotics'), the anxiolytics (antianxiety agents); the antidepressants (the tricyclics, the monoamine oxidase inhibitors, and the 'new generation' antidepressants); the mood stabilisers (antimanic agents), and the anticholinergics (antiparkinsonian drugs).

- The *neuroleptics* (Box 11.5) are used as an important treatment in ameliorating psychotic behaviour. While helping to produce the desired therapeutic effects, this group of compounds has a high incidence of anticipated troublesome side effects. These side effects include sedation, hypotension, anticholinergic effects and extrapyramidal side effects (EPSE). The EPSEs include psuedoparkinsonism, akinesia, dystonia, oculogyric crises and tardive dyskinesia.

- *Antidepressant* drugs (Box 11.6) are used to treat depression. The tricyclics (TCAs) and monoamine oxidase inhibitors (MAOIs) are two common groups. More recently developed compounds include the tetracyclics, such as mianserin (Tolvon), the serotonin-specific re-uptake inhibitors (SSRIS), such as Prozac, and the reversible inhibitors of monoamine (RIMA), such as Aurorix. Lithium carbonate is the *mood-stabilising* drug for clients with bipolar disorders (Box 11.7).

- *Anxiolytics* (Box 11.8) are used to relieve mild or moderate anxiety, or to treat 'psychoneurotic' or psychosomatic conditions. Subgroups include the antihistamines, propanediol dicarbamates, beta-adrenergic blocking agents and benzodiazepines.

- *Anticholinergic* drugs (Box 11.9) are used to control the parkinson-like effects of the neuroleptics.

The appropriate management of a mentally disordered client with any of these agents requires a clear diagnosis of the client's behaviour, objective assessment of the needs of the client, and familiarity with clinical **pharmacokinetics** (interactions between drug and body, as the drug is absorbed, distributed, metabolised and excreted).

The groups listed above will now be discussed in more detail.

## Neuroleptics

This group of drugs are most widely used in treatment of psychotic conditions. They derive their name from their capacity to affect several integrating systems of the brain, including the ability to produce movement disorders.

## $B$ OX 11.5: *Neuroleptics used to treat psychotic behaviour*

The neuroleptics are frequently used in the management of a variety of disturbed behaviours, including behaviour that is classified as psychotic. These compounds were formerly known as major tranquillisers or antipsychotic drugs. The term 'neuroleptic' reflects their ability to selectively reduce emotionality and psychomotor activity (Feldman & Quenzer 1984).

They are palliative, not curative. All classes of neuroleptics are thought to exert their potent antipsychotic action by blocking DA in certain areas of the brain (Snyder 1976, 1980), even though most of them block NE to some extent. More specifically, their antipsychotic potency correlates with their ability to inhibit DA-sensitive enzymes that are required to drive neural pumps (like the Na+ pump in DA-activated neurons in the mesolimbic system of the brain).

As with all pharmacological agents, the neuroleptic drugs have many effects in addition to their principal therapeutic effects, and these can be seen peripherally as well as centrally. For instance, the DA-blocking action which they exert on the mesolimbic system of the brain probably accounts for their antipsychotic effects, while the same DA antagonism on the nigrostriatal pathway probably accounts for the unwanted parkinsonian symptoms that result from prolonged administration (Snyder 1976). This is because there are also cholinergic neurons in the striatum that are normally inhibited by DA. If there is DA deficiency, the cholinergic neurons become overactive and may contribute to the parkinsonism.

These compounds also produce changes in brain electrical activity (measured in electroencephalographic changes), endocrine effects and cardiovascular effects. They do not cause their action by sedation and, although some may cause drowsiness, clients are easily aroused. These sedative effects are secondary to the antipsychotic effects.

## TABLE 11.1: *Examples of neuroleptics*

| GENERIC NAME | TRADE NAME | DOSE EQUIVALENCE[1] | RELATIVE POTENCY[2] | DOSE RANGE (MG/DAY)[3] |
|---|---|---|---|---|
| Chlorpromazine | Largactil | 100 | low | 100–1000 |
| Trifluoperazine | Stelazine | 5 | | 5–60 |
| Fluphenazine | Modecate | 2 | | 2–50 |
| Haloperidol | Serenace | 1.6 | high | 2–40 |

[1] That is, it takes more chlorpromazine than haloperidol to have the same effect.

[2] Low potency is more sedating, more likely to have anticholinergic effects; high potency is more likely to produce extrapyramidal effects.

[3] The range of effective therapeutic doses among neuroleptics varies; these doses indicate possible therapeutic ranges. Note also that parenteral administration may provide much greater bioavailability than oral forms, so parenteral doses are much smaller than those given orally.

*Choice and route of drug.*    Carefully controlled comparison studies have failed to demonstrate substantial differences in the antipsychotic effects of neuroleptic drugs, and/or evidence of specificity effects. Frequently, then, a decision is made according to the knowledge of the pharmacological properties and adverse effects of the various neuroleptics, or the client's past responses to a particular agent. A client who is unresponsive to one compound may respond well to another. Recent trends, however, indicate a preference for the selection of 'high-potency' drugs, rather than the more sedating 'low-potency' compounds, and for the combination of one of the longer-acting benzodiazepines with a high-potency antipsychotic (Table 11.1). The rate at which the desired therapeutic effect is achieved may also determine the choice of compound and the route of administration—for instance, rapid relief for a severely agitated client may require parenteral administration. The choice of the compound may also depend on whether the client is compliant with oral administration. For individuals who have difficulty with oral administration, parenteral maintenance therapy using fluphenazine decanoate, which is a long-acting, depot neuroleptic, is common.

### Clozapine

A compound that is receiving increasing attention in the treatment of schizophrenia is clozapine (Clozaril). First synthesised in 1959, clozapine was withdrawn from unrestricted use in 1975 after eight people in Finland developed agranulocytosis (an acute disease in which there is a sudden drop in the production of white blood cells, leaving the body defenceless against bacterial infection) and died (Chatterton 1994, p.86). Its use has been slowly reintroduced since 1988 for the treatment of schizophrenia unresponsive to other compounds (*treatment-resistant schizophrenia*). Clozapine is contraindicated in the following situations:

- when there is a history of drug-induced agranulocytosis;
- bone marrow disorders;
- circulatory collapse;
- depression of the central nervous system (CNS);
- alcohol or toxic psychoses;
- drug intoxication;
- coma;
- uncontrolled epilepsy;
- severe renal, hepatic or cardiac disease.

Close medical supervision is required for clients taking clozapine because it can lower the seizure threshold, cause cardiac impairment and other serious pathological changes. Due to its toxicity, clozapine is only available in certain hospitals and the white blood cell counts of all patients taking it must be monitored at frequent regular intervals.

The dose for each patient must be individualised. Treatment commonly begins with 12.5mg on Day 1; if well tolerated, the dose is increased to 25–50mg on Day 2; if well tolerated, the daily dose is increased by 25–50mg per day up to 300mg per day within 14–21 days; thereafter the dose is increased by 50–100mg per week up to a maximum of 600–900mg per day. After achieving maximum therapeutic benefit, a maintenance dose is achieved by titrating down to 150–300mg per day. The course of treatment is not commenced until classic neuroleptic medication has been withdrawn for at least one week. Strict conditions apply to the use of clozapine because of its lethal side effects. Readers are referred to Chatterton (1994) for further details of site requirements and for a discussion of the role of the nurse in caring for clients taking clozapine.

## Antidepressants

The applications of antidepressants (see Box 11.6) are more widespread than just the depressive disorders. This is because their pharmacologic activity includes anticholinergic, antihistaminic, hypothermic and antiemetic action. They may be prescribed for adjustment disorders, atypical depression, panic disorder, obsessive-compulsive disorder, chronic pain disorder and eating disorders; also for selective use in substance-related disorders.

Nurses should be aware of the time lag between the initiation of therapy with antidepressants and the clinical effects. This delay has important implications for management of the depressed client and must be taken into consideration by the nurses involved. While clients receiving either TCAs or MAOIs warrant education on the expected effects of their prescription, those receiving the MAOIs require particular consideration because of possible adverse side effects, and the drug's potential for interaction with dietary tyramine.

# BOX 11.6: Antidepressants

These agents consist of several broad groups, of which the tricyclic antidepressants (TCAs) and the monoamine oxidase inhibitors (MAOIs) are commonly encountered in psychiatric–mental health care settings. Neither of these two subgroups is a CNS stimulant; rather, their therapeutic effects are achieved by their influence on neuronal uptake of biogenic amines. Use of the MAOIs relates to their ability to block the degradation of NE and 5HT, which effectively increases the available quantities of these neurotransmitters.

The TCAs are chemically similar to the phenothiazine neuroleptics and possess similar side effects. They have quite different therapeutic effects. The antidepressant effects of the TCAs are believed to be due to their ability to block neuronal uptake of NE and 5HT (uptake would normally terminate the action of these transmitters), while those of the MAOIs relate to their ability to block the degradation of NE. (The enzyme, monoamine oxidase (MAO), metabolises NE, DA and 5HT in brain, heart, intestine and blood.)

The 'new generation' antidepressants—the serotonin-specific re-uptake inhibitors (SSRIs) and the reversible inhibitors of monoamine (RIMAs)—selectively inhibit neurotransmitter function and reportedly have fewer anticholinergic side effects.

The end result of the actions of these groups is that, in the short term, they increase the effective concentrations of targeted neurotransmitters in the brain. The consequence of this short-term increase is an eventual homeostatic *decrease* in responsiveness to neurotransmission (Hollister 1982).

When these agents are administered to those who are clinically depressed, there is a delay of several days before the therapeutic effect is seen. The delay in therapeutic effect may, in fact, reflect the time taken to develop the decrease in neurotransmission referred to above.

*Choice of drug* (Table 11.2).    The TCAs and MAOIs are considered roughly equivalent in efficacy, although individual clients may respond more to a TCA than to an MAOI. The TCAs differ in the degree of sedation and anticholinergic effects they produce, while the MAOIs may sensitise the individual to tyramine—a sympathetomimetic found in many fermented foods and beverages. This interaction can potentiate hypertensive crises.

The serotonin-specific re-uptake inhibitors (SSRIs) and the reversible inhibitors of monoamine (RIMAs) are reportedly better tolerated than the TCAs or MAOIs, with apparently fewer side effects—especially the anticholinergic effects associated with the earlier groups. Side effects can be a limiting factor for many clients, limiting either the dose tolerated or the willingness to take the drug. Thus, the choice of drug is often determined by the adverse effects. Clients should be aware of the anticholinergic effects and impact on psychomotor tasks that these agents will promote.

# TABLE 11.2: Examples of antidepressants

| GENERIC NAME | TRADE NAME | AVERAGE DAILY DOSE (MG/DAY) |
|---|---|---|
| *TCAs* | | |
| Amitriptyline | Tryptanol | 50–250 |
| Doxepin | Sinequan | 75–300 |
| Imipramine | Tofranil | 50–250 |
| *MAOIs* | | |
| Phenelzine | Nardil | 15–60 |
| Tranylcypromine | Parnate | 20–60 |
| Iproniazid | Marsilid | 50–75 |
| *SSRI* | | |
| Paroxetine | Aropax | 20–50 |
| *RIMA* | | |
| Moclobemide | Aurorix | 300–600 |

## Prozac

Although the tricyclic antidepressants are the most widely used compounds in the treatment of depression, they are associated with unsatisfactory side effects. Newer antidepressants, such as Prozac (fluoxetine), have better side effect profiles and longer half-lives. The half-life for Prozac is 2 to 3 days, whereas the half-life for the tricyclics is 10–14 hours. Therefore, Prozac is commonly administered once daily, in the morning. The therapeutic effect of Prozac is attributed to its ability to combine to the cholinergic, histaminergic and alpha-1 adrenergic receptors with minimal affinity. It is a selective serotonin (5HT) re-uptake inhibitor (SSRI) that is particularly effective in the treatment of major depressive disorders where other therapy is inappropriate or ineffective. Clients must not be transferred to treatment with MAOIs within five weeks of ceasing Prozac, nor transferred from MAOIs to Prozac for two weeks after ceasing MAOIs. Adverse effects include CNS disturbances, drowsiness, sweating and gastrointestinal disturbances. Initially 1 capsule (20mg) is given daily in the morning. The dose is increased to 40mg daily after two weeks if necessary. This dose can be divided—20mg in the morning and 20mg at noon. The maximum daily dose is 80mg.

## Lithium carbonate

All clients receiving lithium require regular serum level assessment—at least monthly during maintenance therapy, and more frequently during initiation of therapy. Serum levels of lithium need to be maintained within fairly defined ranges for both acute therapeutic response and long-term maintenance therapy. Representative values are indicated in Table 11.3. Blood samples are obtained 12 hours after the last dose received. If serum lithium results >1.5mEq/L, or if

$\mathcal{B}$OX  11.7: *Mood stabilisers (antimanic compounds)*

Lithium carbonate (LiCO$_3$) is the only specific anti-manic compound available at present. In normal subjects, this compound has no obviously psychotropic action. It is used in the treatment of the manic phase of bipolar disorder and for long-term maintenance therapy, as it reduces the severity and frequency of bipolar episodes. When mania is mild, lithium alone may be an effective treatment but, in severe cases, it is almost always prescribed in conjunction with one of the neuroleptic agents. Once the mania is controlled, the neuroleptic may be ceased and lithium continued as maintenance therapy. It is not always the case that maintenance therapy follows treatment of an acute episode. The decision for lithium maintenance is complex and the benefits of continuation must outweigh the risks of adverse reactions and cumulative toxicity. It is also important to consider the frequency, duration and severity of episodes, as well as the client's insight and compliance.

Lithium is slow to enter cells, so there is a time lag between initiation and therapeutic effect (as much as 7–14 days). There is some evidence that Li also increases turnover of NE and alters the metabolism of 5HT, ACh and GABA.

there is some significant clinical circumstance (such as vomiting, diarrhoea, excessive sweating in hot weather, change in intake–output ratio, intercurrent infection, fever, or non-compliance), nurses should consult the prescriber before administering the next dose.

$\mathcal{T}$ABLE  11.3: *Recommended serum levels for lithium carbonate*

| SERUM LEVELS (mEq/L) | TREATMENT STRATEGY |
|---|---|
| 0.8–1.5 | Acute manic episode |
| 0.6–0.8 | Maintenance therapy |

Lithium accumulates in the body and generates a number of toxic and adverse responses (see Table 11.4). It is an essential nursing skill to be able to detect early signs and symptoms of toxicity and to withhold further medication until the patient's serum level is determined.

$\mathcal{T}$*ABLE 11.4:*  *Toxicity to lithium carbonate*

| SIGNS AND SYMPTOMS OF TOXICITY | SERUM LEVELS (mEq/L) |
|---|---|
| *Early signs*<br>Vomiting, diarrhoea, decreased co-ordination, drowsiness, muscular weakness, slurred speech | when range = 1.5–2.0 |
| *Imminent toxicity*<br>Ataxia, blurred vision, giddiness, tinnitus, muscle twitching or coarse tremor, and large output of dilute urine | when range = > 2.0 |

## Anxiolytics

The use of **anxiolytics** (see Box 11.8) is not restricted to the treatment of anxiety. They are also used in depression and aggressive states, as anticonvulsants, pre-operatively (they are particularly valuable in endoscopic procedures), to manage acute withdrawal, and in skeletal muscle spasm (e.g. cerebral palsy, athetosis, tetanus, and status epilepticus). Some anxiolytics have long-acting hypnotic properties and are thus used to treat insomnia.

$\mathcal{B}$*OX 11.8:*  *Anxiolytics used to treat anxiety disorders*

Anxiolytic is the name given to those compounds that are effective in alleviating the symptoms of anxiety. This group of psychotropic agents includes antihistamines as well as the major anxiolytic class—the benzodiazepines. These all have similar pharmacologic properties—small doses are anxiolytic, larger doses are hypnotic. Hypnotic drugs produce drowsiness and encourage sleep. A sedative drug should reduce anxiety and exert a calming effect with little or no effect on motor function. Hypnotic effects thus involve more pronounced depression of the CNS than sedation, although this can be achieved by most sedative drugs if the dose is appropriately increased. The addition to the anxiolytic group of the beta-adrenergic blocking agents (such as propanolol) is a reflection of their ability to block the peripheral symptoms of anxiety. The beta-adrenergic blocking agents are not anxiolytic in themselves.

   The 'true' anxiolytics, the benzodiazepines, are divisible into those compounds which have long half-lives (and are thus long-acting) and those that are shorter-acting. The site and mechanism of action of these compounds is

*continued ...*

unclear, although they do have significant effects on limbic structures of the CNS. It is proposed that they exert their therapeutic effects by dose-related effects on GABA receptors in the brain. This neurotransmitter appears to be involved in states of arousal and, as it has an inhibitory effect, the benzodiazepines (which potentiate that effect) thus produce a graded dose-dependent depression of CNS function and sedation. (GABA has inhibitory effects on DA and ACh.)

The benzodiazepines also interfere with the metabolism of 5HT, blocking 5HT uptake, which enhances 5HTergic activity in the synapse. The benzodiazepine group provides well-documented rapid, effective and safe anxiolysis. They are almost always administered orally and offer good relief from the more disabling symptoms of anxiety. However, this very attribute presents some risk for excessive self-medication. They ought not to be relied on exclusively for the management of anxiety—other means of anxiety relief must be taught. Tolerance, a decreased responsiveness to a drug following continuous exposure, is a common feature with the benzodiazepines. Psychological and physical dependence is possible with chronic use, but the appearance of characteristic withdrawal syndromes depends on the dose used immediately prior to abstinence.

## T ABLE  11.5:  *Examples of anxiolytics*

| GENERIC NAME | TRADE NAME | APPROXIMATE DOSE EQUIVALENCE (mg) | RAPIDITY OF ONSET |
|---|---|---|---|
| *Long-acting (~24 hours)* | | | |
| Chlordiazepoxide | Librium | 10 | Intermediate |
| Diazepam | Valium | 5 | Fastest |
| Flurazepam | Dalmane | 30 | Fast |
| *Intermediate (~12–15 hours)* | | | |
| Alprazolam | Xanax | 0.5 | Fast |
| Lorazepam | Ativan | 1 | Intermediate |
| Temazepam | Normison | 15 | Slow |
| *Short-acting (~4 hours)* | | | |
| Oxazepam | Serepax | 15 | Slow |

Metabolites of the benzodiazepines are centrally active and, in some cases, quite long-acting (Table 11.5). This may account for some of the daytime sedation produced by these drugs. For those compounds with long-acting metabolites (such as flurazepam and clorazepate) there exists a degree of cumulative effect with multiple doses (Skolnick & Paul 1981). This additive effect is also enhanced by the concurrent ingestion of other CNS depressants (such as alcohol). Others (such as oxazepam and lorazepam) are metabolised directly into inactive compounds. These agents have shorter half-lives and thus shorter durations of therapeutic effect.

## Anticholinergics

These are centrally-acting agents, effective in reducing the parkinson-like side effects of the neuroleptics, especially those with low potency (see Table 11.1).

B OX  11.9:  *Anticholinergics Used for Parkinson-like symptoms*

The actions of these compounds are similar to atropine, and have antihistaminic activity. They reduce cholinergic activity and are thus of value in treating conditions where there is dominance of the cholinergic system (they act by blocking ACh in the CNS)—as in all forms of parkinsonism, and in relieving the extrapyramidal effects (pseudoparkinsonism) of the neuroleptics. They are also commonly used as a supplement to L-dopa therapy.

The anticholinergics have peripheral effects, and toxicity to them produces psychomotor overactivity and hallucinations.

T ABLE  11.6:  *Examples of anticholinergics*

| GENERIC NAME | TRADE NAME | USUAL DOSE (mg) |
|---|---|---|
| Benzhexol | Artane | 1–5 |
| Biperiden | Akineton | 2 |
| Benztropine | Cogentin | 0.5–2 |

## Relevance of pharmacological knowledge to nursing

Nurses often perform a crucial role in the selection and administration of appropriate medication (it is often nurses' history-taking, observation, administration and recommendations that contribute significantly to the selection of the drug and the dosage). It is, thus, important for nurses to maintain an up-to-date knowledge of these agents. High on the list of nursing responsibilities is the recognition that clients with mental disorders frequently display a wide variety of behaviours; some may be quite subtle and require careful observation to identify, and some are much more obvious. Nurses, thus, have a responsibility for the accurate assessment of clients and their behaviours if psychotropic medication is to be used effectively and appropriately.

## Psychoanalytic therapy

This model is usually credited to the Viennese physician, Sigmund Freud. Freud's premise was that all psychological and emotional events, however obscure, were understandable. Freud explained behaviour by analysing childhood experiences, which he believed could cause adult neuroses. Therapy, in this model, consists of clarifying the meaning of events, feelings and behaviours, and, in doing so, gaining insight about them.

Psychoanalytic therapy is based on an alliance with the client which utilises the phenomena of **transference** and **countertransference**. Behaviour is interpreted in the light of apparent earlier traumatic conflicts and experiences, and these interpretations are meant to be considered by the client. The therapist remains aloof from the client to encourage the development of transference. Therapy is, thus, aimed at resolving the conflict and uncovering the roots of that conflict in the unconscious. Psychotherapy is based on the view that release of repressed feelings associated with the conflict will cause the conflict to be resolved and the symptoms will disappear.

### Relevance of psychoanalysis to nursing

Many of the terms arising from Freud's work have passed into common usage. Such expressions as conflict, id, ego, rejection, repression, egocentricity, sibling rivalry, phallic symbol and castration complex are freely used, possibly with no real comprehension of the concepts behind them. Psychoanalytic concepts have permeated the education and practice of some clinicians so widely that they have come to be regarded as a fundamental part of understanding mental disorders. Nurses need to be aware of some of the psychoanalytic language, concepts and speculations about client dynamics in order to participate as equal members of the psychiatric team. Nevertheless, the role available to nurses who practise in a setting where a psychoanalytic framework prevails is probably rather limited. Psychoanalysis requires years of specialist training and is, by nature, a protracted process, proving highly dependent on the development and exploitation of the specific relationship between therapist and client. Interpretation of the hidden meanings and symbolic nature of experiences is usually the prerogative of the therapist and traditionally takes place within the confines of the one-to-one relationship. It is important to appreciate that over the past 50 years there has been a proliferation of post-Freudian psychoanalytical frameworks. A good many of these frameworks underpin contemporary approaches to counselling and group work.

## Cognitive-behavioural therapy

This model draws on both psychology and neurophysiology. To the behaviourist, the conditioned or learned response is viewed as the basic unit of learning, reinforced by the outcome of behaviour. Deviations in behaviour occur because of the power of the association between the undesirable behavioural habit and reinforcement, and are considered to be perpetuated because of the associated reduction in anxiety.

This perspective asserts that human beings are merely complex animals with the power of conceptual thought, propositional language and the ability to attach meaning to hypothetical or metaphorical concepts. These abilities are all fully attributable to complex physiology, rather than to some non-material source. Who we are (self) simply reflects the total of past learning—our behavioural repertoire. Concepts such as 'consciousness' and 'self' can only be inferred from behaviour which can be observed, described and recorded. Behaviour is reinforced by conditions in the environment, so the self is a structure of stimulus–response chains (habits). The symptoms of a disorder are, in fact, the substance of the person's troubles. Since behaviour can be learned, it can be unlearned.

The aim of behaviour therapy is to change behaviour. In many behavioural settings, clients follow prescribed schedules for daily living and are rewarded for desired behaviour. Behavioural deviations are not rewarded; more productive behaviours are reinforced. Thus, acceptable behaviours that reduce anxiety or deviance are substituted for the undesirable ones.

The cognitive perspective broadens this viewpoint. Behaviour does not occur in a vacuum; rather, people think about the stimuli they receive. This thinking may occur rapidly and without awareness. Nevertheless, when sensory stimuli are received, they are processed, interpreted and compared with idealised and stored memories. The cognitive theorists indicate that it is cognitive processes such as thinking, memory and recall that influence behavioural responses.

### Relevance of cognitive-behavioural therapy to nursing

Nurses have a role in teaching cognitive-behavioural principles to clients to enable them to act as their own change agents. Non-professionals can be taught to use behaviour principles effectively to eliminate the chronic, maladaptive behaviour that often accompanies long-term mental disorder. In general, behavioural modification offers a rapid, efficient and effective system of nursing intervention.

## Social-interpersonal therapy

This model developed because of general dissatisfaction with other models. It is a combination of a social model and an interpersonal model. The social model suggests that social and environmental factors create stress, which then causes anxiety. Symptoms develop as a result of this anxiety. However, what has been called 'deviant' behaviour is considered to be merely a reflection of societal views; **labelling** behaviour as deviant is a way of meeting the needs of social and political systems. This view argues that mental disorder is a label earned by certain behaviours that violate the rules of conduct imposed by significant others. The interplay between individuals and their social context is crucial, since it is the social context that labels certain behaviour as deviant. Therapy appropriate to the social model is directed towards helping the client to deal with the social system more effectively. New resources are created when necessary to help the client interact with the social environment more successfully.

The interpersonal view integrates perspectives on the organism and the milieu, and suggests that relationships with other people largely determine behaviour. Positive interpersonal relationships protect against the insecurity, dissatisfaction and anxiety that rejection generates. If we can be helped to improve the quality of our interpersonal relationships, our feelings of security increase. Therapy, according to this model, relies on establishing a trusting therapeutic relationship between client and therapist, thus providing a corrective interpersonal experience.

The combined social-interpersonal model focuses on the larger and more general context of deviance and on the processes by which an individual comes to be labelled as deviant. Therapeutic interventions include programs for social change, political involvement, **advocacy**, community organisation, social planning, family support groups and education. Clients are approached in a holistic way, reflecting the interrelation and interaction of the biophysical, psychological and socioeconomic-cultural dimensions of life. This holistic approach increases the number of factors that must be assessed when caring for a client.

## GUIDING PRINCIPLES OF NURSING INTERVENTIONS

When planning interventions for any client with an enduring and disabling mental disorder, it is necessary to recognise sensitivity to change and failure, and to set realistic goals for client change. Prioritising the most troublesome areas of client functioning, and setting short-term goals that can increment to achieve longer-term goals, is a satisfactory approach that reinforces client involvement and achievement. (See Chapters 13 and 17 for detailed examples of this process.)

There are some general principles that guide the interventions of mental health nurses. It is important that they be applied in ways that respect the fundamental rights and responsibilities of people with mental disorders, as well those without.

### Assistance with grooming and hygiene

Some clients will require help in establishing and maintaining personal care habits, and this may necessitate teaching and motivating clients to use these skills.

### Promoting adequate and appropriate communication

Communication with people with disabling mental disorders such as schizophrenia may, by virtue of the condition, be difficult and exasperating for carers. However, the sufferers, like all other human beings, try to communicate observations about their environment, needs and concerns. While the nature of the disorder may impede communication, lack of respect for clients means the carer is unlikely to make honest attempts to understand their messages and is less likely to respond in a way that enhances those capacities that are intact.

### Promoting organised behaviour

In those clients for whom a mental disorder significantly disrupts appropriate and acceptable behavioural patterns, direction and limit setting may be required to help these clients make their actions more effective and goal-directed.

### Encouraging social interaction

Social isolation is a predominant feature of many mental disorders, especially the severely disorganising disorders, and may be heavily reinforced by past interpersonal relationship difficulties as well as fear of rejection. Therefore, mental health nurses need to respect the client's anxiety about social contact. Giving encouragement to try out new behaviours that are likely to promote success leads to small increments in behaviour change.

### Promoting reality-based perceptions

In some clients, distorted perceptions can be frightening. Reassurance of their safety, maintaining a safe environment, validating accurate perceptions, and helping to distinguish reality from misperception can all help clients attend to real rather than internal stimuli. This reality-grounding helps to orient clients to the real situation, protects them from acting on perceptual disturbances in ways that might harm themselves or others, and reduces impulsive behaviour that may otherwise occur in response to distorted perceptions.

### Promoting compliance with medical regimen

Psychotropic medications play an important part in the treatment of many mental disorders. The range of medication used to diminish the focal symptoms of disorders (e.g. perceptual disturbances, anxiety, mood disturbance, somatic distress) has increased exponentially in recent decades. Many of the 'new generation' drugs have far greater pharmacological effects and fewer troublesome side effects; consequently, the expected therapeutic responses may appear to be ever more predictable. However, individuals may respond in unique ways to such medications. Thus, in addition to administration of medication, it is still necessary to observe clients for evidence of therapeutic and adverse effects, to teach clients about the therapeutic and possible untoward effects, to help them take action to prevent untoward effects (e.g. maintenance of fluid intake to minimise postural hypotension), and to evaluate their subjective response to the medication and attitude towards continued use.

Consistent compliance with a medication regimen presents a problem to many people with a mental disorder. Non-compliance is not solely attributable to cognitive disorganisation in clients that may make it difficult for them to follow instructions. Many clients give accounts of poor instructions on administration procedures, the consequences of medication side effects, the stigmatisation attached to the mental condition (both on the part of clients and other community members, including their peers), problems with the cost involved in acquiring medication, and the lack of acceptable participation in treatment decisions. All these factors may contribute to the client's level of compliance with treatment. Provision of appropriate and clear information on the nature of the medication, the dose ranges prescribed, the effects that can reasonably be expected to occur, the side effects, which side effects might have to be tolerated and which require attention, and the expected duration of the medication regimen are all preventative strategies in which nurses play a significant and accepted part.

### Promoting family understanding and involvement

Many people with mental disorders live with other people—in families, groups and communities. Appropriate sharing of information, encouragement and involvement in current, future and post-discharge planning all require the involvement of clients and their immediate families or carers (see Chapter 12).

### Promoting community contacts

Community support and potential treatment programs available to clients with various mental disorders are vital to the success of treatment. Familiarisation of the client with the support systems available will help the transition from inpatient care back to the community.

## CONCLUSION

According to the biopsychosocial model, the clinician's approach to the client incorporates three interacting dimensions of the client's functioning: biological (physical or organic processes); psychological (aspects of mental functioning, including thought, emotion and behaviour); and social (interactions with others, including family, friends, colleagues at work, professionals and others important to the client). It may not always be necessary or practical to pursue fully all three aspects of the biopsychosocial model with each client. Although clinicians should retain the biopsychosocial perspective, they must also be flexible and individualise diagnostic assessment and interventions. For example, if a client's problems clearly reflect a primary biological process, it is appropriate to focus on the biological dimension in the biopsychosocial assessment. The psychodynamic, cognitive-behavioural, social-interpersonal and biological models provide mental health professionals with the means of organising information about human behaviour, including abnormal behaviour, and a conceptual framework which helps to formulate plans for treatment.

# SUMMARY

- Flexibility is required in the application of stress management techniques and care should be taken to align the expectations of the client with the likely success of the selected intervention.

- Medical-biological interventions derived from extensive research are available for the treatment of mental disorder. Neuroleptics, antidepressants and anxiolytics are among the categories of drugs used to treat mental illness. The choice of drug depends on the person treated, the pharmacological properties of the compound, the clinical effect sought and the ability of the client to comply with treatment.

- Nurses have an important role in observing clients, in order to provide information that may assist with the choice of drug to be prescribed. They also have an important role in ensuring that clients are fully informed about their medication, and in observing for adverse drug reactions.

- Other interventions used in the treatment of mental disorder include psychoanalytic therapy, practised by specialist practitioners, cognitive-behavioural therapy, and social-interpersonal interventions.

- Clients present with a wide range of needs arising from their life experiences and their mental disorder, but there is a set of principles to guide the mental health nurse in planning nursing interventions in most clinical settings. The chief principle is to respect the rights and responsibilities of the client. It should also be remembered that mental health nursing practice extends to providing support to the families and friends of clients.

# DISCUSSION QUESTIONS

1. What factors are taken into account in selecting interventions to assist a client with a serious mental disorder? Answer from the perspective of the treatment of a client with schizophrenia or a client with major depression.

2. What non-physical treatments and nursing interventions can be used to assist a client with florid symptoms of schizophrenia?

3. How may stress management techniques be used by a mental health nurse to help a client with an anxiety disorder? Explain the rationale for your approach.

4. Briefly describe the basic tenets of the biopsychosocial model of mental disorder.

5. Somatic interventions for mental disorders include pharmacotherapy. What limitations are evident in this approach?

6. Outline the guiding principles of mental health nursing interventions for people with mental disorders.

# EXERCISES

1. Interview a mental health nurse about the treatment options and nursing interventions used in the care of a selected client, making sure to collect information on any medication that has been prescribed by the psychiatrist or general practitioner, and note the intended benefits for the client. Interview the client about his or her perceptions of treatment and compare the client's account with that of the nurse. How do you account for any disparities in the perceptions of the nurse and the client?

2. Refer to the boxes and tables on the categories of drugs used in the treatment of mental disorder to draw up a pro forma to note similar information about the drugs in use in the setting where you next undertake clinical experience in mental health nursing.

3. Draw on the principles of mental health nursing practice to conduct a mental status examination on a client who has given informed consent. Use this information to devise a nursing care plan, and to make recommendations for treatment. Modify the nursing care plan and treatment options to take account of additional information which suggests that the client may be thinking about suicide.

# FURTHER READING

The following texts provide detailed accounts of nursing approaches to mental health care.

- Doenges, M.E., Townsend, M. & Moorhouse, M.F. (1995) *Psychiatric Care Plans: Guidelines for Planning and Documenting Client Care* (2nd edn) Philadelphia: F.A. Davis Co.
- Barry, P. (1989) *Psychosocial Assessment and Intervention*, Philadephia: Lippincott.
- Rawlins, R. & Heacock, P. (1993) *Clinical Manual of Psychiatric Nursing*, St Louis: Mosby.
- Wilson, H. & Kneisl, L. (1992) *Psychiatric Nursing*, Menlo Park: Addison Wesley.
- Arthur, D., Dowling, J. & Sharkey, R. (1992) *Mental Health Nursing. Strategies for working with Difficult Clients*. Sydney: W.B. Saunders.

# REFERENCES

Chatterton, R. (1994) 'Clozapine: a new hope for people with schizophrenia', *Australian and New Zealand Journal of Mental Health Nursing* (3)3, pp.86–90.

Feldman, R.S. & Quenzer, L.F. (1984) *Fundamentals of Neuropsychopharmacology*, Massachusetts: Sinauer Associates.

Free, M. & Oei, T.P.S. (1989) 'Biological and psychological processes in the treatment and maintenance of depression', *Clinical Psychology Review* 6, pp.653–88.

Hollister, L. (1982) 'Antidepressants' in B.G.Katzung (ed.) *Basic and Clinical Pharmacology*, Los Altos, California: Lange Medical Publications, pp.302–8.

Human Rights and Equal Opportunities Commission (1993) *Human Rights and Mental Illness. Report of the National Inquiry into the Human Rights of People with Mental Illness*, Canberra: AGPS

Jacobsen, E. (1938) *Progressive Relaxation*, University of Chicago Press.

Oei, T.P.S. & Baldwin, A. (1992) 'Smoking education and prevention: a developmental model', *Journal of Drug Education* f22, pp.155–81.

Skolnick, P. & Paul, S.M. (1981) 'The mechanism(s) of action of the benzodiazepines', *Medical Research Reviews* (1) p.3.

Snyder, S.H. (1976) 'The dopamine hypothesis of schizophrenia: focus on the dopamine receptor', *American Journal of Psychiatry* 133(2), pp.197–202.

Snyder, S.H. (1980) 'Neuroleptics: the correlation between clinical potency and presynaptic actions on dopamine neurons', *Science*, 188, pp.1217–19.

Society of Hospital Pharmacists Australia (1985) *Pharmacology and Drug Information for Nurses* (2nd edition), NSW: Saunders.

# CLIENTS

P EOPLE FACE DIFFERENT mental health problems as they go through life. One way of making sense of these experiences is to consider them in the context of stages in the development of the family. Part V considers the relationship between stages in the development of families and mental health. Rather than examine the mental health problems associated with each stage of family development, two important stages in the life span have been selected—adolescence and old age.

Chapter 12 sets the scene by analysing the concept of 'family' in the light of contemporary social trends in Australia. The chapter also discusses some of the mental health problems experienced by families with children, and families with older members. A model of family assessment that can assist nurses to help families is introduced. The chapter makes the important point that the mental health of all members of the family is affected when a family member has a mental health problem.

Chapter 13 takes up the theme of young people and mental health, reviews relevant research on adolescents, and demonstrates through a case study the important link between nursing theory and practice. Chapter 14 considers the mental health of older people and makes another important point: most older people are neither in poor health nor dependent. The chapter presents two case studies that will assist readers to devise nursing care plans for older people and their families.

# Bonds

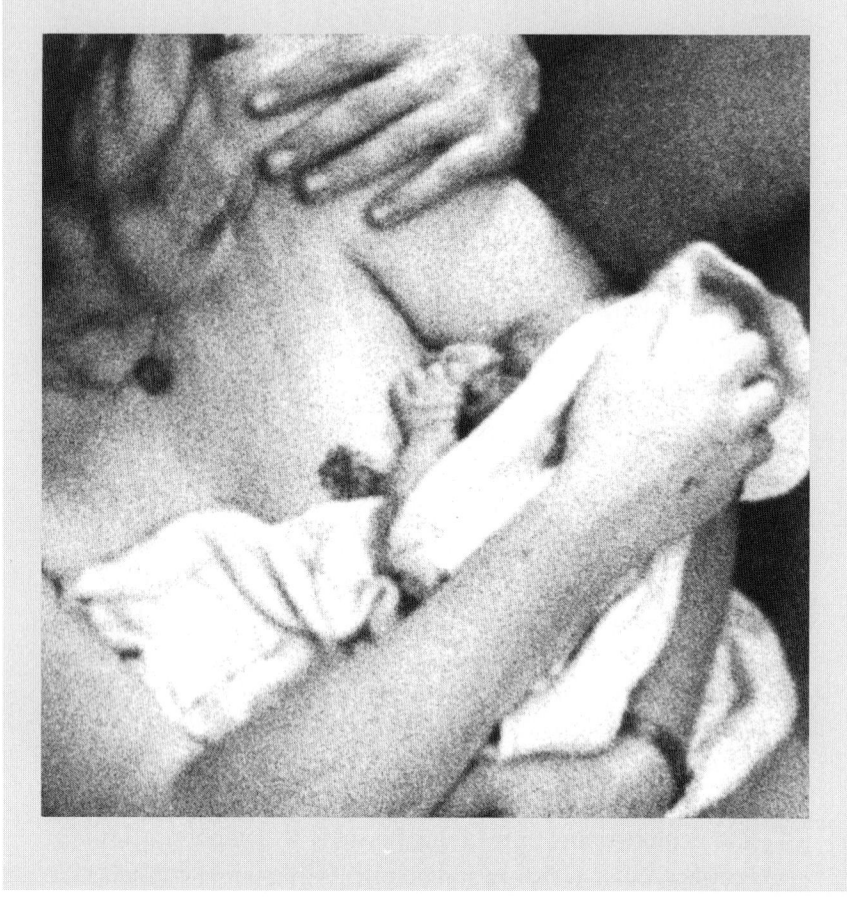

Ties of mutual affection and respect are core values in all types of families.
The key for family nursing is the principle that the family is whatever its members
declare it to be.

BRONWYN JEWELL

## CHAPTER 12

# FAMILY NURSING AND MENTAL HEALTH

Jill Mannion and Helen Edwards

## CONTENTS

# LEARNING OBJECTIVES

This chapter will assist readers to:

- explore definitions of the concept of family;
- discuss current family structures and social trends;
- develop an awareness of how the health of a family member can impact on the mental health of the whole family;
- describe how families can influence an individual's response to a health problem;
- discuss major mental health issues for child-bearing families and families with ageing members;
- outline a model of family assessment;
- describe interventions nurses can use when working with families;
- reflect on the role of the nurse in providing care for individual members of a family, and for the family unit.

# INTRODUCTION

For most of us the notion of family brings forth powerful images and associated feelings. For some, these feelings bring a warm sense of belonging, but for others they evoke sadness, anger or anguish. Nurses working with families need first to acknowledge their own thoughts and feelings in relation to their family experience. Until they can accept these feelings, they will be unable to accept those whose experience of family is different from their own.

Families are recognised as playing a significant role in determining the health and well-being of family members across the life span. It is well recognised that illness and disability of individual family members can have a major impact on the functioning of the family as a whole, as well as an impact on the mental health of other family members. Families also influence how individual family members experience illness and disability, and how they respond to, or engage in, treatment. For nurses to work effectively with families, they must be able to interview the family members and assess the family as a whole to identify strengths and problems, and then offer interventions to assist the family unit.

This chapter will firstly examine the family structures and social trends in Australia. Athough the experience of these changes and the response may differ from family to family, they provide a basis for understanding how illness and disability may impact on the mental health of families in Australia today. This will be followed by a discussion of how the family is defined for the purpose of nursing care. Child-bearing families and families with ageing members are then used as examples of two of the stages in which families may encounter difficulties with mental health issues. It is hoped that the material presented will stimulate thinking about families in other stages of the life cycle, where similiar difficulties are experienced. A case study will demonstrate the use of the Calgary Family Assessment Model (CFAM)) and the Calgary Family Intervention Model (CFIM), developed by Wright and Leahey (1994).

# SOCIAL TRENDS AND FAMILY STRUCTURES

It is important to consider the different family structures and social trends that place families today under considerable pressure. Most of the changes are common to other industrialised countries, but this does not lessen their importance. Social trends such as the reliance on dual incomes for many families, or high unemployment—although at different ends of the employment continuum—have changed the experience of family life in Australia and New Zealand. When reading the following description of Australian families today, consider the impact on the family's ability to adjust and to continue to function effectively if they were faced with the added burden of a sick or disabled member.

The usual way that information is obtained on family structures and social trends is by a census of households. For example, the Australian Bureau of Statistics (ABS) gathers data in the Census of Population and Housing, which is held every five years. The ABS defines a family as 'two or more persons, one of whom is at least 15 years of age, who are related by blood, marriage (registered or de facto), adoption or fostering, and who are usually resident in the same household'. (ABS 1993). Separate families are identified for each married or de facto couple and for each one-parent family in the household. Reports on family trends and structures are usually based on this information. It is important to note that, while this is important information, it does not detect the strong physical, emotional and financial ties that sometimes extend across households (McDonald 1993).

## Family structures

Several kinds of family structures can be found in Australia today.

### Couple families

By far the majority of household families are couple families. In Australia in 1992, 86% of household families were couple families and 13% were one-parent families (ABS 1993). Of the couple families, just over half had dependent children (McDonald 1993). Couples were married in 92% of these families and the remaining 8% were living in de facto relationships (ABS 1993). Of the de facto couples, most were childless young couples with the woman under 24 years of age in 87% of cases (ABS 1993). The number of same-sex couples has increased over the past 20 years, but this group is believed to represent less than 1% of all couples (McDonald 1993).

### One-parent families

In Australia, 13% of all families are one-parent families, with the mother the lone parent in 84% of cases (ABS 1993). This group of families is more likely to have a low income, be unemployed, to live in rented accommodation or share with another family, and to have less access to a car than couple families (McDonald 1993).

### Step-parent families/blended families

The number of step-parent or blended families has increased as the divorce rate has increased, but almost 80% of children under the age of 24 years live with both their natural parents (ABS 1994). Approximately 7% of all couple families with dependent children contain step-children, and half the de facto couple families with children contain step-children (McDonald 1993).

## Social trends

Trends in marriage, divorce and the work and educational environment have a major impact on families.

### Marriage and children

There are several significant social trends relating to marriage and having children. The number of de facto couple families has doubled in the past 20 years. Over half the couples who married in 1992 lived in de facto relationships prior to marriage; two-thirds of these were aged between 15 and 34 years (ABS 1994). The percentage of men and women who marry has been declining since it reached a peak 20 years ago, and the number of women marrying at a young age is the lowest it has ever been (McDonald 1993). Teenage births have halved over the last 20 years, while the age at which first births occur has increased. The number of unmarried women giving birth has been gradually increasing and accounted for 23% of births in 1991 compared to 9% in 1971 (ABS 1994). The number of women choosing to remain childless has also increased (McDonald 1993).

### Divorce

Although for every five marriages registered in 1991 there were two divorces, the average duration of marriage has showed little change in the 20 years to 1991, with 10% of marriages ending in divorce in the first 5 years and 30% by 20 years (ABS 1994). Remarriage rates have decreased as other options, such as de facto relationships, and relationships where partners live in separate households, have increased (McDonald 1993).

### Economic changes

Since the 1980s, the work and education environment in Australia has changed dramatically. As unemployment levels have risen, more young people have stayed at school to year 12, and more have stayed on to do tertiary studies. As a consequence, young people under 25 years of age, even if working part-time or not living at home, may still be financially dependent on their parents. This financial dependence at an age when young people desire independence is seen as one of the tensions facing families today (McDonald 1993). Many couple families today earn dual incomes and rely on both incomes for financial stability. These families experience difficulties when one member becomes sick or disabled. They are also less able to provide support, such as child care or aged care, to the extended family.

## Changes in health care and their effect on families

It is important to consider how the trend to community-based health care, together with the changes in family structures and social trends, could increase the pressure on families and impact on their mental health. The average length of hospital stay for mothers giving birth has decreased significantly, and more families are choosing home births and early discharge programs. Although there are many benefits from these changes, the child-bearing family may need to be self-reliant. Grandparents are often unable to assist because of geographic factors or full-time employment. The new mother, with little or no experience of caring for a baby, may find herself overwhelmed by household responsibilities at a time when lactation is being established and she is experiencing 'baby blues', or postnatal depression.

## VOICE BOX 12.1: Isolated mothering

I had a much more demanding husband when I got home from hospital. I faced a summer of 45°C in a new town 800 kilometres from family, no friends, no visitors. I was on my own. Too hot to do anything, too tired to even get into the wading pool. Baby restless most of the time, I was constantly worried about dehydration. My husband developed glandular fever when the baby was six weeks old. I was constantly running after him when I wasn't with the baby. Where did my time go? Doesn't anybody care about me? I felt I went very near a breakdown. I was embarrassed that I wasn't able to handle things as well as I was sure everybody else could.

More surgical procedures are carried out by day surgery and the length of hospital stays for medical and surgical conditions has also decreased significantly. Families play an important role in assisting recovery and, for short, acute illness episodes, most make satisfactory adjustments. Remember that these families include single-parent families, those experiencing marital breakdown or adjusting to a new blended family, and/or those facing economic hardships due to unemployment or natural disasters such as drought. When the health problem is a severely handicapped child, a family member who is mentally ill, an aged member suffering worsening disability, or a terminally ill member, the family is often expected to take on a long-term commitment for care. Families struggle on, providing what they believe is expected of them, often compromising the physical and mental health of all family members.

## DEFINING THE FAMILY FOR NURSING CARE

If several different people are asked to list the members of their family, it is clear that there are many different ways of defining 'family'. Some will include only those who live in the same household, while others will include those who live in a number of households. From a nursing perspective, it is important to define the family in a way that is responsive to different cultural groups and changing family structures, and in a way that respects the right of individuals to identify those they consider as family members. Friedman (1992, p.9) suggests the family be defined as 'two or more persons who are joined together by bonds of sharing and emotional closeness and who identify themselves as being part of the family'. Wright and Leahey (1994), in their clinical work, use the definition 'the family is who they say they are'. This definition acknowledges the family's belief about its membership rather than focusing on household members.

## NURSING AND FAMILIES ACROSS THE LIFE SPAN

Many illnesses, disabilities and other life events have an impact on the mental health of family members and the function of the family unit as a whole. How families respond, and what nurses can do to assist families experiencing difficulties, has been the subject of considerable research. Families with children, or aged members, are frequently in contact with the health care system, giving nurses the opportunity to identify families experiencing difficulties and to provide help. These two family stages are discussed below. However, many of the difficulties encountered in these stages are common to other stages of the life cycle.

### Child-bearing families

Families at the child-bearing stage of the life cycle can have experiences which have the capacity to compromise their mental well-being. Women have a substantially increased risk of mental illness in the first three months following childbirth (Raphael-Leff 1991). In addition, the emotional difficulties associated with miscarriage, having a baby with a chronic illness or a physical or mental handicap, the death of a baby or young child, or involuntary childlessness mean that many child-bearing families face challenges to their mental wellness. It is a time when women may feel they are being judged as females by their ability to mother effectively. Many women who remain employed until just prior to the birth of the first baby may experience low self-esteem as they stumble through the day, feeling exhausted; they have little sense of achievement, and this may be exacerbated by their loss of ability to contribute to the family finances.

# VOICE BOX 12.2: New parents

> For the first three months after the baby was born, I felt guilty that I didn't feel that overwhelming motherly love I'd expected. While I met all her physical needs, I found I couldn't play and gurgle without conscious effort. My husband did and she began to smile at him and they had obvious fun together while I spent a lot of time crying and needing him to give me lots of love and attention. I began to love her only when she began to respond to me spontaneously. I felt so relieved, I had feared that I would never love her.

## Infertility

Infertility is one of the possible problems, that can place considerable stress on couples. Infertility is usually an unanticipated developmental crisis for couples, where the choice of whether to bear children is taken away. Couples react in a number of ways. For some, the marriage itself takes on an identity of infertility, while for others infertility is just one part of the marital relationship. In some cases, one spouse takes the blame for the infertility, while in others, irrespective of the physiological cause, both spouses share the 'blame' (Olshansky 1988). Sometimes, for those who eventually become pregnant following medical treatment or who adopt a baby, the emotional sequelae of infertility can have profound effects on subsequent parenting. Bernstein (1990) identified increased anxiety during pregnancy or during the pre-adoption period, a prolonged time needed for bonding, separation anxiety, and lack of role models as difficulties associated with the transition to parenthood for couples who had experienced infertility. Decreased self-esteem, stressors within the marital relationship, isolation from family and friends, and unresolved grief and anger related to infertility and dealing with negative feelings about the baby were seen as difficulties associated with effective parenting (Bernstein 1990).

## Loss of a baby

When families experience miscarriages, intrauterine foetal deaths, stillbirths or neonatal deaths, the nurse has a vital role to play in helping the family adjust to the loss. The family may find it difficult to share the loss with friends, because others have few or no bonds or memories of the baby. Siblings may be excluded from the rites and rituals of grief on the advice of health professionals. Nicol (1989), however, argues that children are acutely aware of the feelings within their family, particularly those of their mother. Family adjustment to the loss occurs best when parents openly express their feelings and explain the loss to the children, when children are given accurate information about the death and included in family rites and rituals, and when parents encourage children to express their grief, with the understanding that it may vary in form and intensity to their own grief (Nicol 1989).

### Postnatal depression

Postnatal **depression** is a common psychological disorder following childbirth. Although it is estimated to affect 10–15% of mothers (Kumar & Robson 1984; Cox, Connor & Kendell 1982), it is frequently undiagnosed. Although postnatal depression is a depressive illness, these women, unlike those suffering from the relatively rare condition of **puerperal psychosis,** do not usually experience **delusions** or **hallucinations,** or need urgent admission to a psychiatric hospital. Their behaviour may appear normal and, unless questioned about the presence of depressive symptoms, the disorder may go undetected (Cox 1986). While for some the depression may be short-lived, for others it may continue for several years, with adverse effects on mother–baby bonding (Caplan et al. 1989), the other children and the marital relationship (Morse 1993).

The Edinburgh Postnatal Depression Scale (EPDS) is a 10-item self-report questionnaire that can be used as a screening tool to detect postnatal depression (Cox 1986). Once detected, many women respond to non-directive counselling by the health care worker (Gerrard et al. 1993). In non-directive counselling, the nurse provides a warm, trusting,interested, accepting and non-interfering atmosphere in which the woman is encouraged to explore her feelings, get to know herself better and find solutions to her own problems (Cox 1986). Nurses usually have considerable contact with mothers in the first year following the birth of a baby and, therefore, have the opportunity to detect, counsel or refer women suffering from postnatal depression.

## Families and older people

Social, economic and demographic changes have had an impact on family processes involving older people. For example, at the turn of the century the average length of marriage before one spouse died was 28 years, while in 1983 it was 43 years (Edgar 1991). As well as marriage now being a greater long-term commitment, these days older people are more likely than their predecessors to have adult children and grandchildren. Four- and five-generation families are more likely in the future. While such family networks have the potential to provide support, the networks involved may be complicated by divorce and remarriage (Friedman 1990). With the increase in combined families and step-families, it is possible that grandparents could have several sets of grandchildren. The impact of these changes on older people in the family is discussed below.

### Family caregiving

Family caregiving is two-way. As well as older people providing a substantial amount of child care, adult children provide care for their older parents when required. Family caregiving for older family members has been studied (e.g. Hardy & Riffle 1993; Skaff & Pearlin 1992; Thompson et al. 1993), with an emphasis on family caregiving for dementia sufferers (e.g. Semple 1992; Suitor & Pillemer 1993; Vitaliano et al. 1993). It is interesting to note that little research has examined family caregiving for older people with **depression** (e.g.

Billig 1991; Fadden, Bebbington & Kuipers 1987). The paucity of research in this area probably reflects the underestimation of the incidence and importance of depression in older people.

## Caregiver burden

The research on family caregiving demonstrates that caregivers, and especially those of dementia sufferers, experience stress or burden as a result of caregiving. While most studies have been conducted overseas, Australian research supports the findings of these studies. For example, a study by Wells et al. (1990) found psychological disturbance in 59% of caregivers of dementia sufferers using day care, and in 69% of those about to start day care. Another Australian study (Brodaty & Hadzi-Pavlovic 1990) found that psychological disturbance was greater for those caring for a dementia sufferer at home than for those whose relative was in an institution. However, for the families of dementia sufferers in institutions, the burden of care continues (Clinton, Edwards, Moyle, Weir & Eyeson-Annan 1994).

The documented evidence of caregiver burden has given rise to a number of studies which have explored contributing factors. Important factors identified include the caregiving relationship, caregivers' perception of their role, emotional decline of the older person, and negative behaviours (e.g. wandering, aggressive outbursts) resulting from cognitive impairment (Braithwaite 1990; Deimling & Bass 1986; Morris, Morris & Britton 1988). These factors have been shown to have a greater impact on burden than the physical tasks associated with caregiving. As well as experiencing burden, caregivers feel frustration, anger and guilt, which in turn may arouse negative affect and ambivalence towards the care receiver (Brody 1988; Cohler et al. 1990).

## Interventions to reduce burden

It is important therefore for the health of both caregiver and older family member that interventions to reduce burden are instigated. Social support has been found to reduce caregiver burden more than physical assistance (Morris et al. 1988). However, different types of social support appear to work in different ways. Recent work by Thompson et al. (1993) suggests that providing more opportunities for social participation may be more beneficial for caregivers than intimate, emotional support from family and friends.

Within Australia, intervention studies have focused on caregiver education programs and the use of day care programs. Brodaty and Gresham (1989) randomly assigned caregivers to a full program (caregiver education and memory training for the dementia sufferer), a program for the sufferer only, or to a waiting list. The stress of caregivers in the full program was reduced to a level not seen in the other two programs, and the difference between the groups was strongest 12 months after the program. It is also interesting to note that the full program reduced the demand for residential care. The intervention was an intensive 10-day live-in program and, apart from training and education, it is likely that the caregiver participants engaged in social and recreational activities together. In light of the recent findings by Thompson et al. (1993), future studies in this area will need to separate the effects of the different types of support. Nevertheless, the importance of education and training for caregivers should not be underestimated. In another Australian study of family caregivers, lack of knowledge about caregiving was predictive of high levels of burden (Braithwaite 1990).

Chapter 14 focuses on mental health issues for older people. In that chapter a case study is presented of a husband caring for his wife who has Alzheimer's disease. The care package and nursing interventions suggested for that case draw on the research relating to caregiver burden which has been referred to in this section.

## CASE STUDY 12.1: *Family assessment*

Cheryl and Andrew North, both aged 36 years, have been married for 12 years. Andrew works as a sales representative for a computer firm and Cheryl is a primary school teacher. They planned to start a family after four years of marriage and so Cheryl stopped taking the contraceptive pill at that time. When no pregnancy occurred, Cheryl went to see her family doctor and was referred to a fertility specialist. It took six years of tests, investigations and treatment for Cheryl to become pregnant. Cheryl had an uneventful pregnancy which went to term. When her labour failed to progress a healthy male infant weighing 3800 grams was delivered by caesarean section under a general anaesthetic. Cheryl and Andrew named him 'James'. Andrew was very excited by the birth of a son, but Cheryl was disappointed that she had not had a normal vaginal delivery and was not able to nurse James at birth and put him to the breast. Cheryl experienced wound pain and engorged breasts and was tearful in the first few days following the birth. James was a 'good' baby and breast-feeding was established without any difficulty.

Cheryl, however, seemed to need constant reassurance that her baby was healthy and thriving. Andrew could not understand why his wife appeared so concerned, when he was overjoyed at the long-awaited arrival of their son. Cheryl could not explain why she felt the way she did and thought she would feel much better when she got home, although she was nervous about leaving hospital. Cheryl and James were discharged at six days.

Andrew, Cheryl and James returned three weeks later. Cheryl had continued to feel inadequate and Andrew's leave was finished. He was due to return to work the following week and Cheryl felt she couldn't cope alone. She had visited her family doctor for a check-up for James. The doctor found him to be healthy, and told Cheryl that she was overanxious and needed more time to adjust to parenthood. He had assessed her and ruled out postnatal depression. The doctor focused on the health of James and Cheryl.

A nurse would have assessed the family as a whole. The manner in which such an assessment can be conducted will now be described.

# Family assessment models

A number of assessment models have been developed for nurses to guide and assist them in making sense of the large volume of information generated by the family interview. The Friedman Family Assessment Model (Friedman 1992) and the Calgary Family Assessment Model (Wright & Leahey 1994) are two models developed for nurses working with families. Both models have been modified in response to the changes that have occurred for families.

The CFAM (Wright & Leahey 1994), will be used in this example. The CFAM is based on the theoretical underpinnings of systems theory, cybernetics, communication theory and change theory. Its focus on the reciprocal relationships between the effect of illness on family members, and the effect of the family on the experience of illness, makes it a useful model when issues of mental health and illness are being assessed. The CFAM consists of three main categories of assessment: structural, developmental and functional. Each category has a number of possible subcategories. Wright and Leahey (1994) recommend that nurses include the subcategories they believe are appropriate for each family and each interview.

# Assessment of the North family

The three main assessment categories of the CFAM are now discussed and applied to the North family.

## Structural assessment

Structural assessment, using the CFAM, gathers internal, external and contextual data. The internal data may include the subcategories of family composition, gender, rank order, subsystems and boundaries. The external structural assessment gathers data related to the extended family and larger systems, and the context aspect includes ethnicity, race, social class, religion and environment.

*Genogram.*   The genogram is an extremely useful structural assessment tool. It usually provides a picture of three generations of a family, including much of the information obtained in the subcategories of the structural assessment, in a form that is quick and easy to comprehend. The symbols used are universally accepted. Figure 12.1 shows a genogram of the North family.

Males are depicted by squares and females by circles; the name of the person is written within the symbol. Outside the symbol other important information is noted, such as health status, occupation or other characteristics which the family believes are significant. Family members who have died are indicated by lines drawn into the square or circle (see 'Michael' in Fig. 12.1) and the year of death noted. Miscarriages are symbolised by a rectangle and the sex of the child is noted if known.

Families are usually happy to help complete a genogram of their family, and the process provides a considerable amount of information for the nurse about the family and their interactions.

# FIGURE 12.1: *North family genogram*

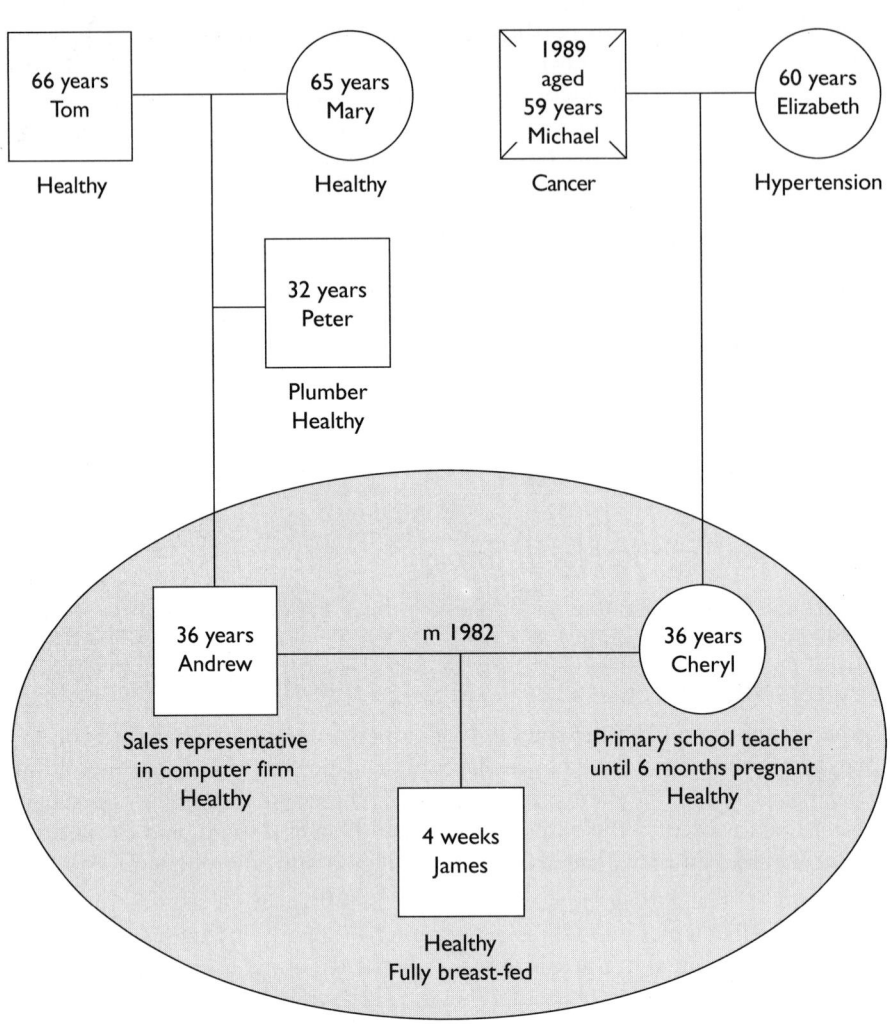

## Developmental assessment

Wright and Leahey (1994) believe that nurses need to consider the developmental life cycle of each family. The **life cycle** depicts the comings and goings of family members; although there may be cultural and ethnic variations for some aspects, for others—such as the starting of school, or retirement—there are general expectations. Wright and Leahey (1994) note that a number of family therapists have identified that family problems frequently occur when families acquire or lose a family member. They recommend that the family

# FIGURE 12.2: *The North's circular communication pattern*

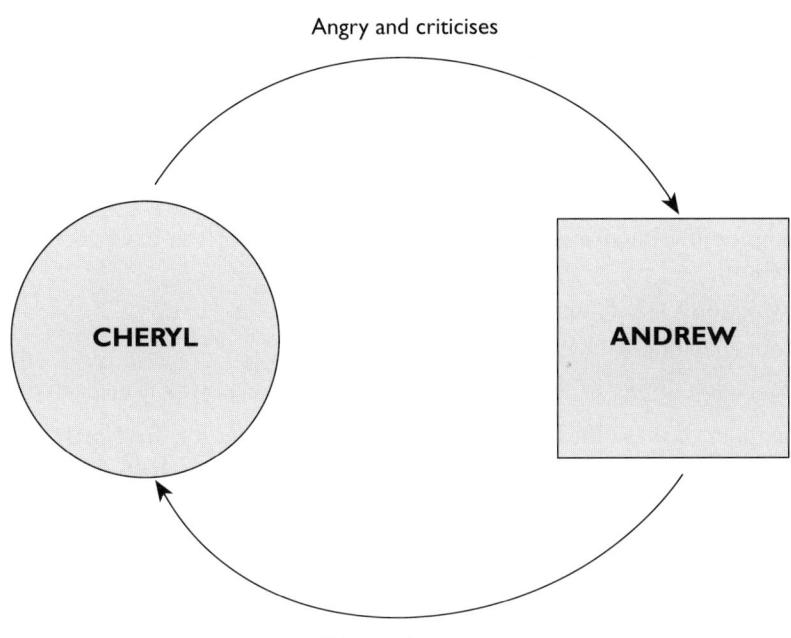

Angry and criticises

CHERYL

ANDREW

Tries to do more

Cheryl believed that she was not a good mother. She had not been able to fall pregnant for all those years; when she did, she was unable to have a normal delivery; and now she couldn't manage to care for her new baby and do all the usual household chores. Her mother had offered to come and stay when Cheryl came home from hospital, but Cheryl believed she should be able to manage without that help and didn't want her mother to interfere or give advice. She had never really got on well with Andrew's mother and was glad she lived too far away to be involved.

## Problem identified

The problem affecting the North family was identified as difficulties associated with the transition to parenthood following a long period of infertility.

## Intervention

The Calgary Family Intervention Model (CFIM) has been developed as a companion model to the CFAM by Wright and Leahey (1994). The CFIM focuses on promoting, improving and/or sustaining effective family functioning in the cognitive, affective and behavioural domains. Wright and Leahey (1994) emphasise the need for a nurse to determine the predominant domain of family functioning that needs changing, and the intervention most likely to bring about this change by its 'fit' for the family. They strongly believe that there is no one 'right' intervention and, although some results may be noted immediately, others take a considerable period of time.

Wright and Leahey (1994, p.105) describe a number of possible family nursing interventions, including:

- commending family strengths;
- offering information;
- externalising the problem;
- validating the client's emotional response when he or she talks about their situation;
- drawing forth family support;
- encouraging family members as caregivers;
- encouraging respite so that family members can take a break from each other.

A number of these interventions could be appropriate for the North family, and the nurse would need to seek the ones with the best fit to help Andrew and Cheryl adjust to their new family member.

Nurses are often those who are most in contact with these families and thus have the opportunity to help. They can intervene to prevent or reduce problems which may compromise the mental health of both the family member principally concerned and the rest of the family. To do this, they must be able to assess a family and intervene appropriately.

## SUMMARY

- Families have an important role in determining the health and well-being of family members.
- The health of family members can have a major impact on the functioning of the family.
- Although a family can be defined in several ways, it is important to use a definition that is responsive to the different cultural groups and changing family structures, and respects the right of individuals to identify those they consider to be family members.
- For nurses to work effectively with families, they must be able to interview the family and use family interventions.
- Child-bearing families can experience events which threaten their mental well-being, and nurses need to be able to assist them to maintain their mental health.
- A significant proportion of older people in the community are cared for by their family and nurses need to work with such families to reduce the incidence and impact of caregiver burden.

# DISCUSSION QUESTIONS

1. What would be the likely benefits and constraints in involving extended family (e.g. grandparents) in promoting family mental health?
2. How can nurses address potential areas of conflict when working with individuals with a mental health problem and their family?
3. 'Care for family members with health problems should be shared more equitably between the family and formal community services.' How realistic is this statement in the current economic climate? Discuss your response.
4. How do moves to community-based care impact on families? Consider mental health, acute services and disability in your discussion.

# EXERCISES

1. Generate a list of questions you would ask to assess the expressive functioning of the North family.
2. How might you evaluate the effectiveness of the chosen family nursing interventions?
3. Observe a family you have got to know in a television program or movie where a member has a health problem. Carry out a family assessment from your observations. What are the issues in relation to the mental health of this family? What interventions would you suggest to help this family?
4. Prepare a genogram of your own family. Consider the life stage reached by each family member, and the mental health issues common to each stage of the life span.

# FURTHER READING

- Friedman, L. (1990) *Why can't I sleep at Nana's anymore? Death, divorce and the grandparents*, Brunswick: Globe Press. This book is written in the form of stories from grandparents, parents, teenagers and children and confirms that, while there may be ex-husbands and ex-wives, there is no such thing as an 'ex-grandparent'.
- Thompson, E., Futterman, A., Gallagher-Thompson, D., Rose, J. & Lovett, S. (1993) 'Social support and caregiving burden in family caregivers of frail elders', *Journal of Gerontology* 48(5), S245–S254. This article reports findings from research which suggest that interventions that focus on caregivers regularly experiencing pleasant activity with friends and other family are more likely to reduce the burden of caregiving.

- Watson, W.L. (producer) (1989) *Families and Psychosocial Problems* (videotape), Calgary: University of Calgary. This educational video demonstrates how nurses can engage, interview and intervene with families experiencing psychosocial problems, using the CFAM model.
- Wright, L. & Leahey, M. (1994) *Nurses and Families: A Guide to Family Assessment and Intervention* (2nd edn), Philadelphia: F.A. Davis. This book provides a conceptual framework for interviewing families, identifying strengths and intervening with problems. It is a practical 'how to' book that reflects the authors' extensive clinical experience with families, and also includes many case examples based on theory and research.

# REFERENCES

Australian Bureau of Statistics (1993) *Australia's Families: Selected Findings from the Survey of Families in Australia 1992*, Canberra: ABS.

Australian Bureau of Statistics (1994) *Focus on Families: Demographics and Family Formation*, Canberra: ABS.

Bernstein, J. (1990) 'Parenting after infertility', *Journal of Perinatal and Neonatal Nursing* 4(2), pp.11–23.

Billig, N. (1991) 'Attitude and burden in families of depressed elderly patients: strategies for care', *Southern Medical Journal* 84(2), pp.225–8.

Braithwaite, V.A. (1990) *Bound to Care*, Sydney: Allen & Unwin.

Brodaty, H. & Gresham, M. (1989) 'Effect of a training programme to reduce stress in carers of patients with dementia', *British Medical Journal* 299, pp.1375–9.

Brodaty, H. & Hadzi-Pavlovic, D. (1990) 'Psychosocial effects on carers of living with persons with dementia', *Australian and New Zealand Journal of Psychiatry* 24, pp.351–61.

Brody, E.M. (1988) 'The long haul: a family odyssey' in L.F. Jarvik & C.H. Winograd (eds) *Treatments for the Alzheimer Patient*, New York: Springer, pp.107–122.

Brown, P., Williams, S., Mitchell, R. & Brown, L. (1992) 'Care givers of institutionalised and non-institutionalised patients with dementia', *American Journal of Ageing* 11,1, pp.8–12.

Bureau of Immigration Research (1991) *Australia's population trends and prospects 1990*, Canberra: AGPS.

Caplan, H., Coghill, S., Alexander, H., Robson, K., Katz, R. & Kumar, R. (1989) 'Maternal depression and the emotional development of the child', *British Journal of Psychiatry* 154, pp.818–23.

Carter, B. & McGoldrick, M. (eds) (1988) *The Changing Family Life Cycle: A Framework for Family Therapy* (2nd edn), New York: Gardner Press.

Clinton, M., Edwards, H., Moyle, W., Weir, D. & Eyeson-Annan, M. (1994) 'Stress in Nurses Caring for Residents with Alzheimer's Disease in a Dementia Unit in a General Hospital', Final Report to Queensland Nurses Council.

Cohler, B.J., Groves, L., Borden, W. & Lazarus, L. (1990) 'Caring for family members with Alzheimer's disease' in E.Light & B.D. Lebowitz (eds) *Alzheimer's Disease Treatment and Family Stress: Directions for Research*, Department of Health and Human Services, Rockville, Md, US, pp.50–105,

Cox, J. (1986) *Postnatal Depression: A Guide for Health Professionals*, Edinburgh: Churchill Livingstone.

Cox, J., Connor, Y. & Kendell, R. (1982) 'Prospective study of the psychiatric disorders of childbirth', *British Journal of Psychiatry* 140, pp.111–17.

Deimling, G.P. & Bass, D.M. (1986) 'Symptoms of mental impairment among elderly adults and their effects on family caregivers', *Journal of Gerontology* 41, pp.778–84.

Donnelly, C., Giblin, R., Oddie, U., Tutty, J. & Veitch, K. (1986) *The Parents Book Collective. Feeling our Way*, Maryborough: Penguin.

Edgar, D. (1991) 'Ageing: everybody's future', *Family Matters* 30, pp.15–19.

Fadden, G., Bebbington, P. & Kuipers, L. (1987) 'Caring and its burdens: a study of the spouses of depressed patients', *British Journal of Psychiatry* 151, pp.660–7.

Friedman, L. (1990) *Why can't I sleep at Nana's anymore? Death, Divorce and the Grandparents*, Brunswick: Globe Press.

Friedman, M. (1992) *Family Nursing: Theory and Practice* (3rd edn) Norwalk: Appleton & Lange.

Gerrard, J., Holden, J., Elliott, S., McKenzie, P., McKenzie, J. & Cox, J. (1993) 'A trainer's perspective of an innovative programme teaching health visitors about the detection, treatment and prevention of postnatal depression', *Journal of Advanced Nursing* 18, pp.1825–32.

Hardy, V. & Riffle, K. (1993) 'Support for caregivers of dependent elderly', *Geriatric Nursing* 14, pp.161–4.

Kumar, R. & Robson, K. (1984) 'A prospective study of emotional disorders in childbearing women', *British Journal of Psychiatry* 144, pp.35–47.

McDonald, P. (1993) *Australian Family Briefings No. 3: Family Trends and Structure in Australia*, Melbourne, Australian Institute of Family Studies.

Morris, R.G., Morris, L.W. & Britton, P.G. (1988) 'Factors affecting the emotional wellbeing of the caregivers of dementia sufferers', *British Journal of Psychiatry* 153, pp.147–56.

Morse, C. (1993) 'Psychosocial influences in postnatal depression', *Australian Journal of Advanced Nursing* 10(4), pp.26–31.

Nicol, M. (1989) *Loss of a Baby: Understanding Maternal Grief*, Sydney: Bantam.

Olshansky, E. (1988) 'Married couples' experiences of infertility', *Communicating Nursing Research* 21, p.47.

Raphael-Leff, J. (1991) *Psychological Processes of Childbearing*, London: Chapman & Hall.

Semple, S. (1992) 'Conflict in Alzheimer's caregiving families: its dimensions and consequences', *The Gerontologist* 32(5), pp.648–55.

Skaff, M. & Pearlin, L. (1992) 'Caregiving: role engulfment and the loss of self', *The Gerontologist* 32(5), pp.656–64.

Suitor, J.J. & Pillemer, K. (1993) 'Support and interpersonal stress in the social networks of married daughters caring for parents with dementia', *Journal of Gerontology* 48(1), pp.51–8.

Thompson, E., Futterman, A., Gallagher-Thompson, D., Rose, J. & Lovett, S. (1993) 'Social support and caregiving burden in family caregivers of frail elders', *Journal of Gerontology* 48(5), S245–S254.

Vitaliano, P., Young, H., Russo, H., Romano, J. & Magana-Amato, A. (1993) 'Does expressed emotion in spouses predict subsequent problems among care recipients with Alzheimer's Disease?' *Journal of Gerontology* 48(4), pp.202–9.

Wells, Y.D., Jorm, A.F., Jordan, F. & Lefroy, R. (1990) 'Effects on care-givers of special day care programmes for dementia sufferers', *Australian and New Zealand Journal of Psychiatry* 24, pp.82–90.

Wright, L. & Leahey, M. (1994) *Nurses and Families: A Guide to Family Assessment and Intervention* (2nd edn), Philadelphia: F.A. Davis Co.

# Youth

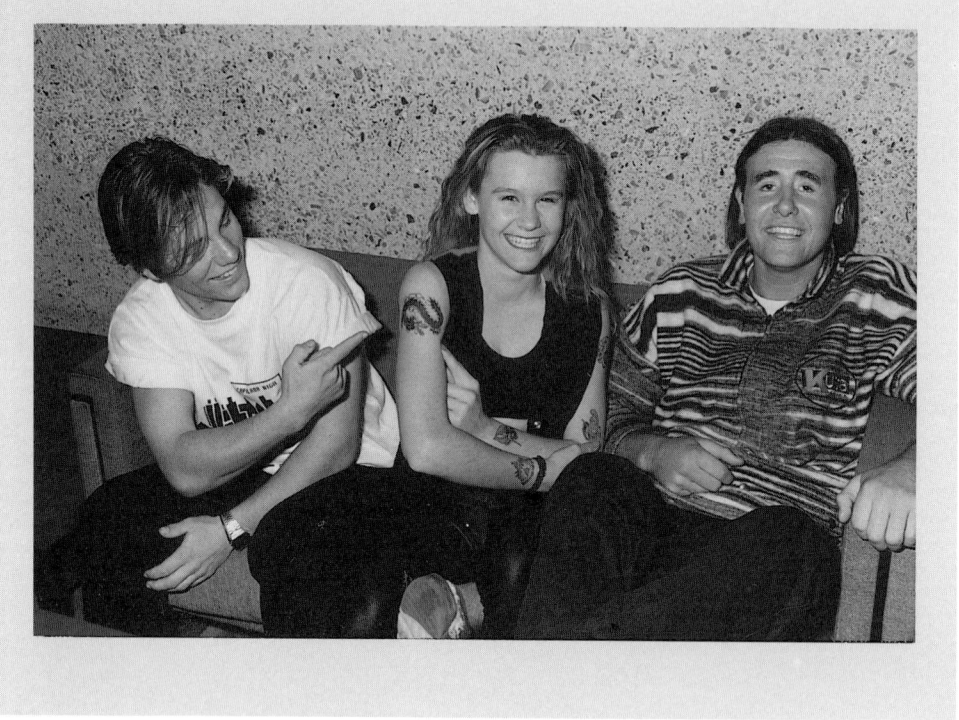

Growing up—a time of healthy irreverence, rebellion and increasing responsibility.

TIM OWEN

## CHAPTER 13

# YOUNG PEOPLE

Debra Creedy and Wendy Patton

## CONTENTS

# LEARNING OBJECTIVES

This chapter will assist the reader to:

- appreciate the complexity of the developmental period of adolescence;
- understand the associated complexity of mental health issues in adolescence;
- review stressors identified by adolescents;
- identify maladaptive behaviour in adolescence, especially the relationship between depression and suicide;
- identify the major categories of data that the nurse should collect;
- recognise concepts and issues to guide the thinking and actions of mental health nurses.

# INTRODUCTION

In western societies, adolescence is a period during which individuals experience considerable change, including the development of a personal identity, increasing independence from the family, increased awareness of personal sexuality, ongoing attempts to define themselves within restricted societal frameworks of femininity and masculinity, and related pressures to conform. All these changes take place within a society beset with contradictions of race, class, religion and sexuality. Within this context, the adolescent is to learn adaptive behaviours to assist healthy functioning through adulthood.

An increasing number of researchers and practitioners have commented on the neglected nature of child and adolescent mental health relative to similar work with adults (Kazdin 1993; Puskar & Lamb 1991). This chapter will review the relevant literature and discuss definitional and theoretical issues that have contributed to the area's relative neglect. It will then present a discussion of current perspectives of adolescent mental health which have emerged in parallel with the field of developmental psychopathology, and review the work on at-risk behaviours and adolescent-identified stressors. Finally, the chapter will review prevention and treatment issues and examine the role of mental health nurses in these aspects of adolescent mental health.

# DEFINITION AND THEORY IN THE STUDY OF ADOLESCENCE

Researchers rarely agree on a clear definition, but adolescence has been viewed historically as a phase between childhood and adulthood. The perception of adolescence as a period has contributed to the view that problems of adolescence are restricted to this stage and will pass with time. Most writers now view adolescence as a transitional process rather than as one or more stages of development. However, it is also recognised that experiences during adolescence can have an important influence on what happens later in life.

The transitional process of adolescence is believed to result from a number of physiological, emotional and cognitive changes, and external pressures originating from changing relations with peers, parents, teachers and others. Three theoretical explanations for these processes are:

1. The *psychoanalytic approach*, which focuses on the psychological factors that underlie the young person's development.
2. The *sociopsychological view*, which focuses on the effects of the social setting in which the young person is engaging.
3. The *life span developmental view*, which argues that these factors interact and that they both have an influence on adaptation.

The multiple and complex changes during adolescence have contributed to its portrayal as a time of emotional disturbance and turmoil. However, empirical research has negated this traditional view and now presents adolescence as relatively stable for the majority of young people. Importantly, the continuing stereotyped view of adolescence as essentially tumultuous may result in the 'normalisation' of many serious disturbances, which thus may not be identified and helped. Although very little Australian and New Zealand epidemiological research on the prevalence of mental health in children and adolescents has been conducted, studies indicate that 14–23% of children and adolescents have mental health problems (McGee et al. 1990; Sawyer et al. 1990). Overseas studies support this finding, indicating that 10–20% of adolescents exhibit some type of severe emotional disturbance, a percentage similar to the adult population (Powers, Hauser & Kilner 1989). Data from a number of major epidemiological studies in America (Robins & Regier 1991) and New Zealand (Wells et al. 1989) indicates that most psychiatric disorders have their onset in adolescence or early adulthood. In discussing the implications for Australia, Rey (1992) affirms that an increased emphasis on identification and treatment is necessary during childhood, adolescence and early adulthood.

In summary, adolescence has only recently been recognised as a phase of transitional processes that does not inevitably result in stress and emotional turmoil for young people. As a result of early theoretical conceptions of the period, the existence of specific mental health problems has been masked. Research findings on the existence of psychopathology in young people are scarce; however, those that exist identify mental health problems in a significant number of adolescents.

## DEFINITION OF ADOLESCENT MENTAL HEALTH

Defining mental illness and mental health in young people is a complex issue, again related to the multifaceted and complex nature of adolescent development. The Australian report of the National Youth Affairs Research Scheme on mental health and young people (Sawyer et al. 1992) presented more than 70 terms that workers in the field use to define mental health problems, 29 terms to define the concept 'psychiatric illness/disorder', and 58 terms used when describing mental health problems. Terms used to define mental health problems illustrated a broad range, including unemployment, poor life skills, and suicide. While the report showed a greater agreement in definition of 'psychiatric illness/disorder', it was also claimed that it was an inappropriate term to use with young people.

In view of the theoretical complexity of the period of adolescence, Powers et al. (1989) maintain that any model of adolescent mental health needs to adopt a multidimensional view and be able to accommodate the interindividual differences in adolescence. They describe adolescent mental health as a model of optimal development and adaptive functioning, and the absence of clinically diagnosed psychopathology, a description endorsed by Kazdin (1993). The focus on elements of positive functioning is important, as so much work concentrates on behaviours that reflect 'abnormal' functioning.

Peters (1988) presents characteristics of mentally healthy children and adolescents. The first characteristic is social competence, described as the ability to relate effectively to others, including peers, family and other adults. Key aspects of social competence include communication and assertion skills, skills in cooperation, self-awareness, and being able to resist negative external influences. A second characteristic is cognitive problem-solving skills, the ability to identify and approach problems in a realistic and systematic way. A third characteristic involves well-developed adaptive and coping skills, particularly in relation to dealing with emotional stress. Finally, well-developed external support systems, including the family, the wider relationship network, and the school, are environmental factors integral to the development and successful operation of these characteristics.

Defining adolescent mental health is a complex issue, and professionals in the field rarely agree on terminology. There are three main points to keep in mind.

1. Adolescent mental health describes optimal development and adaptive functioning, and the absence of clinically diagnosed psychopathology.

2. It is important to adopt a view that accounts for a large array of interindividual differences.

3. A focus on characteristics of mentally healthy young people can assist in our understanding of adolescent mental health.

# POEM

### to the mind
### undeveloped

*in some exclusive place unattainable exists*
*ultimate knowledge*
*yet to be fed*
*to the mind of the being*
*undeveloped*

**Charles Buckmaster**

# ADOLESCENT-IDENTIFIED STRESSORS

Studies that have attempted to elicit stressors identified by adolescents have noted that the understanding of adolescent stress needs to be different from the understanding of adult stress. Stressful life events for adolescents are better viewed as occurring within a framework of complex and ongoing life stresses. Sources of distress in a large sample of New Zealand adolescents from the general population were examined as part of a larger mental health study (McGee & Stanton 1992). Chief stressors identified by this group included problems with friends, parents and school, and problems of self-image, self-determination and competence.

## VOICE BOX 13.1: *Adolescent stress*

I've just finished year 10 and I don't know where to go from here. Sometimes I feel really lonely and I just don't seem to fit in.

Some gender differences were found in the frequency of reported stressors, and in the level of distress reported. In general, boys and girls find the same sorts of things distressing, but they are reported as more stressful by girls. Girls reported more stress about disagreements with parents, not being good enough at sport, feeling left out of things, and being overweight. These differences reflect the often restricted societal options available to girls, and the pressures in relation to body image. Girls did not differ from boys on aspects of positive mental health.

A similar study of adolescent worries in America (Kaufman et al. 1993) also found that six of the ten most frequently endorsed worries were similar for girls and boys. These were terrorism, going out on a date, thoughts about having sex, parents' physical or mental health, getting special recognition at school, and feelings that 'I am a bad person'. The additional four female worries concerned periods, getting bad grades, death or illness of a friend or family member, and 'people being afraid of me'; the additional four male concerns were having too much free time, eating too little or too much, popularity with friends and classmates, and trouble with the law. Stressors associated with relationships with boys or girls, conflict with parents, and changes in relationships with friends, school, finance, leisure and work were also identified by Puskar and Lamb (1991). Gender differences in the area of **body image** were found, with females reporting more concerns. Figure 13.1 presents a model identifying the complexity of stressors during the adolescent period of transition.

F I G U R E   1 3 . 1 :   *Stressors impinging on the adolescent*

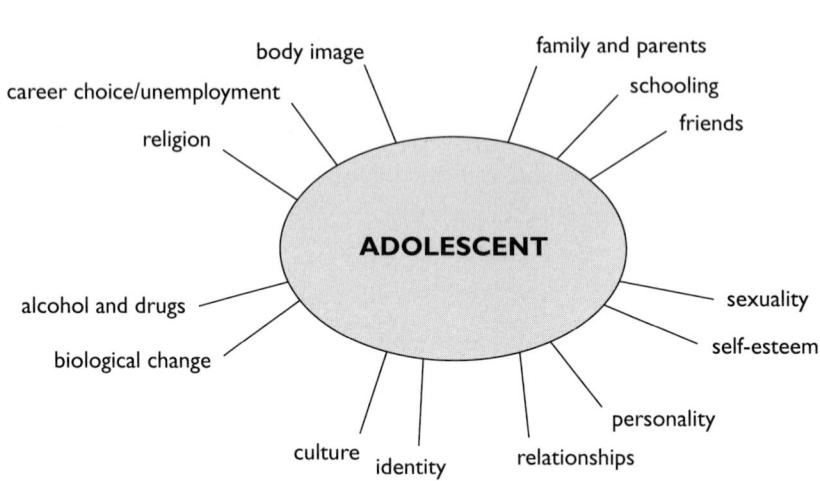

## AN OVERVIEW OF MENTAL HEALTH PROBLEMS IN ADOLESCENCE

The remainder of this chapter will provide an overview of mental health problems in adolescence within the framework of adolescent vulnerabilities and at-risk conditions, and serious mental illnesses which may have their onset in adolescence. Finally, the chapter will present issues of assessment, **prevention** and treatment.

### Factors contributing to adolescent vulnerabilities

Aspects of adolescent development, including the adolescent's personal beliefs about being invulnerable to ill-health and mortality, highlight the difficulty of identifying early signs of mental health problems in this age group. A major irony in this field is that adolescents are acutely vulnerable to certain at-risk factors. The report of the National Inquiry into the Human Rights of People with Mental Illness (HREOC 1993) identified a number of risk factors, which can be categorised as individual factors, parental–family factors, and other factors (see Box 13.1).

Other risk factors include personal issues such as low self-esteem, sexuality and identity concerns. Youth unemployment is also relevant. A major Australian longitudinal study with young people (Winefield et al. 1993) highlighted the poor mental health outcomes for unemployed young people, as well as the importance of satisfying work in promoting mental health.

B O X  1 3 . 1 :  *Identified risk factors in the development of mental illness*

*Parental–family factors*

- infant or childhood physical, psychological, sexual or emotional abuse
- genetic predisposition
- dysfunctional family life and major domestic conflict
- parental mental illness
- parental alcoholism or habitual substance abuse
- prenatal, perinatal and postnatal disease; trauma in mother or baby, or both
- family poverty or unemployment

*Individual factors*

- serious childhood physical illness, or physical or intellectual disability
- alcohol or substance abuse
- homelessness
- being held in protective or corrective custody

*Other factors*

- membership of an Aboriginal or Torres Strait Islander community
- non-English speaking background or refugee status
- living in a rural or isolated area
- other major trauma or disaster

Young people engaging in at-risk behaviour is another example of adolescent vulnerability to conditions that jeopardise optimal mental health. These behaviours are related to, but separate from, the at-risk factors mentioned above. They include alcohol and drug abuse, unprotected sexual activity and its associated risk of sexually transmitted diseases and unplanned pregnancy, antisocial and violent behaviour, dropping out of school and running away from home. While nearly 30% of 15-year-olds have been identified as exhibiting a binge pattern of alcohol consumption, daily tobacco use, and use of cannabis at some time (Cormack, Pols & Christie 1992), specific groups are at particular risk of developing harmful drug-use patterns. These groups include the small percentage of young people with already harmful patterns of use, homeless youth, some Aboriginal adolescents, some adolescent females, young male drink drivers, and adolescents living in homes where there is a parental alcohol or drug problem (Cormack et al. 1992). The use of illicit drugs and alcohol by young people poses a major social problem. Teenagers are starting to drink earlier and are drinking more heavily. Heroin is now claiming five times as many lives as it did 10 years ago. Adolescent sexual activity is difficult to research, but recent Australian data claims activity is increasing. Factors which predict, or correlate with, increased unprotected sexual activity appear to be related to alcohol consumption, social class, unemployment, and family influences such as parental separation. While truanting and homeless youth may be at greater risk of unprotected sex, even less research has been directed at these groups (Kosky, Eshkevari & Kneebone 1992).

It is important to make three points when considering the relationship between mental health problems and adolescence.

1. The relationship between risk factors and mental health problems is unclear. High-risk factors may operate in a correlational manner and may not be causal; that is, the use of illegal drugs *per se* may not predispose an individual to adverse mental health effects.

2. The severity of mental health problems and the associated background conditions may vary. For example, a homeless young person may be more at risk of developing mental health problems from drug taking than a young person living at home.

3. Risk behaviours and conditions rarely operate alone; many problem areas interrelate.


## Clinical dysfunctions, depression and suicide

Until recently, clinical dysfunctions particular to adolescence received scant attention. Over 40 different disorders that arise in infancy, childhood and adolescence have been delineated (Kazdin 1993). However, further research is required to discern developmental differences in the manifestation of dysfunction. Very little data is available to indicate the extent of these disorders in adolescence. From the data available, the leading cause of psychiatric first admissions in the 15–19 age group in New Zealand in 1992 consisted of males with schizophrenic disorders (15% of total admissions) and females with stress and adjustment reactions (17% of total admissions). In the 20–24 age group, 23% of admissions were males with alcohol dependence and abuse, and 12% were females with anxiety and depressive disorders. As with the at-risk conditions and behaviours, many young people experience two or more diagnosable disorders concurrently (Kazdin 1993).

Depressive disorder emerges with higher prevalence rates and significant gender difference in adolescence (Petersen et al. 1993) in clinical and community samples. **Depression** is associated with sad **affect** (feeling state), lack of interest in day-to-day activities, eating and sleeping problems, feelings of worthlessness and other symptoms. While gender differences are not apparent in childhood, the prevalence and severity of depression is greater for female adolescents than for male adolescents.

While **suicide** is related to depression, it warrants separate comment due to its increasing occurrence in the adolescent population. Youth suicide is the greatest killer of young people in Australia after traffic accidents, particularly for males between the ages of 15 and 24. During the past 25 years the suicide rate among 15–19 year old males has increased from 7.3 per 100 000 to about 21 per 100 000; the rate for females has increased twofold (HREOC 1993). Rates of attempted suicide have also increased. The most alarming increase identified in the report of the Royal Commission into Human Rights and Mental Illness was that for adolescent males in rural communities and small towns. While there is no reliable way of identifying young people who may commit suicide, risk factors include emotional disturbance (especially depression), the at-risk conditions and behaviours discussed previously, pressure of societal expectations, media coverage of youth suicide, and poor education or leaving school early (HREOC 1993). Other at-risk factors include chronic family discord, substance abuse and bereavement (Davis 1992).

## MENTAL HEALTH NURSING WITH ADOLESCENTS

The literature suggests that the prevalence of adolescent emotional disturbances is increasing. The demands of promoting adolescent mental health require nurses to be competent in the knowledge and skills necessary to work in this special area. By use of a case study, the following sections will address several considerations of adolescent mental health nursing practice: assessment, crisis intervention, milieu therapy, family involvement in levels of intervention, and promotion of adolescent mental health.

### Theoretical framework

In working with adolescents, mental health nurses need to adopt a framework for assessment, treatment and evaluation that differentiates between (1) psychopathology and medical diagnoses, and (2) the human responses that are of concern to nursing. Diagnosing is not the same as understanding a particular phenomenon such as depression. What it is, how it arises, its general course or form, its long-term effects on the individual's life, and other explanatory aspects of the concept are of interest to, and used by, nurses. When working with adolescents, the adopted nursing framework requires a human developmental focus so that nurses can identify strengths, as well as needs, and potential intervention methods.

The work of Peplau (1952) remains a common frame of reference for many nurses, particularly in mental health nursing, and her theory will be used as a basis of practice in the case study. The interpersonal relations nursing theory of Peplau is based on the notions of growth and change in both the client and the nurse. Her theory has been described as drawing from developmental, interpersonal and learning theories. Peplau (1952, p.16) has defined nursing as

> ... a significant therapeutic, interpersonal process that aims to promote a patient's health in the direction of creative, constructive, productive, personal and community living.

The individual is perceived as someone who has the ability to learn and improve problem-solving skills in order to develop a more productive life. The relationship (interaction) of the nurse with the client is a key influential factor in the outcome for the client. Through this positive interaction, which identifies and uses common meanings, the person and the nurse both develop and grow. The counselling and teaching roles of nursing therefore become an integral part of practice.

Peplau (1952, p.17) conceptualised the nurse–client relationship as developing through phases of orientation, the working phase (subdivided into identification and exploitation) and resolution. The nurse and client have changing goals and roles as they pass through each phase. The phases can be overlapping and interlocking. For example, after initial issues have been resolved during the exploitation phase, the client and nurse may return to problem identification where new issues can be explored.

## CASE STUDY 13.1: Brooke Harris

Brooke was brought by ambulance to the A&E department of a large city hospital at 1am. Police reported that Brooke had arrived home intoxicated at 11pm. and when confronted by her mother began throwing household items and could not be calmed. She locked herself in the bathroom and slashed her wrists. Brooke was not easily roused when her mother entered the bathroom and there was a pool of blood on the floor. The multiple incisions required suturing.

She was admitted to the psychiatric ward of the hospital and, with the assistance of her primary nurse, soon settled. The next morning Brooke was complaining of stomach cramps and was in a state of distress and agitation. Initially, she made vague statements about 'not being able to get into a routine' and how she truants from school because 'it's too hard to cope with'. She had not been eating well, mainly muesli bars, and was sleeping only 'one or two hours a night'. She stated that she felt 'lousy and tired' and was 'fed up being kicked around'.

Brooke, who is 15, recently broke up with her 18-year-old boyfriend, but has now missed a period and is concerned that she may be pregnant. She described erratic use of alcohol and drugs, 'mainly on weekends at parties with friends', but feels she can't talk to her mother about what's worrying her as 'she'd kill me if she ever found out'.

## I. ORIENTATION PHASE: CRISIS INTERVENTION

The orientation phase begins with the first encounter of the nurse and adolescent. In this phase the nurse and client come to know each other as individuals and to understand the role and expectations of each other in the relationship. Consistency and clarity on the part of the nurse are essential in setting the parameters of the nursing role. Commonly, the adolescent will test these parameters in order to establish that the nurse is a trustworthy person. The orientation phase is complete when the patient can begin to identify problems to work on in the relationship.

There are several immediate issues confronting Brooke. Clearly, she is in crisis and has been employing maladaptive coping strategies to deal with her stressors (see Chapter 2). There has been abuse of prescribed and illicit drugs and alcohol. Her inability to regulate her behaviour has resulted in self-harm. School difficulties and the possibility of pregnancy are highly likely to impact negatively on her future life choices, and may be further compounded by a perceived lack of social and family support. The combination of self-mutilation, somatisation, unsafe sex practices, substance abuse and possible suicide attempt indicates a likelihood of childhood neglect and abuse, and requires further investigation.

### Definition

**Crisis intervention** is short-term therapy whereby the nurse actively enters into the life of the person who is undergoing the crisis in order to decrease its impact and to help the client to mobilise personal resources, regain equilibrium and, if possible, move to a higher level of functioning. Crises may be of a situational or maturational nature, and may occur when the individual faces an obstacle that seems insurmountable with the usual coping skills (Rawlins & Heacock 1993, p.393).

Peplau (1952, p.255) suggests that, during a crisis, each person will behave in a way that has worked in relation to crises faced in the past. During a crisis, the nurse must identify the immediate precipitants of the crisis and any longer-standing conflicts and problems. As Brooke is at high risk of further suicide attempts, the role of the nurse is to assess the situation quickly and accurately, and to assist her in a tentative formulation of her problem.

## Areas to assess

Assessing Brooke's developmental functioning as part of the evaluation will give the nurse a clearer sense of her strengths, limitations and characteristic behavioural repertoire. Such information will help to determine whether her behaviour is adaptive or maladaptive, and indicate where and how the nurse can begin to help. The nursing assessment will include:

1. a full psychosocial assessment of Brooke and her family;
2. a determination of developmental progress; and
3. the interrelationship of family and significant others.

There are several good texts that outline formats of psychosocial assessment (e.g. Barry 1989). In association with the psychosocial assessment, Box 13.2 identifies questions that may help the nurse to determine Brooke's developmental progress and subsequent areas for intervention.

## Box 13.2: *Questions raised during assessment*

- Is the behaviour appropriate for Brooke's age and developmental level?
- How isolated or pervasive are the areas of difficulty or problem behaviours?
- How frequently does the difficulty occur?
- How aware or concerned is Brooke about the difficulties, and how much is she suffering?
- What is the pattern of the difficulty/problem behaviour?
- What support systems are available?

Simultaneously assessing family relationships gives the nurse a sense of any previous relationship problems and the resulting coping behaviours. The families of adolescents who attempt self-harm are often those in which chronic marital and parent–child conflict are common (Trautmam & Rotheram-Borus 1988). Genograms, as part of a full psychosocial assessment, are an efficient way of developing a diagrammatic representation of family history and relationships (see Chapter 12) and are an important component of history-taking and assessment. With an understanding of Brooke's psychosocial functioning, unachieved developmental goals, and family relationships, the nurse can discuss with Brooke ways in which she could enhance her sense of effectiveness, and identify the support she will need to achieve her goals.

## Nursing strategies for suicidal behaviour

In this case, nursing interventions need to build self-esteem and good relationships, and assist adaptation to changing circumstances. This is done by providing activities designed to tap Brooke's strengths, improve her resilience and develop her coping skills. Initially, however, the crisis needs to be managed. While in the A&E department, Brooke was given a full physical examination, her lacerations required sixteen sutures and two dressings, a blood alcohol sample was taken, and a urine specimen was taken for a pregnancy test. While mindful of Brooke's physical condition, the nursing strategies discussed here will focus on the psychosocial aspects of her inpatient care. Brooke was hospitalised to provide a safe and contained environment in which she could start to develop more adaptive behaviours and begin to confront the difficulties within herself and her family.

*Definition*
**Suicide** is the act of voluntarily and intentionally taking one's life. Committing suicide involves the individual's conscious wish to be dead and the action required to carry out that wish. Suicidal behaviours are those gestures, attempts, or verbal threats that result in death, injury or pain inflicted upon the self.

The term 'suicidal behaviour' may refer to an attempted suicide, a threatened suicide, or suicidal ideas (Rawlins & Heacock 1993, p.316).

According to Peplau (1987), self-destructive behaviours may result when anger is repressed and turned inward. Feelings of hopelessness are a significant clue in those at risk of suicide. Intense emotional suffering results from the irrational ways people construe the world and the assumptions they make. Assumptions may lead to self-defeating internal dialogue, such as 'I'm worthless; nobody loves me', which has an adverse effect on behaviour. Distorted thinking may produce a depressive episode and contribute to the risk of suicide. Three identifiable cognitive patterns emerge:

1. devaluation of self;
2. negative interpretation of experiences; and
3. a pessimistic view of the future.

## Interventions

Brooke was asked to make a commitment to no further suicide attempts, and to tell nursing staff if she began to think about suicide. This commitment, which includes steps she will take and individuals she will turn to, should suicidal feelings recur, is written as a contract. Such contracts are equally useful in the outpatient setting. Nursing staff need to simultaneously assess suicide potential and to determine an appropriate level of suicide precautions, such as constant observation and no access to sharp implements. Observation of raised spirits is sometimes an indication that a decision to commit suicide has been made. Also important is the need to provide for release of tension, anger and guilt through physical activities and non-directive counselling approaches. The nurse can assist Brooke in identifying experiences of sadness, anger or hostility and in responding to feelings of hopelessness. Brooke may also require prompting to maintain proper nutrition, elimination and rest.

When effective management of the initial crisis is established, Brooke will be afforded more individual freedom and will begin to take part in unit activities. In applying Peplau's framework, emphasis must be placed on the development of a therapeutic environment as a major component of the orientation phase.

## Milieu therapy

**Milieu therapy** is defined as the purposeful use of the environment for therapeutic purposes. Every interaction with the client is seen as having potentially beneficial outcomes in promoting optimal functioning (Wilson & Kneisl 1992, p.995).

An effective therapeutic milieu is intense and involving and aims to counter-act the regressive effects of institutionalisation (such as dependence and loss of contact with peers). Such a milieu is characterised by an equitable distribution of power in that individuals constructively influence their own treatment.

There are open communication, structured activities, involvement of family and community, and adaptation of the environment to meet clients' developmental needs. The focus is on action and solving problems in everyday experiences. Aspects of the milieu include therapeutic relationships, the ward environment, and rules and limits.

## Therapeutic relationship

The closeness of the relationship between the nurse and the adolescent is an essential part of nursing, out of which should come effective therapeutic change. Strategies that may assist in establishing a therapeutic nurse–adolescent relationship are outlined in Box 13.3.

## Box 13.3: *Establishing the nurse–adolescent relationship*

- Provide a safe environment with well-defined and consistently enforced limits.
- Involve adolescents in their own care. Allow choices when feasible.
- Encourage questions about their health status and treatment plan.
- Encourage the open expression of concerns.
- Stress confidentiality.
- Respect privacy and fear of embarrassment.
- Give understandable and reliable explanations.
- Reinforce information that has already been presented.
- Avoid negative criticism.
- Provide positive feedback.
- Serve as a positive role model.

Adolescents who are exceedingly anxious and disturbed are often out of control—that is, they will act unwittingly, or not take responsibility for their acts or for their effects on others. By talking with Brooke directly in counselling, and during brief contact in the ward, the nurse will help to focus her attention. Talking forces thinking and listening and, if this is done consistently and with interest, Brooke will begin to want to focus her attention and understand her behaviour.

If the nurse raises simple questions using short sentences, such as 'When did this happen?', 'Tell me more about …', 'Describe that', Brooke is challenged to exercise useful intellectual competencies and thus develop them for purposes of problem solving and formulating the meaning of experience. Discerning the meaning of experience is generally problematic for adolescents, in that they have an experience but cannot adequately make use of it for learning. Learning from experience is a necessary competence to develop in clients.

Difficulties can arise in the development of therapeutic relationships. The issue of becoming overinvolved, and questions of transference and countertransference, can present problems. **Transference** occurs when the adolescent behaves towards the nurse as though the nurse were a significant person from their past, usually a parent. It is quite possible for the nurse to fall into playing the role, and start feeling and behaving like a mother. Such behaviour is called **countertransference.** Clinical supervision sessions, peer consultation (see Chapter 19) and weekly nurses' groups can help nurses to bring such counselling issues into the open to be discussed, and are a necessary part of the nurse's development and education, as well as underpinning good practice (Hearne 1994). Supervision in nursing has tended to be hierarchical, but peer consultation is a more progressive approach, augmented by similar joint work with other members of the health care team.

## Ward environment

Any ward environment is constantly undergoing change. Its physical, psychological and social maintenance as a contained environment provides stability, without becoming rigid and institutionalised. The nursing of adolescents includes dealing with the small issues of everyday living on the ward. Interactions are occurring all the time and the manner in which nurses handle them is part of their skill in helping the adolescent deal with personal and interpersonal difficulties, change and growth,

For example, Brooke and Sarah (another client) argued about which program to watch on television; this difference quickly escalated to become a much larger issue for those involved, resulting in accusations and violence. The two were brought together and the problem of the outburst sorted out. But while an interim resolution is necessary, the incident also deserves to be examined carefully and in depth. The daily ward group facilitated by the nurses was used to discuss why the incident may have happened, how it happened, and how it was resolved. Other adolescents in the group were invited to comment on how they viewed the incident and ways in which they might have dealt with it. Small issues present nurses with important therapeutic work—how the nursing staff manage, and are seen to manage, such aspects of the community's day profoundly influences the whole milieu.

## Rules and limits

Every inpatient facility has rules that provide a sense of security for individuals in the knowledge that, no matter what happens, the structure will remain intact. Although it is important to provide structure, it is equally important to be flexible in the face of changing circumstances, so that movement can occur for the sake of individual adolescents and for the group as a whole. Brooke needs the security of knowing that her distress, outbursts and challenges will be held within the limits formed by the milieu.

When aggressive or unacceptable behaviour occurs, the use of 'time out' procedures allows nurses to maintain an individual's safety and gives the client the opportunity to regain equilibrium. Short **time out** in a quiet room or bedroom provides a chance for clients to reflect on their actions and decrease alienation from peers as a result of unacceptable behaviour; at the same time it protects them from possible dangerous behaviour towards themselves or others. Structured reintegration into the milieu when appropriate is essential.

## 2. WORKING PHASE

The working phase of Peplau's model incorporates both the identification and exploitation subphases. Identification is twofold. The adolescent begins to identify the purpose of the encounters and also the problems to be addressed. The nurse and client may plan how to address issues, but the actual *doing* signifies movement into the exploitation phase (Peplau 1987). Exploitation occurs when the client is able to make full use of the therapeutic relationship. After plans are implemented, the relationship may involve the identification of further issues, which entails a return to the problem identification or to the resolution of the relationship (Peplau 1952).

During the working phase, the nursing focus will be on interpersonal phenomena such as language, learning and the development of problem-solving competencies. At this time, Brooke directs the content by identifying the issues, while the nurse directs the process by encouraging exploration of issues. Together the nurse and Brooke will plan daily activities and assign structured tasks. Brooke will be helped to identify stressors and explore coping strategies. As problem-solving skills develop, success with tasks will increase. Such activities will enhance her self-concept and reduce the incidence of negative statements about self.

### Family involvement

Adolescent mental health nursing cannot lose sight of the family system and the meaning and implications of separation and admission. Brooke identified her sense of isolation and she decided to involve the family during her inpatient stay and to make contact with one or two friends.

When Brooke was admitted, her mother felt relieved, but it was important that this much-needed relief was not confused with being relieved of responsibility and authority. The nursing staff took care to involve the family in the treatment program. The level of family involvement in the treatment program is an important issue, calling for early discussion and regular review. Questions of authority, responsibility and consent must be carefully negotiated and clarified.

Brooke's parents, who had had an argumentative and abusive relationship, had separated and her stepfather had moved interstate. On meeting her mother it was evident that work was required to enable her to regain authority in her parenting role. From a nursing viewpoint, this was achieved by involving the mother in decisions about Brooke, applying sanctions to some of Brooke's behaviour, and by teaching the mother and Brooke more effective methods of managing conflict.

*Definition*

**Family therapy** involves treatment of the entire family for symptoms that are problematic. Symptoms of family disruption are often displayed in the behaviour of one family member and act as a signal of family distress (Rawlins & Heacock 1993, p.393).

The focus during family therapy is on present feelings and behaviour. Families are helped by the nurse to enact how they usually resolve conflict, support each other, enter into alliances and relieve stress. Dysfunctional communication is investigated and meanings are clarified. Dysfunctional behaviour is relabelled or reframed, so that all members can begin to make sense of the presenting behaviour. For example, Brooke's acting out could be seen as a safety valve for the rest of the family. When pressures in the family build up, a crisis develops, and the attention is focused onto Brooke rather than addressing the real issues within the family.

Brooke and her family tended not to talk about the suicide attempt after a week or two. However, the nurse continued to use the suicide event to produce positive therapeutic effects during therapy. The nurse drew on similarities between this and other situations in which Brooke felt stressed. Questioning Brooke helped her to explore thoughts or self-talk that could lead her to a solution that did not involve self-abuse and harm. In this way Brooke and her family became aware of a number of options for managing stressful situations.

## 3. RESOLUTION PHASE

The resolution phase involves the mutual termination of the relationship. It begins when all plans have been implemented and ends when no further nurse–client encounters occur. Resolution includes planning for alternative sources of support, problem prevention, and the client's integration of illness experiences (Peplau 1952). In particular, the nurse aims to reduce the incidence of dysfunctional behaviour, or minimise its effect, by offering a broad range of services necessary to support normal growth and development (West & Evans 1992). An education program developed with Brooke emphasised the influence of drugs on her behaviour, and safe sex practices. Self-esteem exercises helped to decrease Brooke's use of drugs to alter her feelings.

Nursing interventions are needed that are consumer-oriented and empower young people and their families as they work to manage illnesses and maladaptive behaviours. Case management is the key to client adjustment to the community on discharge from inpatient facilities, as it provides the link between clients and the support services they require. Case management embodies the concepts of continuity and comprehensiveness of care in a personalised manner. The main link between Peplau's theory and case management is the importance of the interactive personal relationship between the nurse and the client (Forchuk 1989). Within this relationship the nurse assumes a number of roles, depending on the client's needs, such as therapist, advocate, teacher, community organiser, and interagency coordinator.

# PROMOTION OF ADOLESCENT MENTAL HEALTH

Adolescents in western societies tend to reject preventive health measures and to take risks with their health. Risk-taking should be seen to have definite functions for young people, related to their development and to the attainment of symbols that seem to confirm adult status. The use of cigarettes and alcohol, for example, serves as a tangible, openly accessible and, not least, culturally promoted prerequisite for developing identity and lifestyle. So, although risk-taking may be medically or psychiatrically hazardous, such practices seem to be elements of coping with developmental challenges in a socially legitimate way. Through risk-taking, the adolescent, striving for identity, attains a sense of participation in the adult world.

A change in nursing perspective is warranted from a focus on problems and vulnerability to a positive emphasis on the young person's active part in growing up and dealing with problems. A variety of interventions and services (e.g. psychotherapy, home-, school- and community-based programs, and residential and hospital programs) is required to treat, manage and prevent the types of problems discussed previously (HREOC 1993). Prevention programs are required to enable adolescents to:

- develop positive self-esteem;
- make friends with themselves;
- maintain social and family relations, form intimate partnerships and cope with their sexuality;
- improve their health knowledge and access to public health services;
- gain meaning from education and employment.

Adolescence is a critical period for the development of self, identity and body image. Although adolescent mental health represents a significant social issue in need of attention and resources, there is very little research being conducted in Australia and New Zealand on adolescence. Further research is required into activities which place adolescents at risk of untoward mental and physical health. In particular, issues such as unemployment and its impact on adolescents mental health need to be captured. Such research has the potential to help nurses work more effectively with adolescent clients.

# SUMMARY

- Adolescence is a distinct and different developmental period. Biological, cognitive, psychological and social growth together fashion the maturational patterns of this age group.
- While these patterns of adolescent development show individual, cultural and socioeconomic influences, there are striking similarities alongside the genetic, racial and national differences.
- The scope of clinical dysfunction and at-risk behaviours to which adolescents are exposed is enormous.
- A comprehensive nursing assessment gathers data about the adolescent's sense of self, strengths and talents, impulsiveness, support systems and sexuality.
- Various intervention strategies for working with disturbed adolescents include milieu, individual, family and group therapies.
- Working with adolescents is demanding, and requires self-awareness and a willingness to confront transference and counter transference.
- The diversity of potential and actual problems, and their prevalence, convey the need for treatment, prevention and multiple services.

# DISCUSSION QUESTIONS

1. Mental health problems are disproportionately borne by the socially, culturally and economically disadvantaged. Discuss this issue in relation to your local community.
2. Discuss possible strategies that could be used to direct mental health intervention to the adolescent years.
3. 'Adolescence is an essentially tumultuous stage of development.' Discuss.
4. Why is it particularly important to have effective mental health promotion programs for children and adolescents? (Refer to Chapter 5.)
5. What are the components of Peplau's interpersonal relationships nursing theory? What are some of the skills that mental health nurses need to apply Peplau's model effectively?

# EXERCISES

1. Assessment skills and level of awareness are sometimes enhanced if practitioners reflect on their own development. Based on your understanding of issues that are confronted during adolescence, undertake a self-assessment of your achievements. Assess yourself according to psychosocial, cognitive, moral and physical domains. Share these insights with your peers.

2. Assess the availability of community resources that aim to address the needs of adolescents who are experiencing difficulty in the areas of anorexia and bulimia, drug abuse and unplanned pregnancy.

3. Ask a fellow student to assist you in a role play in which you undertake a mental status examination of an adolescent client. (Refer to Chapter 9.) Reverse roles and discuss your findings and experiences.

4. Use Peplau's interpersonal relationship model to role play developing a care plan for an adolescent client.

# FURTHER READING

- Kosky, R., Eshkevari, H. & Kneebone, G. (eds) (1992) *Breaking Out: Challenges in Adolescent Mental Health in Australia*, Canberra: AGPS. Presents research reviews and contextual perspectives on particular issues in adolescent mental health, including adolescent sexual behaviour, adolescent drug use, and culture.

- West, P. & Evans, C.L. (1992) *Psychiatric and Mental Health Nursing with Children and Adolescents*, Maryland: Aspen Publishers. Provides an overview of nursing knowledge and practice. Contemporary problems such as eating disorders, substance abuse, sexuality and legal issues are well presented.

- Barry, P. (1989) *Psychosocial Nursing Assessment and Intervention*, Philadelphia: Lippincott. Discusses psychosocial assessment issues. The format of assessment is easily adaptable to a range of settings and is a useful tool for beginning practitioners.

- Marriner-Tomey, A. (1994) *Nursing Theorists and their Work*. St Louis: Mosby. Identifies major nursing theorists, and reviews some of their important ideas and their implications for practice.

# OTHER RESOURCES: MOVIES

John Duigan has written and produced several excellent films, such as 'The Year my Voice Broke' (1987) and the sequel 'Flirting' (1991), which explore adolescence in an Australian context.

# REFERENCES

Barry, P. (1989) *Psychosocial Nursing Assessment and Intervention*, Philadelphia: Lippincott.

Buckmaster, C. (1989) *Collected Poems*, ed. S. McDonald, St Lucia: Queensland University Press.

Cormack, S., Pols, R. & Christie, P. (1992) 'Alcohol and drug use' in R. Kosky,

H.S. Eshkevari & G. Kneebone (eds) *Breaking Out: Challenges in Adolescent Mental Health in Australia*, Canberra: AGPS, pp.61–73.

Davis, A. (1992) 'Suicidal behaviour among adolescents: its nature and prevention' in R. Kosky, H.S. Eshkevari & G. Kneebone (eds) *Breaking Out: Challenges in Adolescent Mental Health in Australia*, Canberra: AGPS, pp.90–103.

Forchuk, C. (1989) 'Incorporating Peplau's theory and case management', *Journal of Psychosocial Nursing* 27(2), pp.35–8.

Hearne, B. (1994) 'Clinical supervision and psychiatric nursing', *Proceedings of Australia's Second International Psychiatric Nursing Conference*, Melbourne, pp.62–93.

Human Rights and Equal Opportunities Commission (1993) *Human Rights and Mental Illness*, Vols 1 & 2. Canberra: AGPS.

Kaufman, K., Brown, R., Graves, K., Henderson, P. & Revolinski, M. (1993) 'What, me worry? A survey of adolescents' concerns', *Clinical Paediatrics* 32, pp.8–14.

Kazdin, A. (1993) 'Adolescent mental health: prevention and treatment programs', *American Psychologist* 48, pp.127–41.

Kosky, R., Eshkevari, H. & Kneebone, G. (eds) (1992) *Breaking Out: Challenges in Adolescent Mental Health in Australia*, Canberra: AGPS.

McGee, R., Feehan, M., Williams, S., Partridge, F., Silva, P. & Kelly, J. (1990) 'DSM-III disorders in a large sample of adolescents', *Journal of the American Academy of Child and Adolescent Psychiatry* 29, pp.611–19.

McGee, R. & Stanton, W. (1992) 'Sources of distress among New Zealand adolescents', *Journal of Child Psychology and Psychiatry* 33, pp.999–1010.

Peplau, H.E. (1952) *Interpersonal Relations in Nursing*, New York: G.P. Putman.

Peplau, H.E. (1987) 'Interpersonal constructs for nursing practice', *Nurse Education Today* 7, pp.201–8.

Peters, R. (1988) 'Mental health promotion in children and adolescents: an emerging role for psychology', *Canadian Journal of Behavioural Science* 20, pp.389–401.

Petersen, A.C., Compas, B. E., Brooks-Gunn, J., Stemmler, M., Ey, S. & Grant, K.E. (1993) 'Depression in adolescence', *American Psychologist* 48, pp.155–68.

Powers, S., Hauser, S. & Kilner, L. (1989) 'Adolescent mental health', *American Psychologist* 44, pp.200–8.

Puskar, K. & Lamb, J. (1991) 'Life events, problems, stresses, and coping methods of adolescents', *Issues in Mental Health Nursing* 12, pp.267–81.

Rawlins, R. & Heacock, P. (1993) *Clinical Manual of Psychiatric Nursing*, St Louis: Mosby.

Rey, J. (1992) 'The epidemiological catchment area (ECA) study: implications for Australia', *Medical Journal of Australia* 156, pp.200–3.

Robins, L. N. & Regier, D. A. (1991) (eds) *Psychiatric Disorders in America*, New York: The Free Press.

Sawyer, M., Sarris, A., Baghurst, P., Cornish, C. & Kalucy, R. (1990) 'The prevalence of emotion and behavioural disorders and patterns of service utilisation in children and adolescents', *Australian and New Zealand Journal of Psychiatry* 4, pp.323–30.

Sawyer, M., Meldrum, D., Tonge, B. & Clark, J. (1992) *Mental Health and Young People* (Report to National Youth Affairs Research Scheme). Research and Evaluation Unit, Child and Adolescent Mental Health Service, Adelaide Children's Hospital.

Trautman, P. & Rotheram-Borus, M. (1988) 'Cognitive behaviour therapy with children and adolescents', *Review of Psychiatry* 7, pp.584–607.

Wells, J. E., Bushnell, J. A., Hornblow, A. W., Joyce, P. R. & Oakley-Browne, M. A. (1989) 'Christchurch psychiatric epidemiology study, 1: methodology and lifetime prevalence for specific psychiatric disorders', *Australian and New Zealand Journal of Psychiatry* 23, pp.315–26.

West, P. & Evans, C.L. (1992) *Psychiatric and Mental Health Nursing with Children and Adolescents*, Maryland: Aspen Publishers.

Wilson, H. & Kneisl, C. (1992) *Psychiatric Nursing*, Menlo Park: Addison-Wesley.

Winefield, A.H., Tiggemann, M., Winefield, H.R., & Goldney, R.D. (1993) *Growing up with Unemployment: A Longitudinal Study of its Psychological Impact*, London: Routledge.

# Health

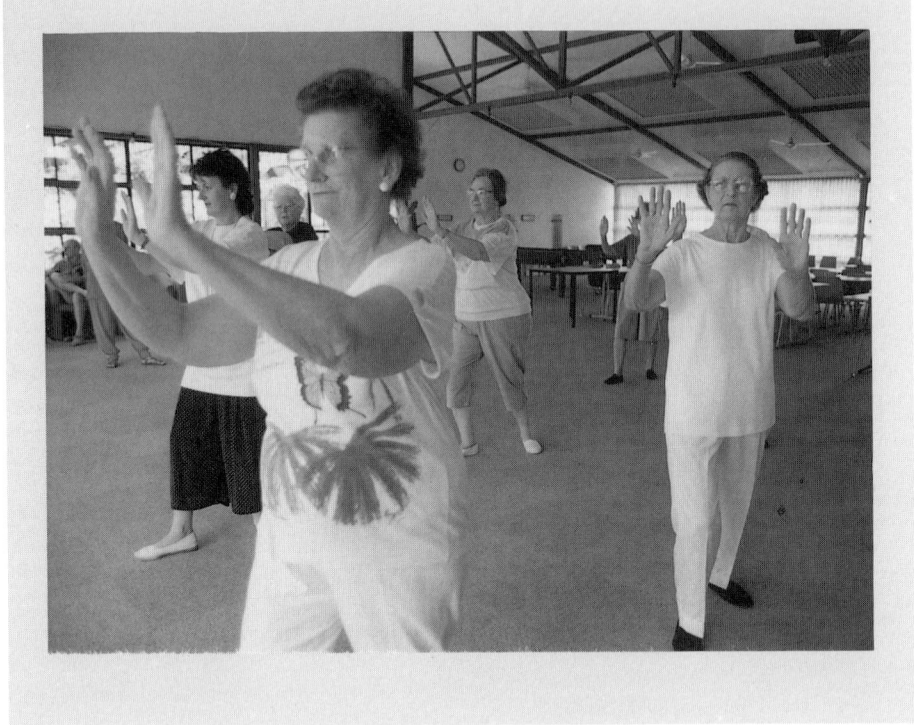

Most people over the age of 65 live full and healthy lives.

TIM OWEN

# OLDER PEOPLE

Helen Edwards

## CONTENTS

# LEARNING OBJECTIVES

This chapter will assist the reader to:

- examine demographic trends relevant to older people and their mental health;
- question the myths and 'problems' commonly associated with ageing;
- explore strategies to promote mental well-being in older people;
- demonstrate an understanding of dementia and depression in older people;
- develop care plans for older people with selected mental disorders.

# INTRODUCTION

The proportion of older people in our communities is increasing to the extent that it is likely that health care professionals of the future will be working predominantly with this group of people. This chapter focuses on the mental health of older people. Strategies to promote mental health are discussed and then two case histories are presented to illustrate the nature of the two **mental disorders** selected as particularly relevant to the older population: **dementia** and **depression**. While a brief review of each disorder is given, the focus of the case histories is nursing care and nursing interventions. As most older people remain in the community with their family, this nursing care usually takes place in the community setting. Sometimes, however, placement has to be considered.

# DEMOGRAPHY OF AGEING

The increasing proportion of older people in the population is commonly referred to as the 'greying' of Australia. In 1900, 4% of the Australian population were aged 65 years and over, compared with 9% in 1961 and 11% in 1989. Between 1989 and 2011, it has been projected that there will be a 60% increase in the older (65 years and over) population. By 2031 it is predicted that 20% of the population will be over 65 years of age (Bureau of Immigration Research 1991). In 1991, 11.3% of the New Zealand population were aged 65 years and over. It is expected that this will increase to 11.9% in 2001 and 19.4% in 2031 (Population and Demographic Department, New Zealand 1991). The increasing proportion of the population over 65 years of age is a common trend in developed countries. As Jorm and Henderson (1993) note, however, the increase will be greater in countries like Australia and New Zealand, which have relatively young populations when compared with countries such as Britain or Sweden.

Of particular concern for health professionals is the growth of the 80 years and over age group, which will increase more rapidly than the 65–80 age group. By 2031, it is predicted that there will be 1.4 million people in Australia aged

80 and over, compared with 357000 in 1989. Based on 1986 census data, it is predicted that the percentage of the New Zealand population aged 85 years and over will increase from 0.8% in 1986 to 1.3% in 2001 and 2.3% in 2031. The large numbers of 'older' old people will have an impact on the health care system, as it is this group that is likely to make the most demands on the system. Over the next four decades it seems inevitable that, regardless of the setting in which they work, nurses in Australia and New Zealand will find themselves working more and more with older people. Therefore, it is imperative that nurses understand both the ageing process and the role of nursing in promoting the physical and mental well-being of older people.

## CRITICAL GERONTOLOGY

Much attention has been focused on the impact that an ageing population will have on society. Governments have examined the economic and social implications and, in particular, have investigated how services need to be reorganised to meet the needs of older people. The media constantly raise concern about the effect of an ageing population on the health care system, the welfare system and families. All these issues are important and need to be considered. However, they are frequently portrayed as 'problems'. By regarding the issues as problems, it is often implied that older people themselves are the cause of the 'problems'. The fact that systems and organisations in society may actually contribute to some of the 'problems' associated with an ageing population is rarely acknowledged.

Phillipson and Walker (1987) suggest that a critical gerontology perspective challenges the myths of old age. This perspective recognises that many of the problems facing older people are created by the systems and organisations that exist in society. Such a perspective disputes the idea that individuals are responsible for their own predicament. Working within this framework, nurses can view ageing as a normal process and recognise that older people can, with support and empowerment, exert control over the quality of their lives.

Many myths associated with ageing can be refuted. For example, Australian data suggests that most people over 60 years of age believe their health to be 'good' or 'fair' (Jones 1989). Most older people live in their own home, with a spouse or a sibling, and only a small percentage (less than 7%) live in nursing homes, hostels or hospitals. Community services such as Meals on Wheels and domiciliary nursing are used by less than 12% of older people (Howe & Sharwood 1989). The majority of older people do not need assistance with their daily living activities, although those over 85 years of age are more likely to require such assistance (ABS 1990). Overall, there is evidence to affirm that older people are independent, busy and positive members of society. It should not be considered anything but normal for an 80- or 90-year-old to be reasonably physically healthy, mentally competent and socially active. Voice Box 14.1 gives a personal account of an older person's view of ageing.

# *V*OICE BOX 14.1: Gwen

My name is Gwen and I am 82 years of age. My husband, Len, died 10 years ago and I have lived on my own ever since. I have two sons who visit or call me on the phone. I have no serious health problems but I'm treated by my doctor for high blood pressure and occasional chest pains. I can still move around and do most of my own housework but because I have arthritis I find it a bit hard to get up and down the stairs and I can't do gardening any more. I think I'm very well because I can get around and do most of the things I want to do.

Since my husband died my neighbours have been very good to me. One set take me shopping once a week and another take me to church every Sunday. I also go to a Senior Citizens Centre once a week and am picked up by the Centre bus. I have a man come in to do my gardening and to mow the lawn, and a woman comes in once a month to do the heavy things around the house. I like living on my own as I can do what I want when I want. My sons have suggested a hostel or retirement village but I think that should be left for those who really need those type of services. I have many friends at the Centre and we ring each other during the week and sometimes we visit each other for lunch. I read a lot and enjoy knitting and making crafts for my grandchildren and the Centre. I look forward to many more happy years in my home.

My only regret is that Len died so young and has not been around for me to enjoy his company. He was very sick though and I didn't want him to suffer. It was hard at first but I've got used to it.

I don't consider myself to be old. I know I'm not as young as I used to be but I think being old is not being able to do what you want to do and not being happy with your life. I'm very happy but I get cranky because I can't do the gardening and some things around the house. I know some people who are worse off than me and I hope I don't get their problems. I still have a very active mind and I listen to discussions on the radio and read about the government in the paper. In my local church we have monthly groups where we talk about issues and often we invite people to hear what we have to say about an issue or we write to our local member. I am also a member of the neighbourhood watch program and my house is a safety house for young children. I know I can't do much in the community any more but I try to do my little bit. I am very content with my life.

*Note*   Gwen lives in a suburb in Brisbane and wrote this in response to a request for her to tell us about her life at present and 'getting older'.

# *S*TRATEGIES TO PROMOTE MENTAL WELL-BEING

Mental disorders in older people are difficult to diagnose, but research has identified some causal factors with the potential to reduce the mental health of older people. A longitudinal study of more than 2000 men, conducted by

Aldwin et al. (1989), concluded that individual lifestyle factors, stressors and coping mechanisms are likely causal factors in the emotional distress of older people. Level of social support and physical health were found to be major determinants of mental disorder in another longitudinal study of people over 65 years of age (Haug, Breslau & Folmar 1989). Another factor which has been demonstrated to influence mental health in older people is increased control and autonomy (Hofland 1988; Reich & Zautra 1989). Research which has specifically examined coping processes in old age has found that older people appear capable of using a wide repertoire of coping strategies, and appear to be able to select the most effective ones for a given situation (Folkman, Lazarus & Pimley 1987; Irion & Blanchard-Fields 1987).

Nurses can use the findings of these studies as the basis for interventions to maintain the mental health of older people and to assist in the prevention of some mental disorders. Below are suggestions of interventions for nurses to use with older people.

- Involve older people in decisions that affect them, and enable them to take control of their lives.
- Ensure that older people have adequate and effective social support and that they use it when needed.
- Assist older people to manage any physical health problems they may have.
- Help older people to examine their lifestyles to identify factors that could affect their physical and mental health.
- Encourage older people to continue to use coping strategies already familiar to them.
- Encourage the use of a wide variety of coping strategies, including some new ones.
- Encourage older people to select the coping strategies they believe will be most effective to deal with their problems.
- Encourage older people to seek advice from professionals when appropriate.

Despite all that nurses can do to promote the mental health of older people, a certain percentage of people aged over 65 develop mental disorders. The next section will examine the incidence of mental disorder in the older population and problems in diagnosing mental disorder in older people.

## MENTAL DISORDER IN OLDER PEOPLE

The estimated incidence of mental disorder in older people varies from 4% to 45% (Hooyman & Kiyak 1995). The discrepancy between rates results from the measurements used, the population sampled and the categories of disorders used (Aldwin et al. 1989). Despite the fact that the incidence of mental disorder in the older population is difficult to determine, it is a serious issue for nurses. The Federal Human Rights and Equal Opportunities Commission Inquiry into the

Mentally Ill (1993) reports that the health care system ignores older people who are mentally ill. The inquiry found that older people with mental disorders are often placed in inappropriate institutions, and are more likely to get drugs, less likely to receive psychotherapy, and less likely to use outpatient services than younger patients. Therefore, even if only a small percentage of older people have a mental disorder, the mental health of this age group is an issue that must be addressed by health professionals, including nurses. In the following section, two case histories will be presented to explore the nurse's role in disorders common in old age: dementia and depression.

## Dementia

**Dementia** is an organic mental disorder in which a person's previous level of functioning declines in multiple cognitive areas, including memory. An important feature of dementia is that, although there is global, progressive deterioration in thinking, judgment, orientation, language, comprehension, behaviour and emotion, consciousness is not impaired. For a confidant diagnosis of dementia to be made, the symptoms and impairments should have been evident for at least six months and be severe enough to interfere significantly with work or social activities or relationships (American Psychiatric Association 1994). Dementia develops across a continuum and is generally described as either mild, moderate or severe.

### Prevalence

While the point has been made earlier that only a small proportion of older people have a mental disorder, the increasing proportion of 'older' old people will result in a substantial increase in the prevalence of dementia. It is estimated that approximately 140 000 Australians have moderate to severe dementia (Alzheimer's Disease and Related Disorders Society (ADARDS) 1990). Jorm et al. (1987) integrated data from 22 studies and found that although prevalence rates differed greatly from study to study, a consistent trend was that prevalence doubled for every 5.1 years of age. It is estimated that one in ten Australians aged 70 and over, and one in four aged 80 and over, will develop dementia (ADARDS 1990). The rise is expected to be greater for **Alzheimer's disease** than for the other types of dementia. An important demographic fact for nurses is that approximately 50% of people in nursing homes in Australia have dementia (ADARDS 1990). Therefore, it is clear that, regardless of the setting in which they work, nurses are likely to encounter older people with dementia.

### Types

Different types of dementia are usually described according to their underlying cause. Four major types and their causes have been identified to date.

1. *Alzheimer's disease* (sometimes referred to as Senile Dementia of the Alzheimer Type (SDAT)), which involves changes to the structure of the brain itself and in the chemical functioning of the brain (50% of dementia).

2. *Vascular dementia* (including multi-infarct dementia), which usually results from an infarction of the brain due to vascular disease (20% of dementia).

3. *Mixed dementia*, which involves features of both Alzheimer's disease and vascular dementia (20% of dementia).

4. *Dementia due to other causes* such as AIDS, Parkinson's disease or severe alcohol abuse (10% of dementia).

The types of dementia defined above can present with different symptoms, and these differences, together with the history of the development of the disorder, enable accurate diagnosis (Mace & Rabins 1991; Woods 1989). Although the causes are not yet fully understood, prevention related to the known risk factors is possible (Jorm 1990; Jorm & Henderson 1993).

# CASE STUDY 14.1: *Dementia*

Mrs Mary Black is cared for at home by her husband, Harry. She was diagnosed with dementia (Alzheimer's disease) 12 months ago and is now considered by her doctor to have moderate dementia. Mary and Harry have two married children who live interstate. They have no other relatives to help them, but their neighbours assist Harry when they can. Harry has been caring for his wife with no formal help but recently his GP became concerned about Harry's ability to keep on caring for his wife and referred their case to the community health nurse. The nurse assessed Mary and the summary below highlights important information obtained during the assessment.

## Summary of Mary's assessment

Mary cannot remember any new information given to her but can remember her name and some of her personal and family details. Most of the time she is disoriented in time and place, and her judgment and problem solving are impaired. Her concentration span is poor and she can perform only simple, well-learned behaviours. She requires assistance with dressing and hygiene and is occasionally incontinent of urine and faeces. While Mary's speech is unaffected, she is frequently incoherent and repetitive. An assessment of her cognitive status revealed that she had a Mini Mental State Examination score of 15 (see Folstein, Folstein & McHugh 1975). During the day Mary either drops off to sleep in her chair or wanders around the house. She has, on occasions, been found down the street or in a neighbour's yard. Harry says the most difficult behaviour he has to deal with is Mary's aggressive and violent outbursts, which are unpredictable but appear to occur when he is showering her. Mary has no other major illness and the only medication she takes is thioridazine (Melleril), 10 mg three times a day, to control her agitation.

## Care package

Following an in-depth assessment of Mary and Harry's situation, the nurse, in collaboration with Harry, organised the following care package:

- Domiciliary nursing services for hygiene, three times a week.
- Home help for domestic assistance, once a week.
- Day Centre care for Mary, to enable Harry to do his shopping and have lunch with his mates at the local RSL, etc. twice a week.
- In-home respite care to enable Harry to keep doctors' appointments, etc. as required.
- Longer-term respite care (three weeks) available for Harry if he wants a break at some stage.
- Volunteer visitors from a local church group.
- Harry to begin attending his local ADARDS group for education, support and counselling.

The nurse developed a plan of care for Harry and Mary. This plan and the related care package focused on maximising Mary's functional ability and helping Harry to cope with her illness. Research suggests that these principles are the most effective for assisting Alzheimer's patients and their caregivers (Brodaty & Gresham 1989; Buckwalter, Abraham & Neundorger 1988; Wilson 1989). There were several nursing diagnoses in the plan of care, and two of these and some selected interventions are listed in Box 14.1. For more suggestions regarding appropriate interventions, readers are referred to Carpenito 1992; Gwyther 1985; Mace and Rabins 1991; Ryden and Feldt, 1992; Wilson and Kneisl, 1992; Woods, 1989.

$\mathbb{B}$ O X   1 4 . 1 :   *Nursing care: Mary and Harry*

**Nursing diagnosis: Alteration in thought process related to memory impairment (secondary to dementia)**

*Independent nursing interventions*

The nurse advised Harry to:

- Provide Mary with clear, simple, step-by-step directions, one at a time.
- Not ask Mary to do things beyond her capabilities.
- Give verbal reminders if Mary refuses or forgets to do something.
- Use supportive statements when Mary fabricates stories (e.g. 'Yes, I know it's hard when things slip your mind').

*continued ...*

- Keep to routines as much as possible, particularly when dressing Mary or attending to her hygiene. A regular daily schedule for meals and showering will also help.
- Provide cues for Mary to aid her memory (e.g. 'It's Monday today, Mary, so the nurse will be here today to give you your shower').
- Encourage Mary to use clocks, calendars, etc. and to read the newspapers.
- Talk to Mary about happy experiences or activities they have shared. (This can be aided by the use of a family photo album or by playing some familiar, relevant music.)
- Talk to Mary about current events in the newspapers or on TV, even if she does not appear to follow all the details.
- Continue to use the strategies and cues that he finds best for helping Mary to use her memory.

### Nursing diagnosis: Potential risk for violence related to aggression/agitation (secondary to dementia)

*Independent nursing interventions*

The nurse advised Harry to:

- Keep to consistent routines as much as possible.
- Identify triggers which appear to elicit aggressive behaviour from Mary (e.g. certain clothes/shoes, as they could be too tight). Often there is another cause for the aggression (e.g. constipation, pain, fear).
- Approach Mary in full view, calling her by name and avoiding touch. Most aggressive behaviour occurs in response to personal touch or invasion of personal space.
- Keep Mary physically comfortable (i.e. dry, clean, warm).
- Try to give Mary some choice and sense of control in activities where this is possible (e.g. which clothes to wear; what to have for dinner). Be careful not to ask too many questions or to give her too many choices.
- Provide Mary with some positive social experiences (e.g. neighbours in for afternoon tea; playing some of her favourite music).
- Try to obtain a balance between overstimulating Mary and understimulating her (e.g. too many visitors/outings versus none).
- Be undemanding, supportive and calm when Mary is aggressive. Leave Mary alone for a while and return later to complete the activity, providing her safety is not compromised.
- Use rocking, holding hands, patting or soothing music to calm Mary when agitated.
- Schedule physical exercise/activity into each day (e.g. walk to the local park, gardening).

## Questions

1. How might the community nurse respond to Harry's statement: 'I don't know how I will manage Mary if she gets any worse'?
2. What other issues are likely to arise as Harry continues to care for Mary?

# Depression

Many of the cognitive impairments that occur with dementia can also occur with **depression**. It has been suggested that 30% of people with dementia could be more correctly diagnosed as having depression (Minichiello, Alexander & Jones 1992). As depression is treatable, it is crucial to identify the underlying cause of any cognitive changes in older people (Miller 1990). When the older person's depressive illness is manifested mainly by a physical symptom (e.g. excessive tiredness, chest pain), diagnosis can be difficult and symptoms may be misinterpreted as a physical illness. Because of poor health and the social and cognitive changes that can be associated with ageing, it is possible that older people may exhibit depressive symptoms without satisfying DSM-IV criteria. All these factors may result in the underdiagnosis and mistreatment of depression in older people.

Another concern when diagnosing depression in older people is the differentiation between types of depression. Older people have to deal with many unhappy and serious life events (e.g. relocation, death of loved ones or thoughts of their own impending death) and it is possible that these may trigger depressive reactions. It is important to distinguish major depression from bipolar disorders, sadness, and grief reactions. Most depressions in older people are unipolar and manic-depressive disorders are rare, while secondary or reactive depressions to significant life events are common in older people.

## Prevalence

The true prevalence of depression in later life is difficult to determine and estimated prevalence rates range from 5% to 44% (Blazer 1986). In an Australian community sample of older people, Kay, Henderson and Scott (1985) found that 23% of 70–79 year olds were depressed and that 38% of those of 80 years and over were depressed. More recent research indicates that depressive disorders are not as common in the older age group as in the younger age group (Feinson 1989; Hendrie & Crossett 1990). Bowers (1991) concludes from the evidence available that the minimum prevalence for major depression in the community may be about 10%. According to Parmelee, Katz and Lawton (1989), 12% of older adults living in nursing homes meet the criteria for major depression, while 30% exhibit minor depressive symptoms. It has also been estimated that depression accounted for 50% of admissions to a psychogeriatric unit (Gilchrist et al. 1985).

The incidence or prevalence of depression in older people makes it a serious health issue. The prognosis for depression in older people is poor compared with that of younger people, and depends on the initial severity of the depression, the older person's physical health, and the presence of serious life events (Williams 1989). Older people are also more likely than younger people to experience further depressive episodes (Blacker & Clare 1987). Older men with severe physical and/or mental illness and a likelihood of institutionalisation are at greater risk of **suicide** than women (Williams 1989). The suicide rate, according to Osgood (1985), is higher for older adults than for any other age group.

## Aetiology

Although the aetiology of depression has been discussed earlier, in Chapter 9, psychological factors are considered to play a major role in the development of depression in older people. Factors contributing to depression in older people include loss of loved ones, social isolation, retirement, and changes in living arrangements (Burvill, Stampfer & Hall 1986). An Australian study by Henderson, Scott and Kay (1986) found that older people who lived alone had more dysphoric symptoms (e.g. agitation, uneasiness) than those who lived in a shared household. There were, however, no differences between the groups in terms of clinical depression.

The role of social support has been identified as a critical factor in the development of depression in older people. Recent research suggests that availability of support may not be as important as the amount or type of support given. Dean, Kolody and Wood (1990) found that low support from an available spouse had a stronger negative effect on depressive symptoms than widowhood. Low support from children who were available to provide support was found to increase the risk of depression, while not having children did not. This study also found that, for older people, support from friends exerted stronger positive effects on depressive symptoms, whereas support from children exerted weak effects, and support from other relatives exerted no effects. These results highlight the need for individual assessment of each older person's situation.

## Management

As discussed in Chapter 11, management of depression can be by pharmacological or non-pharmacological treatments, or a combination of both (Johnson & Wilson 1989). The commonest treatment for the depressed elderly is pharmacological—particularly for those with a major depression. Although antidepressants work well for some older people, the side effects prevent their use in others. These side effects, which include postural hypotension, cardiac arrhythmia, urinary retention, disorientation and dry mouth, may be more detrimental than the depression itself. Because of these side effects, more doctors are suggesting alternative treatments for older people.

Older people with depression have been successfully treated with specific psychotherapy, usually in combination with antidepressants (Johnson & Wilson

1989). Viney, Benjamin and Preston (1989) have demonstrated the benefits of personal construct therapy in reducing depression in a group of older adults. Secondary or reactionary depression in older people appears to respond well to supportive psychotherapy, which allows them to review and come to terms with the stresses in their life and to re-establish control and emotional stability (Hooyman & Kiyak 1995). A study comparing the effects of behavioural, cognitive and psychodynamic therapy for a group of people over 60 found that, after one year, there were no differences between the treatment groups. About half the participants showed no depressive symptoms after the one-year follow-up. From recent reviews of cognitive behaviour theory and empirical evidence from studies involving cognitive behaviour therapy (CBT), it can be concluded that CBT has the potential to be an effective intervention for depression in older people (Beck 1991; Oei & Free 1994). Electroconvulsive therapy has been found to be safe and effective for older people with severe depression (Benhow 1987. However, some psychiatrists avoid using it because of its potentially harmful effects on memory.

## CASE STUDY 14.2: *Depression*

Bill White is a 72-year-old man, admitted as an inpatient to a psychogeriatric unit for treatment of depression. Bill's wife had suffered from a chronic lung disease and he had looked after her, at home, for five years until she died six months ago. During his time as a carer, Bill received an extensive care package which enabled him to provide care for his wife as well as maintain his social and family contacts. His two married children provided as much help and assistance as they could, given their own family responsibilities. The community health nurse kept in contact with Bill for the first month after his wife's death and, according to her, he appeared to be coping 'reasonably well with his loss'. Bill had told the nurse that he was glad his wife's suffering was over. He had maintained his social contact with his mates at the local bowls club and would frequently visit the day care centre his wife had attended.

It appears that Bill was coping with the loss of his wife until about two months after her death. At this time he stopped going to the bowls club and visiting the day care centre. His family also noted that he would not accept their invitations for meals. Over the next three months his children reported that their father:

- lost interest in everything;
- sat around the house all day, sleeping or dozing off in front of the television;

*continued ...*

- refused to join in any social activities or have any visitors;
- was very 'down' and when asked why he wouldn't go out any more, would say 'What's the point?', 'Why would anybody want to talk to me?' or 'I'm too tired';
- appeared not to be able to make any decisions (e.g. forgot to pay bills or go shopping);
- ate very little of the food his daughter provided for him, resulting in a significant weight loss; and
- frequently needed reminding to get dressed or to shower and shave.

Bill's children contacted the community nurse who used to visit his wife. After assessing Bill, the nurse identified depressive symptoms and, knowing the risk of suicide, referred him to his general practitioner who prescribed an antidepressant (Doxepin 75 mg/day). After one month of antidepressant medication and support from the community nurse, there was little change in Bill's behaviour and he was referred to a psychiatrist who organised for Bill to be admitted for assessment.

After one week of assessment it was concluded that Bill did not have any underlying organic factor or other mental disorder which could account for his symptoms. He was diagnosed as suffering from 'adjustment disorder with depressed mood'. The management of Bill's depression included antidepressants (Doxepin 100 mg/day), cognitive behaviour therapy (group and individual sessions), and psychoeducation focusing on coping skills. The nurse caring for Bill developed a care plan to meet his needs and to complement his management plan. Box 14.2 displays one of the nursing diagnoses and accompanying interventions which appeared on Bill's care plan.

Bill remained in hospital for one month. During this time he regained some weight, began to take responsibility for his self-care, became involved in the social activities of the unit, increased his social interactions and began to talk about his wife and their life together. It was decided that Bill could be discharged on antidepressants and that he should attend cognitive behaviour therapy sessions once a week. A discharge plan was formulated in consultation with Bill, his family, and his community health nurse.

## Questions

1. What would be the community nurse's priorities in providing care for Bill?
2. What community services/organisations/activities could the community nurse draw on to assist Bill on discharge from hospital?

B OX 1 4 . 2 : *Nursing care: Bill*

## Nursing diagnosis: Dysfunctional grieving related to loss of wife

*Independent nursing interventions*

Promote a trusting relationship with Bill by:

- Scheduling time to meet and talk with him.
- Communicating simply, clearly and directly.
- Creating a safe and private environment to promote sharing.
- Demonstrating respect for his views on religion and politics.
- Promoting his self-worth by focusing on his strengths (e.g. friends, family, bowling interests).

Promote grief work by:

- Allowing Bill to express his grief—he often starts to cry and then stops saying 'This is silly'.
- Acknowledging Bill's grief (e.g. 'It must be difficult').
- Encouraging Bill to express his feelings (e.g. anger, guilt, denial, fear).
- Encouraging Bill to maintain contact with his family and to discuss his loss with them.
- Encouraging Bill to re-establish contact with his friends and to discuss his loss with them.
- Encouraging Bill to reminisce and review his life and his relationship with his wife.

Assist Bill to use a variety of coping strategies by:

- Having Bill describe how he has dealt with stress in the past.
- Informing Bill of the types of strategies he could use (e.g. focusing on problems and emotions).
- Having Bill create a list of the strategies he would feel comfortable in using.
- Encouraging Bill to use the strategies from his list.
- Reinforcing Bill's use of coping strategies.

S UMMARY

- The majority of older people are independent, active and positive members of society.
- Most of the myths associated with ageing can be refuted.
- The mental health of older people can be enhanced by increasing their control and autonomy and by encouraging the use of a range of coping strategies.

- Older people with mental disorders have been identified as 'at risk' for receiving inappropriate and ineffective care.
- Dementia, especially of the Alzheimer's type, is most common in those over 80 years of age.
- People with dementia can be helped to remain in their family environment through services and care that maximise the individual's functional ability, and provide education and support for the family.
- Depression in older people is a common, treatable disorder which is often misdiagnosed.
- Management of depression in older people can include a combination of therapy (e.g. drug therapy, cognitive behaviour therapy), psychoeducation, counselling and social support.

## DISCUSSION QUESTIONS

1. Identify aspects of the health care system which may contribute to the 'problems' associated with ageing. Suggest ways in which the health care system could promote ageing as a normal and positive process.
2. 'Regardless of context or setting, the promotion of mental health is a primary role for all nurses who work with older people.' Discuss this statement, the constraints that may prevent nurses from carrying out this role, and ways to overcome the identified constraints.

## EXERCISES

1. Consider the data presented in the first case history and suggest other nursing diagnoses that are likely to be included in a plan of care for Mary and Harry.
2. For the diagnoses identified in Exercise 1, complete a full care plan (i.e. expected outcome, outcome criteria, nursing interventions, rationales).
3. Outline other interventions that the nurse could use to monitor Mary's progress and treatment.
4. With regard to the second case study, suggest other nursing diagnoses for possible inclusion in Bill's care plan.
5. For the diagnoses identified in Exercise 4, complete a care plan (i.e. expected outcomes, outcome criteria, nursing interventions, rationales).
6. Outline other interventions the nurse should use to monitor Bill's progress and treatment on discharge from hospital.

# FURTHER READING

- Dean, A., Kolody, B. & Wood, P. (1990) 'Effects of social support from various sources on depression in elderly persons', *Journal of Health and Social Behaviour* 31 June, pp.148–61. This article describes research which examined the effect of expressive support on depressive symptoms in older people.
- Jorm, A.F. & Henderson, A.S. (1993) *The Problem of Dementia in Australia* (3rd edn), Canberra: AGPS. This report provides an overview of the epidemiology of dementia, citing what is known about the incidence, prevalence and risk factors of the problem.
- Minichiello, V., Alexander, L. & Jones, D. (eds) (1992) *Gerontology: A Multi-disciplinary Approach*, Sydney: Prentice Hall. This Australian text addresses practice and public policy issues related to older people. It provides a comprehensive review of the biological, sociological and psychological aspects of ageing.

# REFERENCES

Aldwin, C.M., Spiro, A., Levenson, M.R. & Bosse, R. (1989) 'Longitudinal findings from the normative aging study: 1. Does mental health change with age?' *Psychology and Aging* 4, pp.295–306.

Alzheimer's Disease and Related Disorders Society (ADARDS) (1990) *A Fair Go for Dementia*.

American Psychiatric Association (1994) *Diagnostic and Statistical Manual of Mental Disorders* 4th edn (DSM-IV), Washington: American Psychiatric Association.

Australian Bureau of Statistics (ABS) (1990) *Disability and Handicap, Australia 1988* Canberra: ABS.

Beck, L. (1991) 'Cognitive therapy: a 30 year retrospective', *American Psychiatrist* 46, pp.368–75.

Benhow, S.M. (1987) 'The use of electroconvulsive therapy in old age psychiatry', *International Journal of Geriatric Psychiatry* 2, pp.25–30.

Blacker, C.V.R. & Clare, A.W. (1987) 'Depressive disorder in primary care', *British Journal of Psychiatry* 150, pp.737–51.

Blazer, D.G. (1986) 'Depression: paradoxically a cause for hope', *Generations* 10(3), pp.21–3.

Bowers, J. (1991) *Recognition and Knowledge of Dementia and Depression in the Elderly by General Practitioners*, doctoral thesis, Australian National University, Canberra.

Brodaty, H. & Gresham, M. (1989) 'Effect of a training programme to reduce stress in carers of patients with dementia', *British Medical Journal* 299, pp.1375–9.

Buckwalter, K., Abraham, I. & Neundorger, M. (1988) 'Alzheimer's disease: involving nursing in the development and implementation of health care for patients and families', *Nurse Clinician North America* 23, pp.1–9.

Bureau of Immigration Research (1991) *Australia's Population Trends and Prospects 1990*, Canberra: AGPS.

Burvill, P.W., Stampfer, H. & Hall, W. (1986) 'Does depressive illness in the elderly have a poor prognosis?' *Australian and New Zealand Journal of Psychiatry* 20, pp.422–7.

Carpenito, L.J. (1992) *Nursing Diagnosis: Application to Clinical Practice* (4th edn), New York: Lippincott.

Dean, A., Kolody, B. & Wood, P. (1990) 'Effects of social support from various sources on depression in elderly persons', *Journal of Health and Social Behaviour* 31 (June), pp.148–61.

Feinson, M.C. (1989) 'Are psychological disorders most prevalent among older adults? Examining the evidence', *Social Science and Medicine* 29, pp.1175–81.

Folkman, S., Lazarus, R.S. & Pimley, S. (1987) 'Age differences in stress and coping processes', *Psychology and Aging* 2, pp.171–84.

Folstein, M.F., Folstein, S.E. & McHugh, P.R. (1975) 'Mini-mental state: a practical method for grading the cognitive state of patients for the clinician', *Journal of Psychiatric Research* 12, pp.189–98.

Gilchrist, P., Rozenbilds, U., Martin, E. & Connelly, H. (1985) 'A study of 100 consecutive admissions to a psychogeriatric unit', *Medical Journal of Australia* 143, pp.236–7.

Gwyther, L. (1985) *Care of Alzheimer's Patients: A Manual for Nursing Home Staff*, American Health Care Association and Alzheimer's Disease and Related Disorders Association.

Haug, M.R., Breslau, N. & Folmar, S.J. (1989) 'Coping resources and selective survival in mental health of the elderly', *Research on Aging* 11, pp.468–91.

Henderson, A.S., Scott, R. & Kay, D.W. (1986) 'The elderly who live alone: their mental health and social relationships', *Australian and New Zealand Journal of Psychiatry* 20, pp.202–9.

Hendrie, H.C. & Crossett, J.H.W. (1990) 'An overview of depression in the elderly', *Psychiatric Annals* 20, pp.64–66, 69–70.

Hofland, B. (1988) 'Autonomy in long term care: background issues and a programmatic response', *Gerontologist* 28, pp.3–9.

Hooyman, N.R. & Kiyak, H.A. (1995) *Social Gerontology: A Multidisciplinary Perspective* (4th edn), Boston: Allyn & Bacon.

Howe, A. & Sharwood, P. (1989) 'The old old or the new old? Part 2: Health Status and trends of the population aged 80 years and over' *Journal of the Australian Population Association* 6, pp.18–32.

Human Rights and Equal Opportunities Commission (1993) *Human Rights and Mental Illness: Report of the National Inquiry into the Human Rights of People with Mental Illness* Vols 1 & 2, Canberra: AGPS.

Irion, J.C. & Blanchard-Fields, F. (1987) 'A cross-sectional comparison of adaptive coping in adulthood', *Journal of Gerontology* 42, pp.502–4.

Johnson, G.F.S. & Wilson, P. (1989) 'The management of depression: a review of pharmacological and non-pharmacological treatments', *Medical Journal of Australia* 151, pp.397–406.

Jones, S. (1989) 'Pills, perception and participation: health in older age', *Australian Journal on Aging* 8, pp.13–17.

Jorm, A.F. (1990) *The Epidemiology of Alzheimer's Disease and Related Disorders*, London: Chapman & Hall.

Jorm, A.F. & Henderson, A.S. (1993) *The Problem of Dementia in Australia* (3rd edn), Canberra: AGPS.

Jorm, A.F., Korten, A.E. & Henderson, A.S. (1987) 'The prevalence of dementia: a quantitative integration of the literature', *Acta Psychiatrica Scandinavica* 76, pp.465–79.

Kay, D.W., Henderson, A.S. & Scott, R. (1985) 'Dementia and depression among the elderly living in a Hobart community: the effect of the diagnostic criteria on the prevalence rates', *Psychological Medicine* 15, pp.771–88.

Mace, N. & Rabins, P. (1991) *The 36-hour Day: A Family Guide to Caring for Persons with Alzheimer's Disease, Related Dementing Illnesses, and Memory Loss in Later Life*, Baltimore: The Johns Hopkins University Press.

Miller, C.A. (1990) *Nursing Care for Older Adults*, Glenview, IL: Scott, Foresman.

Minichiello, V., Alexander, L. & Jones, D. (eds) (1992) *Gerontology: A Multidisciplinary Approach*, Sydney: Prentice Hall.

Oei, T. & Free, M.L. (1994) 'Do cognitive behaviour therapies validate cognitive models of mood disorders?: A review of empirical evidence', *International Journal of Psychology* (in press).

Osgood, N.J. (1985) *Suicide in the Elderly*, Rockville, Md: Aspen.

Parmelee, P.A., Katz, I.R. & Lawton, M.P. (1989) 'Depression among institutionalised aged: assessment and prevalence estimation', *Journal of Gerontology: Medical Sciences* 44(1), M22–29.

Phillipson, C. & Walker, A. (1987) 'The case for a critical gerontology' in S. di Gregorio (ed.) *Social Gerontology: New Directions*, London: Croom Helm.

Population and Demographic Department (1991) *Statistics*. New Zealand.

Reich, J.W. & Zautra, A.J. (1989) 'A perceived control intervention for at-risk older adults', *Psychology and Aging* 4, pp.415–24.

Ryden, M. & Feldt, K. (1992) 'Goal-directed care: caring for aggressive nursing home residents with dementia', *Journal of Gerontological Nursing*, November, pp.35–42.

Viney, L.L., Benjamin, Y.N. & Preston, C.A. (1989) 'An evaluation of personal construct therapy for the elderly', *British Journal of Medical Psychology* 62, pp.35–41.

Williams, G.O. (1989) 'Management of depression in the elderly', *Primary Care* 16, pp.451–74.

Wilson, H. (1989) 'Family caregiving for a relative with Alzheimer's dementia: coping with negative choices', *Nursing Research* 38, pp.94–8.

Wilson, H. & Kneisl, C. (1992) *Psychiatric Nursing* (4th edn), Menlo Park, California: Addison-Wesley.

Woods, R.T. (1989) *Alzheimer's Disease: Coping with a Living Death*, London: Souvenir Press.

# PART VI

# PRACTICE SETTINGS

Mental health nursing practice takes place in all settings where nurses work, from the community to the psychiatric unit and general hospital ward. The introduction of the National Mental Health Policy and Plan in Australia in 1992 will ensure the mainstreaming of mental health services and the integration of hospital and community care. As a consequence of this reform, more nurses will be caring for patients with complex physical and mental health needs. Chapter 15 takes up this theme by considering holistic nursing practice in acute hospital settings. The chapter draws attention to important mental health needs in people with physical illnesses and recognises the complexity of caring for people with a mental illness and a concurrent physical illness. The discussion of these issues emphasises the importance of holistic care.

The theme of holistic care continues in Chapter 16, as the challenge of mental health nursing practice in rural communities is examined from the perspective of the generalist community nurse. An extended case study illustrates the special needs of rural communities and considers nursing interventions at the level of the community and the individual.

Chapter 17 continues the holistic theme and considers specialised nursing practice in integrated mental health services from within the framework of the biopsychosocial model of care. The important concepts of biological primacy and social and psychological supremacy are introduced. Nursing and multidisciplinary team interventions are strongly emphasised, and two case studies illustrate the link between community and hospital services and the intersectoral collaboration required in mental health care.

# Typhoid fever ward at the Royal Brisbane Hospital, circa 1898

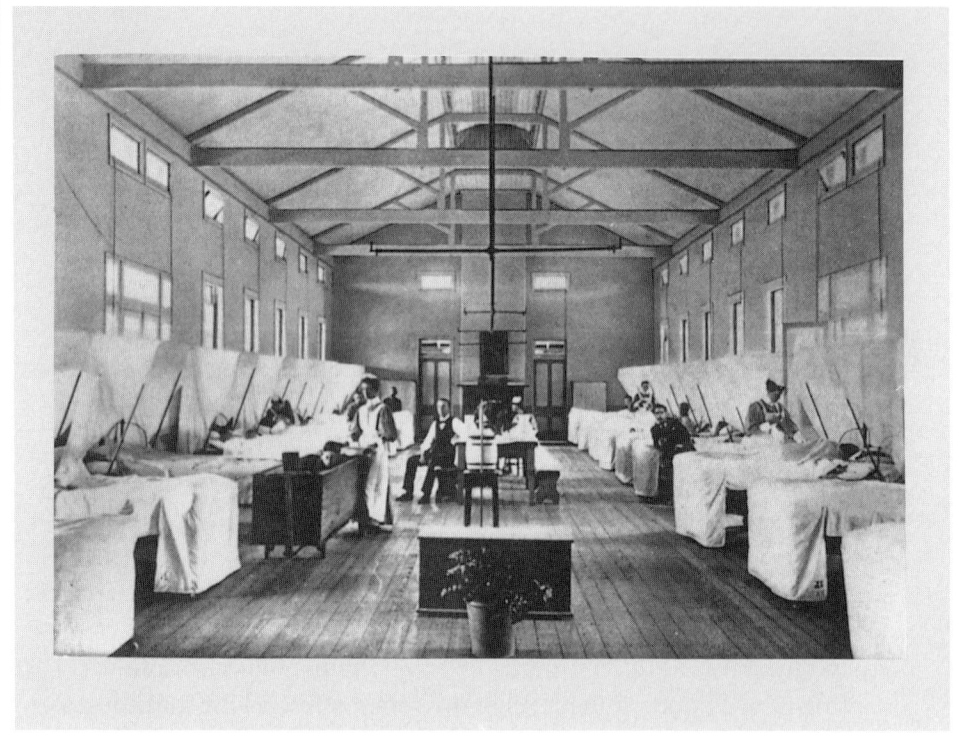

Mental health nursing is an integral part of the nursing tradition.

## CHAPTER 15

# THE ACUTE GENERAL HOSPITAL

Robyn Nash and Helen Edwards

# CONTENTS

# LEARNING OBJECTIVES

This chapter will assist the reader to:

- develop increased awareness of the needs of clients with mental health problems in the general hospital setting;
- discuss clinical manifestations of delirium and panic disorder;
- describe nursing interventions used in the management of delirium and panic disorder;
- reflect on the role of the nurse in holistic patient care.

# INTRODUCTION

Although the incidence of mental illness in Australia has been difficult to establish estimates have been made. *The Better Health Commission Report* (1986) notes that 25% of the population are likely to experience emotional or psychological disturbance at any one time, while the United States Epidemiological Catchment Area Study (ECA) found that the lifetime incidence of one or more of the major psychiatric disorders was one in three, and one in five had an active disorder at the time of interview (Rey 1992). These figures demonstrate the magnitude and seriousness of mental health problems in Australia, and justify initiatives introduced in response to concerns about the mental health of Australians. These initiatives include the introduction of the *Mental Health Statement of Rights and Responsibilities* (1991), the implementation of the *National Mental Health Policy* (1992) and the publication of the *Human Rights and Mental Illness* report (HREOC 1993). A common issue highlighted by these policies and reports is the degree of overlap between mental and physical ill-health. It has been estimated that approximately 30% of patients in acute general hospital beds have a coexisting **mental disorder**, and that 30–50% of psychiatric inpatients have a concurrent physical illness (HREOC 1993).

To ensure that both groups of patients receive the most appropriate form of treatment, a policy of integrated health care has been adopted for Australia (see Chapter 8). This policy will enable most health problems (including mental health problems) to be treated within the same health service. Separate, designated-specific psychiatric facilities will be reduced as mental health services are incorporated into mainstream general health services. The possibility of mainstreaming psychiatric care has, however, raised concern that mental health care could become more closely aligned with the 'medical model' of care (HREOC 1993). It is also recognised that some mental health specific services will still be needed (e.g. long-term care of people with chronic mental disorders such as **dementia**).

Regardless of the degree to which health services become integrated, it is clear that nurses in general hospitals will be caring for an increasing number of patients with mental health problems. Some nurses will find this situation challenging and may need to update their knowledge and skills. As well, many patients seeking treatment for a specific mental health problem require care for a physical illness, and patients with a physical illness often need help with a mental health problem. Increasingly, therefore, nurses working in general hospitals must be prepared to care for patients with complex health needs. To perform this care, the nurse must develop an understanding of the mental health issues implicit in many nursing situations. For instance, stroke patients may experience periods of depression as they alter their lifestyle and adapt to any residual deficits—for example, paralysis or impaired speech (see Chapter 4). Similarly, a person with multiple injuries who faces a long period of hospitalisation may experience a variety of emotions while adapting to hospitalisation, rehabilitation, and financial and social disruption. Nurses working in all hospital settings will continue to encounter situations where patients and/or their families experience loss and grief (e.g. amputation, miscarriage, death).

In addition to caring for patients with a physical illness that has significant impact on their mental health, many people with a pre-existing mental illness are treated in general hospitals. As well as being admitted for treatment of physical health problems, patients with a mental illness often seek treatment at a general hospital. In an acute situation, access to psychiatric services is often limited, particularly at night or weekends, and the Accident and Emergency Departments of general hospitals are used. Collection of data about the use of emergency departments by psychiatric patients has only recently begun in Australia. Preliminary data from a two-month period at a large, metropolitan public hospital indicates that 5% of patients who presented to the emergency department were treated for a psychiatric condition (Richardson & McDowell 1995, personal communication). The conditions treated included severe psychotic episodes, drug and alcohol problems, and attempted suicide.

Recent Australian research also confirms that nurses in general hospitals have to deal with a variety of difficult and aggressive behaviours. Brayley et al. (1994) found that 78% of calls for assistance from a 'violence management team' in a general hospital involved patients with organic mental disorders, substance abuse and personality disorders. These examples highlight the complex health problems managed by nurses in general hospitals.

The examples cited earlier demonstrate how a physical illness can result in a mental health problem, and how people with a mental illness can have a separate physical illness. It is important, therefore, to recognise the interaction of physical and mental health, and not to consider health problems from a separate mind or body perspective. For example, many mental health problems have an organic basis or occur because of physiological changes (see Chapter 9). It follows that nurses in general hospitals must be able to care for patients 'holistically'. The following case studies of a patient with delirium and a patient experiencing a panic attack will demonstrate how this is possible.

# DELIRIUM IN A PATIENT WITH CANCER

The most common mental disorders that present as complications in people with cancer are delirium, anxiety and depression (Massie & Holland 1992). Importantly, early symptoms of delirium are often unrecognised by medical and nursing staff or misdiagnosed as symptoms of anxiety or depression (Massie & Holland 1992; Patchell & Posner 1989). Recognition of delirium is important as the underlying cause may be a treatable complication of cancer (Fleishman & Lesko 1989).

Failure to recognise and/or effectively manage delirium can impact significantly on the patient's quality of life. Apart from its possible impact on the sufferer's personal safety and the disruption it may cause for other patients, delirium can result in significant distress for patients and for their families. The nurse thus has a crucial role to play in the early diagnosis of delirium, in the implementation of supportive interventions and in the education of patients and their significant others (Zimberg & Berenson 1990).

**Delirium** is an organic mental disorder which manifests in impaired cognitive functioning and perceptual, emotional and behavioural alterations (Zimberg & Berenson 1990). It is characterised by 'global cognitive impairment of abrupt onset and relatively brief duration (usually less than one month) and by concurrent disturbance of attention, sleep–wake cycle and psychomotor behavior' (Lipowski 1983). The DSM-IV criteria for delirium are shown in Box 15.1. Delirium should be suspected in any patient who shows acute onset of agitation, impaired cognition, altered attention span or a fluctuating level of consciousness (Massie & Holland 1992).

## BOX 15.1: Delirium

**Diagnostic criteria for 293.0 delirium due to ....**
**(Indicate the general medical condition)**

A.  Disturbance of consciousness (i.e. reduced clarity of awareness of the environment) with reduced ability to focus, sustain, or shift attention.

B.  A change in cognition (such as memory deficit, disorientation, language disturbance) or the development of a perceptual disturbance that is not better accounted for by a preexisting, established, or evolving dementia.

C.  The disturbance develops over a short period of time (usually hours to days) and tends to fluctuate during the course of the day.

D.  There is evidence from the history, physical examination, or laboratory findings that the disturbance is caused by the direct physiological consequences of a general medical condition.

*continued ...*

**Coding note:** If delirium is superimposed on a preexisting Dementia of the Alzheimer's Type or Vascular Dementia, indicate the delirium by coding the appropriate subtype of the dementia, e.g. 290.3 Dementia of the Alzheimer's Type, With Late Onset, With Delirium.

**Coding note:** Include the name of the general medical condition on Axis I, e.g. 293.0 Delirium Due to Hepatic Encephalopathy; also code the general medical condition on Axis III (see Appendix G for codes).

Associated Features and Disorders

Delirium is often associated with a disturbance in the sleep–wake cycle. This disturbance can include daytime sleepiness or night time agitation and difficulty in falling asleep. In some cases, complete reversal of the night–day sleep–wake cycle can occur. Delirium is frequently accompanied by disturbed psychomotor behaviour. Many individuals with delirium are restless or hyperactive. Manifestations of increased psychomotor activity may include groping or picking at the bedclothes, attempting to get out of bed when it is unsafe or untimely, and sudden movements. On the other hand, the individual may show decreased psychomotor activity, with sluggishness and lethargy that may approach stupor. Psychomotor activity can shift from one extreme to the other over the course of a day.

The individual may exhibit emotional disturbances such as anxiety, fear, depression, irritability, anger, euphoria, and apathy. There may be rapid and unpredictable shifts from one emotional state to another, although some individuals have a constant emotional tone. Fear often accompanies threatening hallucinations or transient delusions. If fear is marked, the person may attack those who are falsely perceived as threatening. Injuries may be sustained from falling out of bed or trying to escape while attached to intravenous lines, respiratory tubes, urinary catheters, or other medical equipment. The disturbed emotional state may also be evident in calling out, screaming, cursing, muttering, moaning, or other sounds. These behaviours are especially prevalent at night and under conditions in which stimulation and environmental cues are lacking.

In addition to laboratory findings that are characteristic of associated or etiological general medical conditions (or intoxication or withdrawal states), the EEG is typically abnormal, showing either generalised slowing or fast activity.

Delirium is caused by altered cerebral metabolism which impairs neuronal functioning. A variety of factors can affect cerebral functioning, either directly— for example, primary brain tumours, brain metastases, or indirectly—for example, electrolyte imbalance, drug or radiation side effects, infection (Patchell & Posner 1989). Readers are referred to Foreman (1986) for a complete list of physiologic, psychologic and environmental risk factors for delirium. In a study of terminally ill cancer patients, over 75% developed a delirium that was most often multifactorial in nature—for example, caused by the combined effects of hypoxia, analgesics and haemorrhage (Massie & Holland 1983). In many instances the precise cause of delirium remains unknown (Lipowski 1983; Stiefel, Fainsinger & Bruera 1992).

Delirium is common in patients with cancer, and those with advanced or terminal cancer are at particular risk (Fleishman & Lesko 1989). Whereas delirium is estimated to be present in 25–40% of patients with cancer at various stages of their illness, it affects up to 85% of patients who are terminally ill with cancer (Massie, Holland & Glass 1983; Fainsinger, MacEachern & Hanson 1991). However, the presence of delirium may be missed by medical and nursing staff, especially when the patient is suffering from a delirium of the quiet, hypoactive-hypoalert type (Stiefel et al. 1992). Case Study 15.1 demonstrates the occurrence of delirium in a patient with cancer, and outlines nursing interventions to be considered in the planning of patient care.

## *C*ASE STUDY 15.1: *Delirium*

Mr Green, a 65-year-old man, was admitted to hospital for further investigation of multiple myeloma, a primary malignant tumour of plasma cells, usually arising in the bone marrow. Until then he had been living at home with his wife, Gwen, aged 63. Eric, as he preferred to be called, had been diagnosed with this condition 12 months previously, and had been treated with chemotherapy. During this time his major problems were fatigue and mild loss of weight. Subsequent to feeling 'unwell', he was admitted to hospital for re-evaluation of his clinical status.

Although he appeared a little restless on admission, Eric settled easily into the ward. The nurse who was responsible for Eric's care noted in her assessment that he appeared alert, oriented and able to perform self-care activities. Advice was given regarding the use of support measures to help reduce Eric's back discomfort, and the prescribed analgesic medication was administered. During the next 24 hours, Eric became increasingly restless. He had not cleaned his teeth or combed his hair. Gwen indicated to the nurse that this was 'not like Eric', but was reassured that there did not appear to be anything in particular to worry about.

At about 8 o'clock that night, Eric was found beside his bed; he had taken off his pyjamas and was looking through his bedside locker. On speaking with Eric, the nurse established that he was disoriented in time, place and person. He thought she was his wife, that he was at home and that it was time to go to bowls.

*continued ...*

While talking to the nurse, Eric continually moved clothes in and out of the drawers and the nurse found it difficult to maintain his attention. She quietly and calmly encouraged Eric to put his pyjamas on and get back into bed. Eric continued talking incoherently to himself and was pulling at his clothes and the bedclothes. While talking with Eric, the nurse also noted that his lips and tongue were dry. The nurse reminded Eric that she was a nurse and that he was in hospital. She placed a small night-light by his bed and arranged for another nurse to stay with Eric to ensure his safety while the on-call doctor was contacted.

By the time the doctor arrived, Eric was trying to remove his pyjamas again, and was calling for Gwen to get his clothes for him. After examining Eric and consulting with the nurse, the doctor prescribed midazolam (a short-acting sedative) to be given immediately, and ordered blood tests, including haematocrit, electrolytes, blood urea, nitrogen and creatinine levels. The results revealed that Eric had a higher than normal haematocrit and that his serum calcium was elevated. The doctor noted Eric's provisional diagnosis as delirium, secondary to dehydration and hypercalcaemia, and commenced intravenous therapy—normal saline (0.9%), 1 litre, 6 hourly. Eric's incoherent speech and agitated behaviour subsided and he eventually went to sleep. The nurse documented the events on Eric's chart and began a plan of care focused on his delirious behaviour, his fluid deficit problem and his self-care needs, including mobility. Box 15.2 lists the nursing interventions that were planned to address Eric's delirious behaviour. (See Carpenito 1992; Wilson & Kneisl 1992 for other nursing interventions.)

Next morning Eric was still disoriented and agitated but he was no longer trying to get over the bedrails. When his wife arrived she was very distressed when she saw her husband. While the nurse was explaining what had happened, Gwen commented that Eric may not have been drinking the fluids they gave him as he hadn't been feeling well, and he didn't like them—'He never drinks tea or coffee at home, only water and fruit juices'.

With encouragement from the nurse, Eric's fluid intake gradually returned to normal. His delirium resolved with no apparent residual cognitive deficits, and he was caring for himself. After further assessment and review of his treatment by medical and nursing staff, a plan for his continuing care was developed and he was discharged home.

## Exercises

1. Identify at least three things that foreshadowed the possibility of Eric's hypercalcaemia and subsequent delirium. Consider also what other assessment data would have been useful for the early identification of Eric's problem.

2. Suggest other nursing interventions that could be used to assist patients who are disoriented.

3. Describe possible intervention strategies for the nursing diagnosis: fluid volume deficit related to decreased oral intake (Carpenito 1992).

4. Suggest ways by which Eric's episode of delirium might have been prevented.

5. What other problems might need to be addressed in a comprehensive nursing care plan for Eric and his wife (e.g. management of his back pain)?

## $B$OX 15.2: *Nursing interventions in Eric's care plan*

*Nursing diagnosis*

Altered thought processes related to disorientation of person, place and time secondary to dehydration and hypercalcaemia (Carpenito 1992)

*Interventions*

- Enhance Eric's sense of integrity:
  - Approach him in a calm manner
  - Maintain a consistent approach
  - Show patience and understanding (i.e. don't argue with him)
- Help Eric to differentiate between reality and his own thoughts:
  - Address him frequently by his name
  - Orient him frequently to time, place, relevant nursing staff, activities about to occur
  - Maintain environmental cues to orient Eric (e.g. familiar objects on bedside table, use a night-light)
- Protect Eric from injury:
  - Remove hazardous objects
  - Place bed in low position with the siderails down, as Eric is ambulant
  - Ensure close observation; assign an individual nurse to Eric's care if necessary
- Assist Eric's wife to orient him to time, place, purpose of hospitalisation etc., (by talking with him about familiar events, people, objects)

## $A$GORAPHOBIA AND PANIC ATTACK IN A SURGICAL PATIENT

A **phobia** is defined as an irrational fear of an object, activity or situation (Wilson & Kneisl 1992). Many people have phobias about things (e.g. snakes, heights) at some time during their lives. However, for some people, phobias interfere with their daily lives and prevent them from carrying out the routine activities they must or would like to perform (see Chapter 10). Phobias are usually classified as simple phobias (fear of specific things, such as spiders or mice), social phobias (fear of situations that may be humiliating or embarrassing) and **agoraphobia** (fear of being alone or in public places) (DSM-IV 1994). More than 50% of people with phobias presenting for treatment have agoraphobia (Evans 1991) and it is estimated that agoraphobia afflicts about 4% of the population (Joyce et al. 1989). Despite a widely held misconception that agoraphobia is found in women exclusively, about 25% of those treated for it are males (Evans 1985).

Whether agoraphobia is a syndrome in its own right, a form of depression, a severe anxiety state or a true phobia is still being investigated. However, evidence suggests that agoraphobia has a biological aetiology which is, to some extent, genetically predetermined (Evans 1991). Agoraphobia usually develops from panic disorder where the person has spontaneous panic attacks and over time becomes phobic about places where the panic attacks have occurred. **Panic attacks** are defined as discrete periods of apprehension or fear, with at least four of twelve possible symptoms present during each attack (DSM-IV 1994). These symptoms include dyspnoea, palpitations, choking sensations, sweating, trembling and fear of dying. It is really the panic attack that is feared, not the situation, and this 'fear of fear' is characteristic of agoraphobia (see Chapter 10). That is why many agoraphobics are frightened to be alone. Agoraphobia without panic attacks can occur but is rare.

As a result of public awareness and a decrease in the **stigma** attached to phobias and panic attacks, people these days present earlier in the course of their illness. A variety of treatments has been used in agoraphobia, including drug treatment, behaviour therapy, cognitive therapy, psychotherapy and family involvement. The drugs most commonly used include benzodiazepines, tricyclic antidepressants and monoamine oxidase inhibitors (see Chapter 11). Combinations of treatments are common and particularly effective. For example, Evans, Holt and Oei (1991) report long-term benefits for patients with agoraphobia with panic attacks who undertook a (brief) two-day intensive group cognitive and behavioural treatment program. This time-saving and cost-effective treatment had long-term benefits for about 85% of the patients involved. After reviewing available treatments, Evans (1991) concluded that drug treatment is important but that the most effective treatment is the use of drugs together with other forms of therapy, especially cognitive behavioural therapy. These days, 70–80% of agoraphobics return to full activity after appropriate treatment. Given the prevalence of agoraphobia in the community, nurses working in hospitals can anticipate that a small proportion of their patients will have agoraphobia. Providing effective care for these patients, and management of their physical health problems, is contingent on the management of their agoraphobia. In some cases, this will involve the nurse assisting and encouraging the patient to continue preventive strategies. At other times the nurse will need to intervene during a panic attack. Case Study 15.2 illustrates how a panic attack in a surgical patient with agoraphobia can be managed, and discusses nursing interventions.

# CASE STUDY 15.2: Panic attack

Maureen Gester, 46, had been admitted to hospital for an abdominal hysterectomy. Several months prior to admission it was discovered that Maureen had a fibroid uterine tumour and, after discussing the situation with Maureen and her husband, the gynaecologist recommended surgery. The date for the surgery was booked two months in advance, giving Maureen time to prepare herself and her family. Maureen was admitted to the ward the day before surgery. She was accompanied by her husband, David, and shown to her bed in a six-bed unit. The nurse told Maureen that she needed to explain the preparation for surgery and talk about her care following surgery, but that this would be done after her husband had gone home. Noticing that Maureen appeared tense (rigid posture, holding husband's hand tightly), the nurse decided to leave the couple alone to allow Maureen time to settle into the ward. Two hours later, the nurse noticed that David was still with Maureen, who looked even more apprehensive. The nurse asked David when he would be leaving but Maureen answered for him, saying, 'I want him to stay as long as possible. You can come and talk to me with David here—he might even remember some things for me.'

## Summary of nurse's assessment

Maureen and David have three children aged 16, 13 and 9, who are all still at school. David has his own carpet-cleaning business and Maureen 'helps him a little bit' but is not in any paid employment. They believe themselves to be financially 'okay' and consider themselves an 'average family' with no major concerns. Maureen's parents live near them and intend helping the family during Maureen's hospitalisation and recovery. When asked about her health, Maureen said that, apart from her current gynaecological problems, she was 'physically well'. Maureen admitted to being a 'bit of an anxious person' when the nurse asked her how she coped when things got on top of her. On further questioning from the nurse, Maureen revealed that over the past six years she had been seeing a psychiatrist who was treating her for agoraphobia with panic attacks. Maureen had only had one panic attack during the last year, but admitted she avoids going out in public unless accompanied by a member of her family. She manages her condition through medication and regular relaxation exercises, and by practising thought-stopping, conscious breathing control and positive self-talk. Maureen admitted to feeling a little anxious 'about being in hospital with strangers all around' and hoped that she would not 'disgrace' herself by having a panic attack.

In order to prevent an exacerbation of Maureen's anxiety and the development of a panic attack, the nurse recognised the importance of helping Maureen to maintain her usual management strategies. In consultation with Maureen and David, the nurse developed a care plan which included the interventions set out in Box 15.3. More detailed information about interventions for agoraphobia and panic attacks is presented in Chapter 11.

*continued ...*

The preoperative interventions were successful, as Maureen did not have a panic attack and said that, although she still felt 'a little anxious about the surgery', she also felt that she was managing her feelings. She went to theatre the following morning and returned to the ward at 1pm. On return to the ward, Maureen was conscious but drowsy, her vital signs were stable and there was no visible ooze at the operation site. Intravenous therapy had been commenced in theatre and was to continue for 24 hours. A continuous intravenous infusion of pethidine had also been started.

During the first four hours following her return to the ward, Maureen slept intermittently, her vital signs remained stable and she reported no pain, only some mild discomfort. With the assistance of another nurse, Maureen's primary nurse gave her a postoperative sponge and changed her out of her theatre gown, ready for her husband's expected visit. While the nurses were threading the intravenous therapy line and bag through her nightie, Maureen became very concerned that 'it would all come undone'. Despite their explanations that this would not happen, the nurses noted that Maureen's body posture became very tense, she began sweating and shaking and kept mumbling 'All come undone, all come undone'. Increased pulse and respiration rates were observed .

Recognising the onset of a panic attack, the primary nurse asked her assistant to leave while she conveyed control of the situation by adopting a calm, firm and authoritative manner. The nurse then engaged Maureen in distraction and breathing control exercises. The distraction was achieved by the nurse sitting on the bed, maintaining eye contact and holding Maureen's hands, while saying, 'Just keep looking at me and breathe slowly with me.' Breathing control was established by the nurse talking Maureen through her 10 to 1 technique: 'Take a deep breath in, 10, 10, 10, 10. Now slowly let it out, out, out, out. Breathe in again, 9, 9, 9, 9 and out, out, relax, relax.' The cycle was continued through to 1 and physical contact was maintained throughout. *The nurse simultaneously observed Maureen for signs of postoperative complications.*

At the end of the breathing cycle, the nurse assessed Maureen to be a little less tense (pulse reduced, face and shoulders more relaxed) but considered it necessary to keep Maureen distracted from her physical environment (especially the intravenous line) and to keep her focused on her breathing. The 10 to 1 cycle was repeated and, during this, Maureen's husband arrived. After explaining the onset of the attack, the nurse offered David the opportunity to assist in Maureen's care. He suggested playing one of her favourite music tapes while he reassured her and helped her to gain further control of her breathing. During the rest of the evening Maureen's environment was kept quiet with minimal interruptions. She progressively became more relaxed and slept intermittently. No postoperative complications were noted by the nurse. Before he left for the night, David massaged Maureen's neck and shoulders and took her through a relaxation exercise from one of her tapes.

*continued ...*

Maureen had no more panic attacks during her stay and the nursing staff continued with the interventions described in Box 15.3. Physically, Maureen progressed after her surgery as expected, and as it was considered appropriate for Maureen to return home as soon as possible, she was discharged four days post-surgery.

## Exercises

1. Identify the factors that could have contributed to Maureen's anxiety.
2. Explain why, after the panic attack, the nurse actively involved David in Maureen's care.
3. Consider what the nurse did to help Maureen and identify some of the other things she could have done, giving a clear rationale for each of your suggestions. (Refer to the Further Reading section of Chapter 2.)

## B O X  1 5 . 3 :  *Nursing interventions included in Maureen's care plan*

- Place Maureen in a single room
- Assign a primary nurse to Maureen and keep other staff contact with her to a minimum
- Visitors and visiting times to be as requested by Maureen
- Staff working with Maureen to maintain a calm, unhurried approach
- Staff to explain aspects of care when requested by Maureen
- Maureen to verbalise any concerns or feelings of increasing anxiety as they develop
- Provide Maureen with the opportunity to carry out her progressive relaxation exercises at least once a day and as needed (Carpenito 1992)
- Encourage Maureen to continue her thought-stopping and thought-substitution activities (Wilson and Kneisl 1992)
- Encourage Maureen to continue the use of her conscious controlled breathing (10 to 1) technique when experiencing periods of hyperventilation (Carpenito 1992)
- Assist Maureen to use anxiety interrupters when elements of her care increase her feelings of anxiety (Grainger 1990)
- Help Maureen to maintain her bedtime activities to promote restful sleep (warm shower, warm drink of Milo and listening to music of her choice)

# CONCLUSION

Currently, a substantial proportion of patients in acute care settings have a coexisting mental health problem, and many psychiatric patients have concurrent physical illnesses. To ensure that both groups of patients receive the most appropriate treatment, a policy of integrated health care has been adopted for Australia. Nurses working in acute hospitals can therefore expect to encounter an increasing number of patients with both physical *and* mental health problems. The provision of quality patient care will require nurses to have a repertoire of assessment and intervention skills that can be used effectively to promote optimal physical and mental health for their patients. The current trend toward increasing acuity (level of dependency) and shortened length of stay in acute care settings underscores the need for nurses to develop sophisticated and flexible approaches to care. Indeed, the challenge of providing care which is truly holistic has, perhaps, never been greater.

# SUMMARY

- Approximately one third of patients in acute general hospitals have a coexisting mental disorder.
- Nurses working in general hospitals care for patients whose physical illness threatens their mental well-being, and psychiatric patients who have a physical health problem.
- Delirium is one of the most common psychiatric complications of cancer, particularly in the advanced or terminal stages.
- Patients who are admitted to hospital with a pre-exisiting mental health problem need to be encouraged to continue with their usual preventive strategies (e.g. relaxation exercises, positive self-talk).
- If a hospitalised patient has a panic attack, the nurse should convey control of the situation and assist the patient with appropriate interventions (e.g. breathing control, distraction).

# DISCUSSION QUESTIONS

1. How can nurses ensure that the mental health problems of patients in general hospitals are managed effectively?
2. What factors influence the quality of care provided in general hospitals for patients with a mental illness who also have a physical illness?
3. What implications does the mainstreaming of psychiatric care have for holistic nursing practice?

4. 'Effective management of any patient's physical condition is contingent on the effective management of any coexisting mental illness or mental health problem.' Discuss this statement.

# EXERCISES

1. Nurses must be able to distinguish between panic attacks and other conditions that present with similar symptoms. What are some of the conditions that a panic attack could mimic?
2. Prepare a nursing care plan, including nursing interventions, for Maureen (Case Study 15.2), assume she has a pre-existing mental health problem *other* than phobia.
3. List the possible causes of delirium and suggest one or more nursing interventions for each cause.

# FURTHER READING

- Evans, L. (1991) 'The treatment of panic disorder', *Australian Journal of Psychopharmacology* 5, pp.11–15. This article gives a clear description of panic disorder. A summary of treatments is given, including behaviour therapy, cognitive therapy, family involvement and psychotherapy.
- Grainger, A. (1990) 'Anxiety interrupters', *American Journal of Nursing*, February, pp.14–15. This very practical article describes interventions that can be used to reduce anxiety. Suggested interventions to interrupt the anxiety pattern include looking up, lowering the shoulders, slowing the pace of thoughts and changing the sculpture of the face.
- Pasacreta, J.V. & Massie, M.J. (1990) 'Nurses' reports of psychiatric complications in patients with cancer', *Oncology Nursing Forum* 17(3), pp.347–53. This article presents the results of a survey of all nurses (n=100) working on 15 inpatient units in a 565-bed cancer research hospital on one day, regarding psychiatric problems presented in 475 patients under their care. The findings indicated that significantly more patients exhibited symptoms requiring psychiatric consultation than did not.
- Steifel, F., Fainsinger, R. & Bruera, E. 'Acute confusional states in patients with advanced cancer', *Journal of Pain and Symptom Management* 7(2), pp.94–8. An overview of the occurrence of delirium in cancer patients is presented and treatment guidelines, particularly with respect to psychotropic medications, are discussed in detail.
- Zimberg, M. & Berenson, S. (1990) 'Delirium in patients with cancer: nursing assessment and intervention', *Oncology Nursing Forum* 17(4), pp.529–353. A useful overview of the nursing management of cancer patients experiencing delirium from a variety of causes.

# REFERENCES

American Psychiatric Association (1994) *Diagnostic and Statistics Manual of Mental Disorders* (4th edn), Washington.

Better Health Commission (Australia) (1986) *The Better Health Commission Report*, Canberra: AGPS.

Brayley, J., Lange, R., Baggoley, C., Bond, M. & Harvey, P. (1994) 'The violence management teaman approach to aggressive behaviour in a general hospital', *Medical Journal of Australia* 161(4), pp.254–8.

Carpenito, L.J. (1992) *Nursing Diagnosis: Application to Clinical Practice* (4th edn), New York: Lippincott.

Evans, L. (1985) 'Phobias and how to treat them', *Practical Therapeutics*, July, pp.49–57.

Evans, L. (1991) 'The treatment of panic disorder', *Australian Journal of Psychopharmacology* 5, pp.11–15.

Evans, L., Holt. C. & Oei, T. (1991) 'Long term follow-up of agoraphobics treated by brief intensive group cognitive behavioural therapy', *Australian and New Zealand Journal of Psychiatry*, 25, pp.343–9.

Fainsinger, R., MacEachern, T. & Hanson, J. (1991) 'Symptom control during the last week of life on a palliative care unit', *Journal of Palliative Care* 7, pp.5–11.

Fleishman, S.B. & Lesko, L.M. (1989) 'Delirium and dementia' in J.C. Holland & J.H. Rowland (eds) *Handbook of Psychooncology: Psychological Care of the Patient with Cancer*, New York: Oxford University Press, pp.342–55.

Foreman, M.D. (1986) 'Acute confusional states in hospitalised elderly: a research dilemma', *Nursing Research* 35, pp.37–8.

Grainger, A. (1990) 'Anxiety interrupters', *American Journal of Nursing*, February, pp.14–15.

Human Rights and Equal Opportunities Commission (1993) *Human Rights and Mental Illness: Report of the National Inquiry into the Human Rights of People with Mental Illness* Vols 1 & 2, Canberra: AGPS.

Joyce, P. R., Bushnell, J. A., Oakley-Brown, M. A., Wells, J. E. & Hornblow, A. (1989) 'The epidemiology of panic symptomatology and agoraphobia avoidance', *Comprehensive Psychiatry* 30(4),pp.303–12.

Lipowski, Z.J. (1983) 'Transient cognitive disorders (delirium, acute confusional states) in the elderly', *American Journal of Psychiatry* 140, pp.1426–36.

Massie, M.J. & Holland, J.C. (1992 'The cancer patient with pain: psychiatric complications and their management', *Journal of Pain and Symptom Management* 7(2), pp.99–109.

Massie, M.J., Holland, J. & Glass, E. (1983) 'Delirium in terminally ill patients', *American Journal of Psychiatry* 140(8), pp.1048–50.

*Mental Health Statement of Rights and Responsibilities* (1991) Report of the Mental Health Consumer Outcomes Task Force. Canberra: AGPS.

*National Mental Health Policy* (1992) Canberra: AGPS.

Patchell, R.A. & Posner, J.B. (1989) 'Cancer and the nervous system' in J.C. Holland & J.H. Rowland (eds) *Handbook of Psychooncology: Psychological Care of the Patient with Cancer*, New York: Oxford University Press, pp.327–41.

Rey, J. (1992) 'The epidemiological catchment area (ECA) study: implication for Australia', *Medical Journal of Australia* 156, pp.200–3.

Richardson, D. & McDowell, L. (1995) Accident and Emergency Department, Princess Alexandra Hospital, Brisbane (personal communication).

Stiefel, F., Fainsinger, R. & Bruera, E. (1992) 'Acute confusional states in patients with cancer', *Journal of Pain and Symptom Management* 7(2), pp.94–8.

Wilson, H. & Kneisl, C. (1992) *Psychiatric Nursing* (4th edn), Menlo Park, California: Addison-Wesley.

Zimberg, M. & Berenson, S. (1990) 'Delirium in patients with cancer: Nursing assessment and intervention', *Oncology Nursing Forum* 17(4), p.529.

# Birdsville 1927

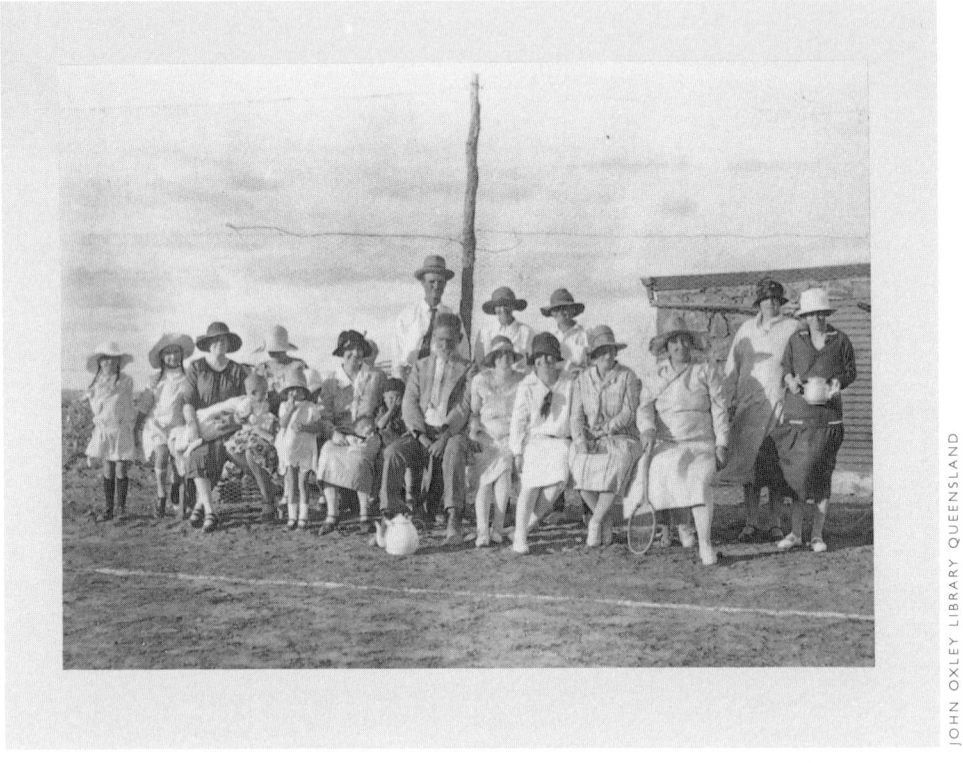

Crowd at opening of Birdsville Tennis Season Easter Sunday.

People are the key resource for nursing in the community. For rural and remote nurses they are sometimes the *only* resource.

## CHAPTER 16

# *T*HE RURAL COMMUNITY

Fran Sanders and Barbara Tooth

## *C*ONTENTS

# LEARNING OBJECTIVES

This chapter will assist the reader to:

- understand the concept of the generalist community nurse addressing mental health issues;
- implement the primary health care approach to community nursing practice;
- understand the diversity of generalist community nursing practice directed at meeting mental health needs;
- summarise current issues in the health of rural communities.

# INTRODUCTION

Although some nurses will undertake postgraduate education in the area of mental health and psychiatric nursing, many nurses working in the community will not have these specialist skills. Major changes in the way care is provided to people with serious mental illness are being implemented. These include the move towards community rather than institutional care and the mainstreaming of services, so that acute psychiatric units are located within general hospitals rather than separately (see Chapter 8). These changes can be expected to flow on to the community with the result that generalist agencies, which previously rarely provided services to people with a serious mental illness, will receive increasing numbers of requests for such care. As well, the need to address mental health issues for all clients is being accepted as a vital aspect of a holistic approach to health and the provision of nursing care.

The basic principles of community nursing are the same whether the nurse is practising in an urban or rural community. The circumstances, the people, the issues, the resources, and the supports available will vary. Although a sound knowledge base is important, nurses can never hope to know everything they will need to know to assist the spectrum of clients encountered. Effective community nurses are those who:

- develop and use networks;
- learn where to obtain resources to address specific issues or problems;
- get to know the community well and respect its members;
- collaborate with other professionals and services to facilitate the solutions the client chooses;
- work with the community and clients rather than just delivering a service;
- seek out new information and take opportunities to update their knowledge; and
- keep the 'big picture' in mind.

Because of issues of isolation and restricted access to resources and specialist services, these skills come under the greatest pressure in rural community practice.

As nursing in a rural community not only poses special challenges but also provides many rewards, it has been chosen as an ideal medium through which to explore the basic principles of community nursing.

## THE COMMUNITY SETTING

The generalist community nurse provides primary, secondary and tertiary level nursing services to clients from a variety of age and ethnic groups, who are facing many different health issues for themselves or their families, and dealing with varied personal, economic, work and life circumstances. Clients will include people coming to terms with chronic or terminal illness, caring for an aged or disabled relative, dealing with relationships within the family or at work, coping with **stress** of whatever cause, attempting to alter behaviour to prevent health problems, adjusting to living in a new country, recovering from illness, accident or surgery, dealing with mental illness, or coping as a single parent. For these and many other clients, nurturing mental health is a vital factor in any nursing approach.

In addition, broad mental health issues arise from time to time, requiring nurses to work with the community as a whole. Some examples of broader issues are addressing community attitudes and stigmatisation in relation to mental illness, assisting groups to lobby for additional facilities or services, and working with the community to address factors that may be having a negative impact on the mental health of the population.

There are also wider community issues, such as unemployment, the rural crisis, and discrimination on the basis of gender, race or sexuality that have significant impact on the mental health and emotional well-being of community members. Within a primary health care framework, such issues need to be recognised and ultimately addressed.

The generalist nurse practising in a rural community setting, including smaller towns any distance from major provincial centres, will be faced with the additional problems posed by distance, a lack of resources, the frequent need for people to obtain specialist help away from their home town, and, on occasions, particular sets of local beliefs and attitudes.

## PHILOSOPHY OF CARE

There is little doubt that mental health problems are prevalent in settings where generalist community nurses work. Epidemiological studies have found that the lifetime prevalence of serious mental disorder is one in three (Rey 1992). However, a substantial number of mental health problems in primary care settings remain unrecognised or inadequately diagnosed. The majority of these disorders in the community are not transient or self-limiting. Current treatment is often inadequate or unavailable but, when properly identified, many of these disorders can be treated effectively (van den Brink et al. 1991).

The inadequacies of mental health care in the community have been further compounded by the process of deinstitutionalisation. Many people suffering the more serious mental health problems are now residing permanently in the community. Unfortunately, it is a well-recognised problem that the majority of available resources have remained tied up in institutions, rather than following clients out into the community (see Chapter 8). This lack of resources to improve community services is one of the factors associated with increasing demands on existing services, both government and non-government. It is an issue that must be addressed as a matter of urgency by policy makers, managers and governments.

Another significant issue impacting on generalist community nurses is the change in care provision in general hospitals. For a variety of reasons, mental health care in the general inpatient setting has traditionally been poor. Early discharge and the introduction of case-mix to the health care system are placing greater responsiblity on community workers to respond to a range of client needs, including mental health care needs. Given these changes in policy and service delivery, it is almost inevitable that mental health care needs will more frequently be considered in generalist community settings as opposed to general hospital settings. This is congruent with the holistic approach to care inherent in the primary health care model, which is increasingly being adopted in such settings. The changing face of service delivery includes the **mainstreaming** of services to cater for mental health needs in generalist facilities (see Chapter 8), and this increasing reliance on community care makes it imperative that primary health care workers rethink their roles in relation to mental health care.

Because of social factors and changes in service delivery, the need for mental health care to be addressed in the community is perhaps greater than ever before. The challenge for the community nurse is to provide intervention strategies that will benefit diverse client groups, while at the same time developing links with the growing number of community services, including those for the seriously mentally ill. Nurses will need to identify their roles within this complex network. This is likely to be easier for the generalist nurse because the philosophy of primary health care is strongly reflected in the current philosophy of care for people who have serious mental health problems. The **prevention** of mental health problems is also a predominant feature of current trends in mental health services but, with the scarcity of resources in the community, few specialist mental health workers can devote much time to this 'luxury'. The close liaison of primary health care workers with specialist mental health workers will enable early detection of mental health problems. Prevention is also a cornerstone of primary health care and closer ties between service providers will be mutually benefical.

## THE PRIMARY HEALTH CARE MODEL

Primary health care is one of the most misunderstood concepts in contemporary health care provision and practice, yet a primary health care approach incorporates a set of principles that are central to the provision of quality services for all groups in our community. As a global concept, primary health care was conceived in the Declaration of Alma-Ata (WHO 1978), and has since undergone considerable development and refinement into a truly comprehensive model for health service delivery within the community. This does not mean that no service delivery based on similar principles existed prior to Alma-Ata. However, for the first time, this Declaration focused international attention on the failure of the predominant technological/biomedical approach, and the urgent need to reorient health services to take into account a social model of health. It provided a serious challenge to the biomedical model, which was generally accepted as providing an adequate explanation of illness, and a rationale for the provision of health services and treatment approaches.

It is a common misperception that primary health care concerns prevention only. This is not so. In the words of the Declaration of Alma-Ata, '[primary health care] addresses the main problems in the community, providing promotive, preventative, curative and rehabilitative services accordingly' (WHO 1978, p.3). The major challenges of primary health care are:

- achieving genuine community participation and empowerment;
- effectively utilising **intersectoral** and interdisciplinary collaboration;
- addressing social justice issues and the social causes of illness;
- actively promoting community mental health rather than merely treating mental illness;
- developing a sustainable, integrated and comprehensive system which is able to address client and community needs holistically; and
- implementing systems which ensure accountability to the community.

# RURAL ISSUES

Australian researchers (Dunne et al. 1994) have identified widespread serious health problems in rural and remote areas as a result of socioeconomic conditions. The authors state that these have arisen because of the economic recession and unemployment, pre-existing lifestyles, cultural attitudes to health, low educational levels, isolation and lack of transport. These and other factors typical of rural communities create special issues for the provision of mental health care, which differ from those in urban centres.

The enormity of mental health problems in rural regions is well documented in the *Report of the National Inquiry into the Human Rights of People with Mental Illness* (Human Rights and Equal Opportunities Commission 1993). The high incidence of youth suicide in rural regions has received particular attention. In New South Wales, youth suicide (10–19 years) was significantly higher in rural as opposed to urban regions (Dudley et al. 1992). This trend in rural–urban differences has been noticed worldwide (Crombie 1991). In Queensland the rates of youth suicide are generally higher than the national average, regardless of locality. The incidence of rural youth suicide is higher than in urban areas, but not significantly so (Cantor & Coory 1993). The suicide rate of Australian males 15–29 years ranked second of nineteen countries (Diekstra 1989).

Youth suicide in Australia highlights the seriousness of mental health problems in our society. Apart from the identification of the suicide trends, formal research into the mental health needs of rural communities has only just begun. Yellowlees and Kaushik (1992) conducted an extensive study in rural New South Wales and found that alcohol abuse among men was four times the national average, and significantly high among women. These authors concluded that this is related, at least in part, to higher rates of domestic violence, sexual assault and incest in rural communities. These rural problems may contribute to higher incidences of anxiety, depression, and abuse of prescribed and non-prescribed medication, and to higher rates of childhood disturbances. However, the rates of major functional psychiatric disorders do not fluctuate between rural and urban regions (Yellowlees & Kaushik 1992).

Many people in rural areas choose to stay there because they consider the advantages of country life outweigh the disadvantages. However, as Collingridge (1991) suggests, it now appears that the problems in rural communities, while different from those in urban areas, are just as severe. These include poorer physical health, a high incidence of domestic violence, lower educational standards and opportunities, poverty and unemployment. All these problems are in addition to the problems of isolation, poor service provision, a high cost of living, poor access to services, and poor communication and transport services (Cheers 1990). The impact of **stigma** can also be particularly acute in small communities (Reed 1992).

The provision of mental health care in rural areas has its own set of difficulties. Rural settings have limited resources coupled with specific social problems. Many people in rural communities have lived there for most of their lives, and may be reluctant to move elsewhere. This factor, together with generally lower educational attainment, has major implications for employment opportunities (Reed 1992). In industrialised countries, rural communities have been under pressure for some time. This has been associated with a decrease in the marketability of traditional work skills, and with a steady decline in opportunities for social and economic mobility (Hargrove 1982). The crisis of the agricultural industry, due to factors such as technological change, the economic downturn and drought, has created its own set of problems. The wealth of rural communities has been eroded. Depression and loss of self-esteem, which frequently accompany such life changes, are common.

One-third of Australia's population lives outside city centres, and is spread throughout rural and remote regions, yet the mental health needs of these people have been neglected, as have those of rural dwellers worldwide (Yellowlees & Hemming 1992). Not only are specialist services inadequate but, for a number of reasons, staff taking up appointment in rural regions frequently stay for only a short time. In addition, the volunteer sector, traditionally strong in rural regions, has been eroded by the economic recession and the return of women to the workforce (Collingridge 1991). The problem of attracting medical practitioners to rural regions has begun to be addressed by the establishment of Rural Training Units, where practitioners undertake specialist training in areas such as obstetrics, surgery, anaesthetics, medicine, and the care of acutely ill people (Strasser 1994). While Strasser notes such benefits of rural practice as community status, a relaxed lifestyle, continuity of care of patients, family treatment, and a sense of belonging in the community, the absence of discussion of mental health issues in rural communities is striking.

Unfortunately, the promotion of rural practice as a 'lifestyle' belies the extent of mental health problems in rural communities. The specialist training of nursing staff for rural practice is still not formalised. The comprehensive training of undergraduate nurses does go part way to addressing this issue, but the availability of opportunities take a rural focus at postgraduate level is also vital. An emphasis on 'localisation', as opposed to the 'specialisation' that occurs in urban regions, is important for the provision of health care to rural communities.

People requiring acute mental health services in rural areas are generally responded to in one of three ways, each of which has numerous disadvantages.

First, if people are admitted to a general hospital ward, they frequently find themselves without access to care by staff with specialist knowledge in mental health and are usually placed in wards (such as geriatric wards) inappropriate for their needs. They may feel humiliated or uncomfortable in this environment and their behaviour may not be understood by staff unfamiliar with mental illness. Judgments are easily made, but not so easily forgotten, and in small towns, where people are known, prejudices built up in this way can have long-term implications for both the sufferers themselves and their family members.

Second, because of the absence of appropriate facilities in many areas, the only option in emergency situations is to place people in police cells, or even in jail. The trauma, disruption and embarrassment associated with such an experience is severe.

Third, people often have to be admitted to distant city facilities, separated from their communities, their everyday lives and their support networks. Frequently, when they do return home, the only transportation available is in the back of a police wagon.

The report, *Human Rights and Mental Illness* (HREOC 1993), highlights the distinction that exists between the way health services in rural areas respond to people who are physically ill compared with those who are mentally ill. In the event of serious physical illness or trauma requiring emergency care, a team of experts is dispatched by aircraft to stabilise and transport the person to a city facility. This is not the case for those people with serious mental health problems. The result of such inequalities is an exacerbation of the effects of prejudice (which are already pronounced) and further damage to self-esteem. While large cities still have major problems in the provision of mental health care, they do at least have the advantage of affording a degree of anonymity.

Likewise, the after-care and follow-up provided for people with mental health problems in rural areas is poor. Visits by specialist teams are still sporadic or unavailable in many areas, despite recent efforts on the part of some authorities to address this deficit. Continuity of care, one of the hallmarks of appropriate mental health care, is of major concern in rural and remote areas. However, as the *Report of the National Inquiry into the Human Rights of People with Mental Illness* (HREOC 1993) found, it is possible to overcome such obstacles.

An example of one successful attempt is the Far West Mental Health Team in New South Wales, which services a population of approximately 33 000 over an area of 150 000 square kilometres. The team is extremely isolated, with the nearest psychiatric facility 800 kilometres away. The approach of this team has been to integrate members into local communities to foster the development of trust between the worker and the community. A fundamental premise of the team's practice is the need for individual team members to take responsibility for particular communities, to enable those communities to get to know the health professional very well. This allows sensitivity towards local issues to develop. Team members also visit local organisations such as hospitals and schools to provide support and assistance to resident professionals (Yellowlees 1990).

Community nurses in rural regions need to be familiar with health care services available in adjoining regions. Because of the sensitivity of people in rural areas to the stigma attached to mental health problems, and concerns about confidentiality, it may be preferable to refer people to appropriate services in neighbouring towns. This issue highlights the need to raise the awareness of people in rural communities in relation to mental health problems, as part of the process of breaking down the marked prejudice existing in many areas.

Isolation is not only a problem for clients but also for professionals. The development of intersectoral links can be used not only to provide back-up and support in care provision, but to break down professional isolation and foster valuable networking. Such networking requires formal development to ensure its recognition and establishment as an integral aspect of practice. Until such structures are in place, health workers will be faced with having to initiate and develop their own networks. However, for most practitioners, the benefits are well worth the effort. Clearly, in rural areas nurses need to be able to identify a mental health specialist or specialist service to be available for consultation and back-up when necessary. The devolution of power from specialist medical staff to nursing staff is a necessary precursor to successful teamwork and the appropriate use of resources, not only in rural and remote regions but also in urban settings.

An additional strain on rural community resources is the transient population of young adults with chronic mental illness. This group of clients is known to be highly mobile and as a result individuals frequently arrive in rural communities with which there may be no previous affiliation. However, there are usually limited resources available to cater to their needs and they are often very conspicuous. The strong kinship ties in rural communities make it much easier (in terms of acceptance) for someone who has grown up in the community and later develops a mental illness, than it is for a transient immigrant. In such instances, the social characteristics of rural communities are likely to exacerbate rather than reduce the person's illness.

An issue that is rarely discussed is the way in which newly arrived health professionals fit into the local community, and the impact of this on the way they are able to practise. Martinez-Brawley (1990) reports that people in rural communities often have greater concerns about, and commitment to, the welfare of their town or region, and hold stronger moral perspectives about what will benefit their community, than do urban dwellers. The credibility of health professionals, including nurses, will depend in part on perceptions of their commitment and contribution to the community. The message for nurses moving to work in a rural area is to spend a lot of time listening and learning, and making sure that actions are compatible with the individuals or groups concerned. Consideration of the context of practice is essential, and this makes it imperative that nurses make themselves familiar with the social, health and service issues facing rural communities.

Case Studies 16.1 and 16.2, and the examples of nursing interventions, highlight many of the issues raised.

## C A S E   S T U D Y   1 6 . 1 :   *Mental health nursing in a rural community*

Jenny works as a generalist community nurse in Stonesfield, a rural town with a population of approximately 2000 (including the town itself and surrounding station properties). Jenny transferred to a newly created position in Stonesfield almost a year ago. Her role includes working with clients on a one-to-one basis, as well as working with families and the community as a whole. Consistent with the current directions in health care being taken at policy and service delivery levels, Jenny practises within a primary health care model that emphasises:

- a holistic approach based on a social view of health;
- a focus on health promotion;
- multidisciplinary and intersectoral collaboration;
- the inclusion of treatment, rehabilitation and support services;
- the participation of individuals and the community as a whole in their health and health services;
- addressing access and equity issues;
- facilitating skills development and access to information; and
- *working with* the community rather than *providing services* to the community.

In recent years Stonesfield and its population have been quite severely affected by both the rural crisis and the drought. The town is about 400 kilometres from the nearest provincial centre, and access to specialist health services of all kinds is limited.

*continued ...*

The community has been shattered by the suicides of two residents in recent months. The first was a 16-year-old boy who lived with his family in the town, and the second a 36-year-old farmer and father of three young children, who had been experiencing severe financial problems. Neither had sought nor received any assistance, but in hindsight their families and friends realised that there had been a number of signs that things were going wrong for them.

Shortly after taking up her position in Stonesfield, Jenny started devoting time to getting to know the community and its people, and giving them the opportunity to get to know her. She met with staff at the tiny hospital and at the Council Office; she met local business people such as the chemist, bank manager and publican, as well as police, teachers, the local Aboriginal community, and the Country Women's Association. When representatives of various services, such as social welfare, family services, the visiting magistrate, or health authorities were in town, Jenny ensured that she made contact with them, to learn what might be made available to the community and to tell them about her role. Once she established these contacts, she continued to devote energy to maintaining them. As a consequence of this process, Jenny has learned a lot about the district and its history, local issues, strengths and problems, the people and their attitudes and concerns, and where the most pressing needs are.

People began coming to her for advice or information shortly after she set up the community centre in shop-front premises in the main street. This was partly out of curiosity about the new arrival in town, and partly to find out what she could do for them. A number of callers were concerned about family members, friends or neighbours whom they believed needed some assistance. Others came to her attention by chance. Some examples were: a 70-year-old woman living in a dilapidated farmhouse 12 miles out of town, caring for three adult intellectually handicapped and sometimes violent sons; women who were the victims of domestic violence; the young mother of a toddler and a three-month-old baby who 'wasn't coping'; the teenage daughter of one of the town's business people who suffered from an eating disorder; the carers of elderly relatives with dementia who were exhausted and stressed; Aboriginal families and two recently arrived Asian families who were clearly subject to racist attitudes and discriminatory practices; people with alcohol problems; seemingly widespread levels of depression; a lonely middle-aged man with a physical disability; and several individuals who had been diagnosed with schizophrenia.

Jenny soon realised that there was a strong stigma attached to mental illness in the community. The health authority had initiated discussions about a proposal to develop the underutilised hospital into a multipurpose centre, which could serve as the base for a number of permanent and visiting health services. The possibility of siting a specialist mental health worker in the centre was floated. There was considerable concern on the part of many community members, who felt that people would not want to use other services in the building because of the fear that it might be thought they were visiting the mental health worker.

*continued …*

Doubt was expressed that such a service would be generally utilised because of the reality of stigma. As the months passed, Jenny came to know a number of families who were caring for relatives with mental illness in total isolation. In some cases, even those who had frequent contact with these families were unaware of their situation. She realised that this prejudice was a crippling factor that she would need to address if effective services and supports were to be established.

Jenny divides her time between assisting individuals and families, and working on whole community issues using a community development approach. She has been successful in bringing the community together to start to address issues affecting mental health and emotional well-being, although she is still only at the beginning of a lengthy process.

Jenny has searched for as much information as possible that may be useful both for herself and for people in the community. This has included developing contacts with community groups and organisations in the city that have been established specifically to help people with mental illness. Many of these groups have invaluable resources and will post out information. She has also built up her own collection of leaflets, booklets and literature from various sources so that she has a range of materials to refer to. In this way, even though she does not have specialist education in the area of mental illness, she has developed a good understanding of the issues people face, and can provide appropriate support for clients and families in collaboration with the mental health professional or service managing their treatment and care.

Another activity that Jenny undertook, with the support of the local community, was lobbying the health authority to provide a visiting mental health worker on a regular basis. This need is now being addressed.

## Interventions

Nursing interventions in the rural community need to be carried out at two levels: with the community as a whole, and with individuals and their families.

### Community level interventions

As part of her work in the community, Jenny undertook a community needs assessment to identify community needs, concerns and priorities. The interventions available to her at community level cover a range of possible activities such as community education, facilitating the establishment of **self-help** or other community support groups, lobbying for improved facilities or services, stimulating community awareness and discussion of issues through the use of the local media (including radio), community development, and getting professionals and community leaders involved. The success of such activities depends to a large extent on the commitment and involvement of the local community, so the identification of priorities and interventions must be done with the community rather than by the professional.

Box 16.1 describes the activities Jenny initiated in order to reduce the stigma attached to mental illness.

## BOX 16.1: *Community intervention: Addressing the stigma of mental illness*

In her contacts with people in Stonesfield, Jenny became aware that the fear of being stigmatised was causing considerable distress, and forcing people and their families to hide mental illness. Over the course of a few months, Jenny drew together a small group of people who wanted to do something to change the situation. The group set out to implement a number of activities over a period of time that would contribute to informing the community and opening up the issue of mental illness for discussion. Activities included:

- establishing a self-help group, so that those directly affected could share experiences, information and support;
- inviting speakers from recognised organisations such as the Association of Relatives and Friends of the Mentally Ill (ARAFMI), the Schizophrenia Fellowship and local health authorities to visit the area to address public meetings;
- speaking on local radio and getting regular information into the local newspaper;
- speaking to service clubs; and
- obtaining the support of general practitioners, the hospital staff and the council.

These activities continue, but already there have been some very positive results. There is much more awareness in the community about the issue of mental illness, and the topic is no longer taboo. Some community members have become involved and offered their assistance to sufferers and their families. Most importantly of all, the isolation of many who were previously coping alone has been reduced, and their sense of being able to do something constructive about their situations has been a very positive outcome. An issue as pervasive as stigmatisation is not easily resolved, and efforts must be long-term.

### Individual level interventions

It is just as important for the nurse to be able to work effectively with individuals and families as with the community as a whole. The principles of primary health care can be applied in different ways at both levels of practice. Box 16.2 illustrates the promotion of mental health in an individual with diabetes, while Case Study 16.2 looks in depth at nursing intervention on an individual and family level, involving bipolar disorder.

$B$OX 1 6 . 2 : *Individual intervention: mental health promotion*

Fred is a 53-year-old diabetic who has lost both legs because of his disease. He lives alone in a shack on the fringe of town. Since his second amputation, two years before Jenny's arrival, he has hardly left his home. Jenny visited him at the request of the general practitioner to see if he needed any help. She found a man living in housing that lacked many of the amenities, such as running water and adequate cooking facilities. He appeared to be neglecting his diet and other aspects of self-care, and talked about the fact that his best mate had died, and now no one visited him. His wheelchair was in disrepair. Jenny began visiting regularly and Fred started to look forward to her visits. With his agreement she arranged for his wheelchair to be repaired, and for the local meals-on-wheels service to call.

In conversation, Fred revealed that what he wanted to do most was to be able to get down to the wharf and do some fishing. With the help of the local publican, who was a keen fisherman, Jenny organised people to take Fred to the wharf and bring him home again on a couple of days each week. The publican also helped by organising bait and tackle. This arrangement was the turning point for Fred. The wharf was a centre for lots of passing traffic and he met people he had not seen for years. Within a few months Fred was much brighter, taking better care of himself, and seeking information about moving into a council flat where he would have better facilities. The help Jenny was able to give Fred in managing his diabetes was important, but without the simple strategy of enabling him to pursue an activity he was really keen on, and which enhanced his mental health, its impact would have been lost.

$C$ASE STUDY 1 6 . 2 : *Individual family/intervention: Bipolar disorder and depression*

Peter Casey is a 34-year-old married man with one child, and has a small business in the local community. He was diagnosed with bipolar disorder six years ago. The disorder developed after the birth of his child and before he came to live in Stonesfield. He had experienced four manic phases of his illness, necessitating hospitalisation, but he was stabilised on his current medication and lifestyle changes. He moved to the country 18 months ago in search of a less stressful lifestyle. Peter and his wife bought the local newsagency, a business that was well established and provided a steady income. Lately, however, the impact of the recession has been taking its toll. In recent weeks, Peter's wife Susan has noticed that he was becoming withdrawn and no longer taking an active interest in the business.

*continued ...*

He would frequently wake in the early hours of the morning and just sit in the bedroom. When Susan asked what was troubling him, he would express concerns about the business and their future. He was unable to see any way out of their troubles. His appetite had decreased, he was losing weight, and showed no interest in his usual activities. Susan was becoming increasingly concerned about Peter, as he frequently expressed feelings of helplessness and hopelessness.

Susan approached Jenny for assistance because Peter refused to see the local GP and she thought that a nurse might be able to persuade Peter to seek medical assistance. The many issues that were raised for Jenny by Susan's request are discussed below.

## Assessment and monitoring of Peter's mental status

Such a situation draws on many of the rural nurse's skills. Jenny needed to establish trust and rapport with Peter to enable her to obtain a psychosocial history and make a preliminary assessment of his mental status. It appeared that Peter was going into a depressive phase of his illness and a priority was to assess the risk of suicide. Nurses need the support of other specialist health professionals to deal with serious mental health problems. Potentially suicidal clients (which includes all people suffering major depression) should not be dealt with by any one health professional alone. It is essential to have the support of other professionals with whom to share concerns, assessment and information, in order to provide maximum safety for the client and health professional.

Jenny spent time with Peter, establishing rapport and encouraging him to talk about how he was feeling and what he wanted help with, as well as giving him appropriate information. In the course of conversation, she found an opportunity to ask him whether he had thought about suicide. Fortunately, in Peter's case this was not so. It is a common misconception that asking someone about suicide may actually make them commit suicide. It is essential to ascertain a depressed person's suicide risk; asking sensitively will usually elicit an answer and also give the person permission to talk about an issue that is often seen as taboo.

## Liaison with the local GP and the nearest specialist mental health service

Since arriving in Stonesfield, Peter's medication had been monitored by the local GP. Jenny needed to ensure that Peter saw his general practitioner and, after lengthy discussion and reassurance, Peter agreed to let her bring the GP to his home. There are no specialist mental health services available locally. It is essential for a nurse in this situation to have established links with the local GP and nearest mental health service, even if the specialist service is at a considerable distance. Such links will enable the nurse to contact specialist health workers to discuss the management of clients with serious mental health problems, and to use such health workers as a general resource. Fortunately, Jenny had already established such links.

If Peter had been assessed as suicidal and had refused to see the GP, Jenny would have been obliged to ensure his safety under the appropriate mental health act. This would have entailed the GP's assistance in admitting Peter to hospital as an involuntary patient or placing him under a community treatment order. In such circumstances, the nurse's liaison with the specialist mental health service is paramount in facilitating the process as effectively and comfortably as possible. The nurse also needs to be sensitive to the confidentiality of the client and his family. Being involved in such an event is traumatic for everyone but is sometimes unavoidable. The trauma will be minimised if positive relationships have already been established.

## Access to specialist support

The trialling of Telemedicine in Australia by Yellowlees and his colleagues is an important development and should improve the provision of health care in rural areas. Telemedicine is 'telecommunication that connects a patient through live, two-way audio, two-way video transmission across distances and permits effective diagnosis, treatment and other health care activities' (Preston, Brown & Hartley 1992, p.25). These authors note that this mode of specialist service provision has been successfully used by psychiatric services in America who found it to be popular with consumers. This technology has the potential to alleviate many of the problems associated with rural practice—it enables the practitioner to link into specialist advice, reduces professional isolation, and can be used for the provision of education.

### Addressing the information needs of Peter and Susan

Both client and family need full and accurate information about the disorder and its treatment. Studies consistently report that health services frequently fail to provide adequate information to clients and their families. Jenny's role was to ensure that Peter and Susan were fully informed about his disorder and its treatment. She also aimed to help Peter maintain wellness and prevent relapse, and to assist him and his family to identify early warning signs and strategies for dealing with them.

### Providing support for Peter and his family

The extent and type of support needed will vary with differing family and other circumstances. Being there to discuss concerns and provide information, as well as to facilitate access to the health system, is often the most important aspect of support. Depending on availability, referral to other services which can meet needs such as transport or child care may be necessary.

### Linking Peter and his family with NGOs such as ARAFMI

There are several **non-government organisations** which provide excellent information and support for sufferers of mental illness and their families (see Chapter 1). Even if such organisations do not exist locally, some have a free telephone line for advice and information, and will provide printed material by post. Knowing about such resources, their role and the assistance they can provide, and being able to give this information to clients and families, is a vital aspect of the nurse's role.

### Helping Peter and his family deal with the fear of stigmatisation

The stigma associated with mental illness is an unpleasant reality for many sufferers and their families, especially in rural areas. Helping people affected by mental illness to discuss and understand what is happening to them is vital. Enabling them to be open with trusted people will help reduce the stress of the situation, and the nurse's support can facilitate this process. Non-government organisations, such as the Schizophrenia Fellowship and ARAFMI or equivalent bodies, can often help with information on how to tell family, friends and neighbours about a diagnosis of mental illness.

### Helping Susan identify ways of running the business while Peter is ill

For Peter and Susan this was not a major issue as a friend was able to help out initially. Jenny found that she was able to assist Peter and Susan to plan how, during his recovery phase, Peter could undertake activities in their business that did not cause him excessive stress. In this way his sense of achievement and competence was fostered, and he was able to support Susan. It also made it easier for him to resume his full role as he recovered. However, this process may sometimes take longer or be more difficult than it was in Peter's case. Local service organisations or other resources may be able to assist with such problems.

### Providing a link with specialist mental health services

People often require some interpretation of the 'system'. Being able to call on the local nurse's links with the specialist treatment facility can be helpful. Well developed communication between the specialist facility and local health professionals is an important factor in facilitating continuity of care.

Jenny was able to provide support, information, links with services, assistance with treatment, and the reassurance of being available in the local community when Peter or Susan needed help or just someone to talk to. There is no single recipe of actions to be taken. Each person, family, group and community should be regarded as unique, and care planned jointly, using the nurse's skills, knowledge and resources, and the needs, priorities and resources of client and family. A summary of the important issues for the generalist nurse assisting people with major mental illness is provided in Box 16.3.

$B$ O X  1 6 . 3 :  *Serious mental illness and the generalist nurse*

- Take a holistic approach. Although it is important to obtain medical or specialist mental health service treatment as quickly as possible, in the long term assisting with social, support and information needs is just as important.
- Listen to clients; develop comfortable non-threatening communication. Don't be afraid to ask how they are feeling, including any suicidal thoughts.
- Get in touch with other professionals or services as appropriate. Seek advice and help to make any referral or admission as comfortable as possible for the client and family.
- Get as much useful information as possible for the client and family, including details of self-help and non-government organisations. Explain this information when passing it on and leave the door open for people to come back to you to clarify issues.
- Remember that often one of the most useful things you can do is simply to be there for the client and the family. Convey acceptance and a non-judgmental attitude.
- Treat clients as individuals and do what you can to help them cope in their own situation, within the context of family, social group, work and community.

## Postscript

Not everything Jenny attempts within the community works. She has to treat each situation on its own merits, look at issues and needs holistically, reach out to draw in resources, continually evaluate the effects of interventions, and always be willing to work with the priorities of the clients and the community itself. This is what primary health care practice is all about.

$S$ U M M A R Y

- Current changes in the delivery of mental health services include the location of acute treatment units in conjunction with general hospitals and services (mainstreaming), the movement of people from long-stay institutions back into residence in the community (**deinstitutionalisation**), and a growing emphasis on the treatment of mental illness within the community.
- These changes mean that many health professionals in generalist agencies are seeing more clients with major mental illness. In this context it is important for generalist community nurses to know how to help these clients. In addition, most clients and families face situations and stresses which have the

potential to impact on mental health. A holistic approach to health requires that the mental health needs of all clients be considered.

- There is a growing emphasis on the importance of promoting community mental health rather than merely addressing the treatment of mental illness.
- Contemporary community nursing practice should be based on a primary health care model which includes interdisciplinary and intersectoral collaboration, client and community involvement, a holistic approach, a focus on health promotion, community development approaches, and the provision of health promotion, preventive, curative and rehabilitative services.
- Rural communities face particular issues and problems due to distance, limited resources, socioeconomic factors, and cultural attitudes and mores. The stigma associated with mental illness exists in both urban and rural communities, but the effects can be more damaging in small communities where people are known and easily identifiable.
- Working as a community nurse in a rural area can be challenging and frustrating, but also extremely rewarding. Nurses who move to such a setting need to invest time and energy in getting to know the community, the people and the issues. They will derive benefit from building networks with other nurses and health workers within and outside the immediate community. The establishment of such networks can facilitate the meeting of client needs, provide back-up and support for the nurse, and prevent feelings of isolation.

## $D$ISCUSSION QUESTIONS

1. What principles of mental health nursing practice are the same, irrespective of whether the nurse is working in an urban or rural community?
2. What is the difference between delivering services and working with the community to address mental health problems?
3. Why are rural communities experiencing an increase in mental health problems, and what is the role of the nurse in helping to address the causes of these problems?
4. What are the principles that underpin the primary health care approach to working with rural communities? How do these principles inform holistic nursing practice?

## $E$XERCISES

1. Locate a rural community to which you can gain access. If you or someone you know lives in a rural area, this would be ideal; or you might utilise a clinical placement. Arrange to visit local community-based services and talk with staff about how they help clients to address their mental health needs.

Use your research to answer the following questions.

(a)  Is there collaboration between the services you visit and others?

(b)  Do staff access resources outside their immediate community?

(c)  In what ways are clients and families supported?

(d)  How are clients helped to address needs such as housing, income, employment and recreation?

(e)  Are there any groups with specific needs? Some examples could be Aboriginal or Torres Strait Islander communities, people from non-English speaking backgrounds, or people from minority religious groups. How are services made sensitive to the needs of these groups of people?

2.  Taking the same community as your example, outline the ways in which you could assist a 20-year-old schizophrenia sufferer and his mother, with whom he lives. Contact relevant community agencies within the local community and in regional centres, and obtain any available information, including brochures and resource information, that you could give to this family.

3.  What are the attitudes towards mental illness in this community? Talk with community health professionals and workers; if possible, talk to people who have experienced mental illness and/or their families and friends. Do these people believe they have been stigmatised? Are there any activities aimed at educating the community about mental illness?

# FURTHER READING

- For a comprehensive Australian text on primary health care practice, see:

  McMurray, Anne (2nd edn 1993) *Community Health Nursing. Primary Health Care in Practice*, Melbourne: Churchill Livingstone; or

  Cooney, Cheryl (ed.) (1994) *Primary Health Care. The Way to the Future*, Sydney: Prentice Hall.

- For a detailed discussion of the mental health issues confronting rural communities, see:

  Cheers, B. (1990) 'Rural disadvantage in Australia', *Australian Social Work* 43(1), pp.5–13;

  Yellowlees, P.M '(1990). Bush psychiatric services', *Australian and New Zealand Journal of Psychiatry* 26, pp.191–6;

  Yellowlees, P. M. & Hemming, M. (1992) 'Rural mental health', *Medical Journal of Australia* 157, pp.152–4.

- For a discussion of workforce issues, trends to multiskilling generalist health workers and the impact of these issues, see: Cheers, B. (1992) 'Some thoughts on multiskilled rural welfare practitioners', *Rural Society Journal*, 2(1), pp.5–8.

# REFERENCES

Cantor, C.H. & Coory, M. (1993) 'Is there a rural suicide problem?' *Australian Journal of Public Health* 17(4), pp.382–4.

Cheers, B. (1990) 'Rural disadvantage in Australia', *Australian Social Work* 43(1), pp.5–13.

Cheers, B. (1992) 'Some thoughts on multiskilled rural welfare practitioners', *Rural Society Journal*, 2(1) pp.5–8.

Collingridge, M. (1991) 'What is wrong with rural social and community services?' Paper presented to the Rural Downturn Strategies Workshop, Bendigo, Victoria, 20 August.

Crombie, I.K. (1991) 'Suicide among men in the highlands of Scotland', *British Medical Journal* 302, pp.761–2.

Diekstra, R.F.W. (1989) 'Suicide and attempted suicide; an international perspective', *Acta Psychiatrica Scandinavia* 354, pp.1–24.

Dudley, M., Waters, B., Kelk, N. & Howard, J. (1992) 'Youth suicide in New South Wales: urban rural trends', *Medical Journal of Australia* 156, pp.83–8.

Dunne, P., Patterson, C., Kilmartin, M. & Sladden, M. (1994) 'Qualitative research: health service provision in rural and remote areas: a needs analysis', *Medical Journal of Australia*, 161, pp.160–2.

Hargrove, D.S. (1982) 'The mental health needs of rural America' in H. Dengerink & H.J. Cross (eds) *Training Professionals for Rural Mental Health*, Lincoln, Nebraska: University of Nebraska Press.

Human Rights and Equal Opportunities Commission (1993) *Human Rights and Mental Illness: Report of the National Inquiry into the Human Rights of People with Mental Illness*, Canberra: AGPS.

Martinez-Brawley (1990) *Perspectives on the Small Rural Community: Humanistic Views for Practitioners*, Silver Springs, Md: NASW.

Preston, M.D., Brown, F.W. & Hartley, B. (1992) 'Using telemedicine to improve health care in distant areas', *Hospital and Community Psychiatry* 43, pp.25–31.

Reed, D.A. (1992) 'Community psychiatric practice. Adaption: the key to community psychiatric practice in the rural setting', *Community Mental Health Journal* 28(2), pp.141–50.

Rey, J. (1992) 'The epidemiological catchment area (ECA) study: implications for Australia', *Medical Journal of Australia* 156, pp.200–3.

Strasser, R. (1994) 'So you want to do rural practice?' *Australian Family Physician* 23(4), pp.725–6.

van den Brink, W., Leenstra, A., Ormel, J. & van de Willige, G. (1991) 'Mental health intervention programs in primary care: their scientific basis', *Journal of Affective Disorders* 21, pp.273–84.

World Health Organization (1978) *Primary Health Care: Report of the International Conference on Primary Health Care*. Alma-Ata, USSR. 6–12 September, Geneva.

World Health Organization (1986) *Ottawa Charter for Health Promotion.* Charter for Action developed at the International Conference for Health Promotion, Ottawa, Canada.

Yellowlees, P.M. (1990) 'Bush psychiatric services', *Australian and New Zealand Journal of Psychiatry* 26, pp.191–6.

Yellowlees, P.M. & Hemming, M. (1992) 'Rural mental health', *Medical Journal of Australia* 157, pp.152–4.

Yellowlees, P.M. & Kaushik, A.V. (1992) 'The Broken Hill Psychopathology Project', *Australian and New Zealand Journal of Psychiatry* 26, pp.197–207.

# $\mathcal{T}houghts$

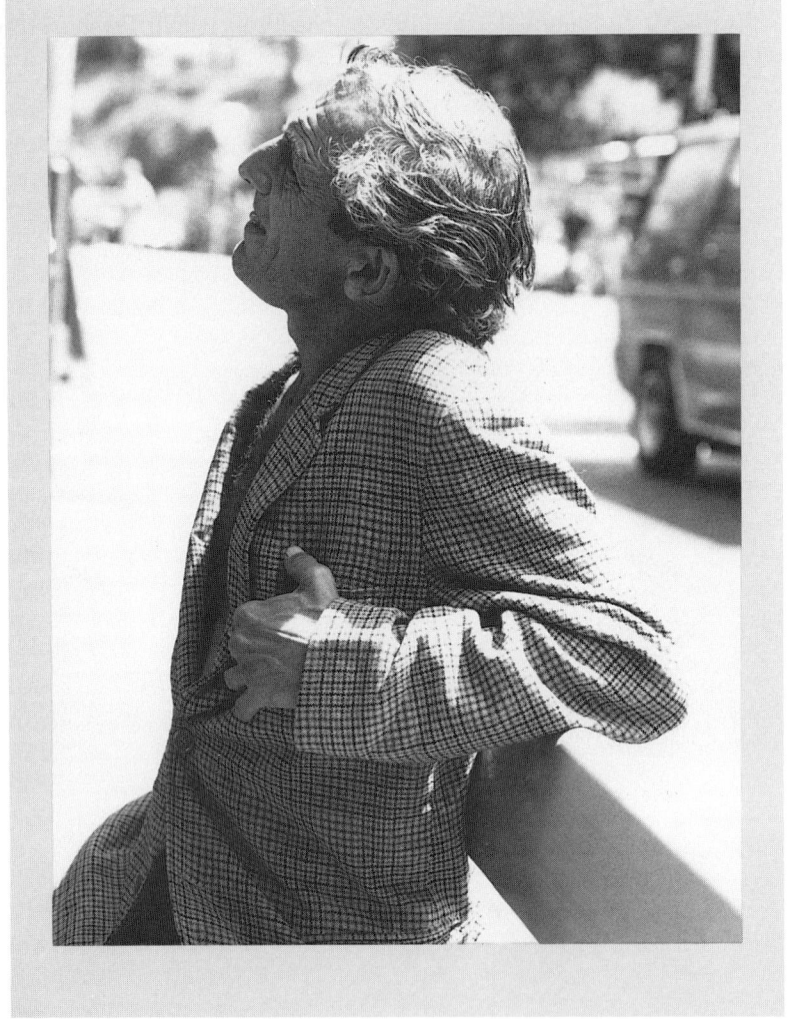

Community mental health nurses work with clients where and as they are.

## CHAPTER 17

# COMMUNITY MENTAL HEALTH NURSING

Tania Yegdich and John Quinn

## CONTENTS

# LEARNING OBJECTIVES

This chapter will assist the reader to:

- explore community mental health nursing care for people with mental illness;
- discuss a conceptual model for community mental health nursing practice;
- explain case management from a community mental health nursing perspective;
- identify factors that promote continuity of care in integrated mental health services;
- examine specific interventions in therapeutic nurse–patient relationships.

# INTRODUCTION

Deinstitutionalisation has seen the dispersal of mental health, social and disability services for people with mental illness from, in Goffman's (1961) words, 'under one roof and under one authority' to various government and non-government agencies in the community. The often pervasive effect of long-term mental illness on a person has accentuated the need for a coordinated multidisciplinary approach to deal with the impairments, disabilities and social handicaps associated with severe mental illness. Today, mental health services, and the mental health nurses who provide them, are part of a community infrastructure that offers a comprehensive range and variety of services for people with mental illness.

# CONCEPTUAL FRAMEWORK FOR COMMUNITY MENTAL HEALTH NURSING

People with mental illness have diverse needs that can be met through biological treatments, supportive social environments, and complex psychological interventions. The combination of interventions based on these approaches to mental health care is known as the biopsychosocial model of care (see Chapter 11). The different components of care are introduced at appropriate need-related intervals in the course of a person's illness. These intervals reflect the rich variability in the interplay between personal vulnerability and biological predisposition to illness, coping and social competency and the environmental social stressors (Anthony & Liberman 1986).

The biological components of treatment focus on pharmacotherapy for acute symptoms or impairments, such as the **delusions** and **hallucinations** that are common manifestations of mental illness. The mental health nurse's role is to administer medication, to monitor progress and to educate patients and their families about pharmacotherapy treatments. Usually the symptoms of the **mental disorder** need to be stabilised before the client's complex social and psychological needs can be addressed. While biological aspects of care always take priority in treatment, the social and psychological remain important and must be addressed (Sabelli & Carlson-Sabelli 1989).

Psychosocial aspects of care are concerned with the effects of the illness on the person, and with societal response to deficits in the person's social and personal functioning. The resulting personal disabilities and social handicaps may be addressed when patients are more able to respond to the demands of their social environment.

Chapter 8 explains how mental health care spans a number of health and social welfare agencies. The needs of mentally ill people are met by the cooperation of different service providers through **intersectoral** links. Within the social components of the biopsychosocial approach to care, mental health nurses advocate 'barrier-free' access to housing and work, and social, vocational and recreational activities to help overcome social **handicaps**. These interventions may offer protection against **stress**. However, people may relapse with symptoms of acute mental illness should the stress of the social environment overwhelm their personal coping skills (see Chapter 2).

Personal coping skills and other social and work competencies help to buffer the course of mental illness and diminish the social handicaps associated with personal disabilities (Anthony & Liberman 1986). Within this aspect of the biopsychosocial model, the mental health nurse develops a therapeutic relationship with the patient. This is the cornerstone of nursing interventions, not only with individuals but also with their families and caregivers.

# CASE MANAGEMENT

While a conceptual understanding of biopsychosocial models helps to articulate and prioritise nursing interventions, case management enables the coordination of different services to achieve continuity of care. Definitions of case management range from brokerage to clinical models (Bachrach 1989). *Brokerage case management* refers to establishing intra- and inter-agency linkages that meet the diverse needs of the person (Bachrach 1989). *Clinical case management* involves the nurse or other team members in direct patient care. A combination of both models is usually adopted.

Case management assists the integration of hospital and community care through the operation of one person, frequently the nurse, who coordinates health and social services in both settings. The main components of case management can be understood in Kanter's (1989) terms as:

- specific patient interventions, including counselling/therapy, social skills training, and **psychoeducation;**
- patient and environment interventions, including crisis assessment teams, outreach follow-up, and monitoring.

Therapeutic tasks in clinical case management are related to engaging the person in a relationship that is special and dependable over time (Harris & Bergman 1988). Case management does not replace direct services, but is based on an adequate infrastructure of community supports for people with a mental illness, such as rehabilitation programs, social skills training, psychoeducation programs and outreach services (Lehman 1989).

Anthony et al. (1988) describe case management as the human link between mental health services and the chronically ill population. Chronicity and the disturbance associated with severe mental illness are major indicators of the need for this type of intervention (Bachrach 1992a). Therefore, the unifying principle that underlies case management is participation in the patient's environment (Kanter 1989). As the individual's needs change between acute and long-term aspects of care, mental health services must be experienced by the person as 'seamless', with the same quality of service available across components of care in 'undisrupted continuity' (Holloway, McLean & Robertson 1991, p.145). Case management emphasises the importance of providing 'tailor-made' interventions for the person within an individualised treatment plan (Minkoff 1987).

## Initial engagement

Establishing rapport with the client is an important part of all nursing care, but it is particularly important in community mental health nursing practice. The primary task during initial interview is to establish sufficient rapport for an assessment to be conducted. In-depth knowledge and understanding of the person will only develop over time as trust in the relationship increases.

### Referrals

Referrals for the assessment of people with mental health problems come from a variety of sources which include self-referral and referral by relatives, friends, hospitals, general practitioners, non-government agencies and other health professionals. Information collected during initial assessment establishes which services may be most appropriate to meeting the person's needs. Many community mental health centres focus on providing intensive case management to support people who are disabled by their illness and unable to access other forms of mental health services effectively.

### Initial assessment

The aim of assessment in community mental health is to match the capacity of patients and their identified needs to optimal interventions. This is achieved by monitoring psychiatric symptoms (impairment), appraisal of social resources (handicap), and observation of level of functioning (disability).

In assessing psychiatric symptoms, standard diagnostic instruments are used. The *Diagnostic and Statistical Manual* DSM-IV (American Psychiatric Association 1994) is universal, as is the mental state examination (see Chapter 10). The Brief

Psychiatric Rating Scale (Overall & Gorham 1962) is a widely used measure of psychopathology. Functional assessments are the domain of mental health nurses, who often undertake them in the person's home. This has the added aim of engaging the family's help from the start. Assessment includes observation of clients in their environment and the collection of collateral information from relatives and caregivers. Self-report instruments are also used in areas such as self-care (personal appearance and hygiene), social competency, family interaction, social isolation, interpersonal conflict, budgeting, housekeeping, use of recreational time, and environmental safety hazards. A variety of instruments is available for this purpose, and include the Australian-formulated Life Skills Profile (Rosen, Hadzi-Pavlovic & Parker 1989).

## Goal setting

Interventions are specifically targeted towards clients' impairments and disabilities. Treatment or rehabilitation is doomed to fail unless it is linked to clients' needs and desires as well as their strengths. The critical aspect in treatment planning is to promote cooperation through active collaboration in setting mutual goals. This establishes a partnership in mental health care between nurse and patient, while fostering a sense of self-responsibility. The therapeutic alliance is strengthened and rapport deepened by communicating to clients a respect for their wishes and belief in their capacity to make decisions. Once goals are articulated, adaptive skills such as an awareness of mental illness, ability to cope with stressful situations, capacity to form interpersonal relationships both with family and friends, and self-care abilities are encouraged. Possible obstacles are acknowledged and may include psychiatric symptoms, medication side effects and limited independent living skills, as well as a lack of social supports and networks, financial resources, social skills and housing.

People with mental illness usually want to achieve the same goals as everyone else (Anthony et al. 1988). These goals include decent accommodation, satisfying work, education, friends, and relief from emotional suffering.

# Environmental interventions

The social environment often has an important influence on the course of mental illness. Deinstitutionalisation has meant that many individuals have families as their primary caregivers.

## Working with families

Families and caregivers are the natural allies of mental health nurses and play a crucial part in supporting the person with mental illness. In undertaking this role, many families and carers experience extreme stress. They require professional support and recognition, both to reduce their stress and perceived burden of care, and to develop more realistic expectations and coping strategies. By engaging families and caregivers in treatment, their expertise is also openly acknowledged by health professionals.

...ation with families and caregivers has three main goals:

...nforce family social networks to maintain the person's adaptation in ...ommunity.

...entify prodromal symptoms, or early warning signs, that may suggest the ...son is relapsing into an acute episode of mental illness. Early interventions might then prevent further disruption to the mentally ill person's life.

3. To involve families in a comprehensive approach to the care of the patient as part of a strategy to encourage treatment adherence and continuity.

Hooley's (1985) critical literature review confirms that the least stimulating environment is a necessary condition to settle acute phases of mental illness. Environments with high expressed emotion (EE), which have a predominantly negative or critical ambience, contribute to the mentally ill person's stress and may diminish personal coping skills. Leff et al. (1982) have demonstrated that education for relatives and carers can be useful in reducing EE, and in preventing relapse. The social interaction model of EE recognises the relationship between the mentally ill person's behaviour and the family's reactions, rather than attributing blame to any member (Tarrier 1991). However, the concept of EE has attracted much criticism from families of people with mental illness, as the concept can be taken to imply (falsely) that families cause mental illness.

## Self-help groups

**Self-help groups**, started by current or former patients (**consumers**), also need professional encouragement, interest and support. Group members can offer hope and inspiration to patients and often have knowledge and experience that professional staff do not have. The focus of these groups is to help individuals to take responsibility for their own care, as well as to advocate for inclusion in decision making about health care provision. Self-help groups advise service planners and providers by evaluating the extent to which existing services meet consumer needs, as well as providing information about what consumers want from health, social and disability services (National Health Strategy 1993) (see Chapter 1).

## Social factors

There are complex interactions between clinical and social factors in mental illness. Acute symptoms may be exacerbated by social factors such as homelessness. Social disadvantages can be demoralising for any individual, but for people with a mental illness they may increase the biological susceptibility to relapse. However, the correction of a social handicap may not necessarily improve **quality of life** or reverse the potentially disabling effects of illness. Indeed, some individuals fall apart when confronted with the everyday stress associated with independent living, work and relationships (Lamb 1988). Nurse case managers establish service links to social and welfare agencies, who cooperate to ameliorate

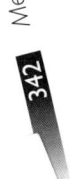
these effects. Service use is also monitored by case managers to est
towards defined goals and to ensure adequate community support.

Just as biological events impact on social events, so social even
the person and may generate psychological disabilities. These disabi.
more specific nursing intervention.

# Nurse–patient interventions

The therapeutic nurse–patient relationship is the basis for successful engagement
in therapy and treatment. Nursing management focuses on the use of therapeutic
skills to enhance the individual's social skills and interpersonal relationships.

## Patient psychoeducation

In both individual and group settings, psychoeducation is effective in alleviating
concerns about taking medication, correcting treatment misconceptions and
providing essential information about mental illness itself. With shorter hospital
admissions, patients may have been prescribed medications in the acute phase
of mental illness when their ability to process information accurately was
limited. Community interventions reinforce the continuity of hospital-initiated
treatment, thereby integrating mental health care. Non-compliance with
treatment by people with mental illness may often be associated with lack of
information and consultation about interventions.

## Groups

Whereas psychoeducation groups are specifically structured and focused on
predetermined content, many pertinent and personal issues are often raised by
group members. Patients in groups may talk about the psychological pain of
needing to take medications for much of their lives. The associated losses to
individuals' sense of self and the effects on their lifestyle are acknowledged and
worked through. (See Chapter 4 for discussion of the concept of loss.) This
ability to adapt to the patient's changing needs, in spite of a predetermined plan,
is an important quality of nursing care directed to the person, not at the illness.

## Individual counselling

Both group and individual therapy, regardless of theoretical orientation, occur
within nurse–patient relationships. The therapeutic value of relationships can
never be overemphasised when offered to patients in ways that assure continuity.
A problem-solving focus based on collaborative goal setting enables the patient
to retain reasonable optimism and pride in adapting to a potentially disabling
mental illness.

## Rehabilitation

Rehabilitation aims to help patients attain a level of functioning beyond their
disabilities, and to enable realistic choices about how to live. This process
involves a long-term vision that Bellack & Mueser (1986) insist must replace

the current 'quick fix approach'. Clinical data indicates that people with a mental illness are not a homogeneous group: they differ in their abilities to handle stressors and demands, and in their wishes and desires (Bellack & Mueser 1986; Kanter 1989; Minkoff 1987). Therefore, the individual's capacity for change and desire for rehabilitation must be assessed by the mental health nurse.

Some people with mental illness may lack the rudimentary social and self-care skills required to live independently in the community. Social skills training addresses deficits in budgeting, shopping, cooking, housekeeping and use of transport, as well as teaching techniques to create social support networks and recreational opportunities. **Cognitive** behavioural techniques help the person to rehearse social situations to build confidence and self-esteem.

## Patient and environment interventions

One of the most important impediments to caring for people with mental illness in the community is the *fluctuation* of insight into mental illness (Minkoff 1987). Individuals may develop a **psychotic** illness and lose judgment and reality-testing capacities. Subsequently, others may intervene on their behalf, sometimes against their consent. After recovery, they may not recall the experience. Some people remain intensely ambivalent about the need for professional help (Bellack & Mueser 1986). It is important to recognise this clinical fact as it poses inherent problems for appropriate intervention.

The essential dilemma in professional ethics is balancing the 'risk of neglect in the name of liberty and the delivery of adequate care with over-controlling paternalism' (Holloway, McLean & Robertson 1991, p.147). This is especially pertinent to clinical judgment for deciding treatment delivery in the psychotic phases of mental illness. This phase of illness may carry powerful ideas that will counteract measures taken by relatives and professionals alike. (See Chapter 19 for an extended discussion on paternalism in mental health nursing practice).

### Acute admissions

Hospital admission is considered in the acute phase of illness to help contain the person in a safe, secure and less stimulating environment. Many consumers will not wish to enter hospital and, when community resources are adequate in providing intensive care, their wish is respected. In the acute phase of the illness, the community mental health team increases the therapeutic contact with the person on a daily basis, sometimes with several visits throughout the day.

### Community treatment orders

As treatment is best provided in the least restrictive environment, involuntary treatment in the community without hospitalisation is recognised by legislation. Precise conditions vary according to individual State and Territorial legislation for community treatment orders (CTOs). Clinical case management that utilises assertive outreach is used in implementing these orders.

*Assertive outreach strategies* enable more active follow-up of the patient. So as not to overwhelm the person, this approach needs careful and sensitive management to counteract the potential for intrusion into the person's privacy. Studies confirm the long-term benefits of preventing possible deterioration in the patient's functioning by implementing early outreach intervention (Torrey 1986; Borland, McRae & Lycan 1989).

When a person cannot or will not attend outpatient appointments or rehabilitation programs, a home visit may determine the nature of the problem. Essentially, assertive services extend geographically and psychologically to 'no matter where the patient is … and no matter what the patient's need' (Torrey 1986).

### Extended hours and crisis teams

In the acute phase of mental illness, extended hours and mobile crisis teams help maintain continuity of care. These teams provide substantial support on a 24-hour basis that can prevent further disruption and hospitalisation. With a mentally ill person's collaboration, this support will assist adjustment to community living. Mobility and quick response to crises at all hours of the day and night are essential features in resolving psychiatric emergencies, such as outbursts of disruptive behaviour or attempts at suicide. Patients, their relatives and carers may rest assured that 'someone is there' and that help is never far away when they need it.

### Continuous care and mobile intensive treatment teams

Mobile intensive teams are used for the longer-term social and psychological care of mentally ill people who have experienced repeated hospitalisations, and unstable accommodation, and displayed non-compliance with medication, disruptive behaviours and poor living skills. The teams aim to prevent homelessness and rehospitalisation while seeking to improve the quality of life for patients, their families and caregivers. Intensive teams follow cohorts of patients across locations and components of care (Torrey 1986). Taube et al. (1990) postulate that a workable ratio of staff to patients in intensive case management is generally 1:10.

## CURRENT CHALLENGES IN COMMUNITY MENTAL HEALTH NURSING

Co-morbidity from substance abuse, plus the problem of loneliness present major challenges to the community mental health nurse.

## Co-morbidity

Co-morbidity (or the existence of more then one mental health problem) is increasingly relevant to mental health. Alcohol- and drug-related problems are ubiquitous. The exact prevalence of alcohol- and drug-related problems in individuals with mental disorder has not been clearly established, although Mueser, Bellack & Blanchard (1992) conclude that estimates vary from 10% to over 65% in schizophrenia. Zisook et al. (1992) found that the drug most commonly used by people with schizophrenia is marijuana, followed by alcohol. The use of amphetamines and hallucinogens is not as common, though poly-drug use is increasing.

As in all substance abuse, the reasons for use and misuse are varied. Some mentally ill people may feel more comfortable being identified with drug-related problems than being perceived as 'mental patients', due to the greater stigmatisation associated with mental illness (Lamb 1988). Social and environmental factors contribute to drug abuse. Both marijuana and alcohol use occur in a social setting and may be a way to satisfy needs for belonging and relating (Dixon et al. 1990). Substance abuse may serve to 'mask' mental illness and Khantzian's (1985) 'self-medicating' theories may be understood as abortive attempts to forestall symptoms. The 'pleasurable' effects of 'getting high' are common to all people and Dixon et al. (1991) suggest that the mentally ill are no exception.

The mentally ill person risks an exacerbation of symptoms by superimposing the cognitive deficits of decreased attention, judgment and processing abilities related to substance abuse on pre-existing impairments (Bellack 1992). The alcohol or drug problem will need to be addressed first as a biological priority, through detoxification. For effective intervention in this area, Drake, Osher and Wallach (1989) recommend a coordinated approach by mental health and alcohol and drug services.

## Homelessness

A connection between mental illness and substance abuse in the homeless population has been confirmed by numerous research studies. This subgroup of dually diagnosed people is often the most disadvantaged and under-served, with the complexity of treating and housing such people frequently commented on (Drake, Osher & Wallach 1991). There are multiple other factors involved in homelessness for the mentally ill, ranging from high unemployment, and limited education and skills, to the loss of family networks, as well as a complex array of other social and welfare stressors (Cournos 1992).

The increasing prevalence and visibility of homeless mentally ill people throughout the western world has driven a highly charged political debate about what are appropriate mental health services and policies (Baumohl 1992). Political arguments have probably influenced service directions more than 'best practice' policies and the interventions of clinicians. Bachrach (1992b) comments that the homeless mentally ill need what other mentally ill people and, in fact, what other poor people need. Moreover, social, psychological and biological needs may be more intense in the homeless mentally ill.

The development of intersectoral links with other government and **non-government organisations** is a welcome approach designed to address these issues.

Advocating for wide-ranging community-based services, and for the access of the homeless mentally ill to them, is an important element of brokerage case management.

The hallmark of a successful mental health service is continuity of care, achieved by the integration of community and hospital services (Bellack & Mueser 1986). Case management is a mechanism that coordinates services across different components of care. It is based on an adequate infrastructure of mental health and other services and does not substitute for direct services themselves. Different aspects of biopsychosocial models of care are used to intervene at different stages of mental illness. In this way a cohesive, varied and comprehensive approach is used to address the diverse needs of the person with a mental illness. A conceptual framework that embraces the principles of biological priority and psychological supremacy offers a prioritising process for the effective planning of nursing interventions and the delivery of an optimal blend of services. The following two case studies demonstrate the application of the biopsychosocial model of care in the community setting.

## CASE STUDY 17.1: *Patrick*

Patrick is a 65-year-old man with a 40-year history of schizophrenia. He has experienced multiple hospital admissions and, in the earlier years of his illness, received treatment as an outpatient. In more recent years he has refused help, and limited attempts made by the community mental health centre to engage him in treatment have failed. For the past seven years, Patrick has been living in a public toilet block near an inner-city church. On several occasions, he has been taken to hospital by the police for his disturbed public behaviour.

Patrick has a complex delusional system which involves (false) beliefs that satanists and constables have inserted a machine inside his brain. He can frequently be seen rubbing his head to ease the pain, and he speaks of a man who has been thrown out of heaven for running a 56-year rebellion against God. While he often sees this man at the local TAB, he never speaks to him. When Patrick is approached, he often responds: 'Patrick is not my name, pensioner books, invalid pensioner.' He hears voices, believes foreign thoughts are placed in his mind and, conversely, that his own thoughts are stolen or can be heard out loud.

The parish priest referred Patrick to the community mental health centre because of these symptoms (and the fact that Patrick had abused some of the parishioners). The mental health nurse and the doctor assessed Patrick at the toilet block. He was irritable, verbally abusive and preoccupied with satanic influences and his 'brain pain'. He stated he was forced to do things he didn't want to do. The doctor suggested he recommence a depot dose of fluphenazine

*continued ...*

decanoate (Modecate), a neuroleptic medication that would help with his thoughts, but he refused and began yelling loudly. Patrick was also at risk of being run over, as he sometimes slept in long grass beside the public car park near the church throughout the day. Functional assessment identified significant deficits in Patrick's self-care and social abilities.

Engaging Patrick in treatment failed due to his overriding psychotic symptoms. As efforts failed to enlist Patrick's cooperation, goalsetting was undertaken by the team in view of Patrick's illness impairments and the need to stabilise his condition. To ensure Patrick's safety and welfare, involuntary hospitalisation was arranged with police assistance. The community mental health nurse accompanied Patrick to hospital and stayed with him to promote engagement and continuity of care. Patrick screamed loudly about the nurse being a satanist, but was not physically aggressive.

Three similarly traumatic admissions occurred over the next three years. The length of each hospital stay averaged two weeks. Patrick always improved with hospitalisation. With the effects of medication his psychotic beliefs would significantly reduce in intensity. He would cooperate and be amenable to further interventions. However, he always stopped taking medication on discharge.

More assertive efforts to improve Patrick's living situation and quality of life were made by the hospital social worker and the community mental heath nurse by finding supportive accommodation. Placements were attempted with his cooperation but ended in failure. On his last admission, he was placed on a three-month community treatment order to ensue continuity of treatment. Unfortunately, he could not be found immediately after discharge and, consequently, it was impossible to ensure ongoing treatment.

Significant connections with Patrick have been established by the mental health team through his admissions to hospital. The community mental health nurse visited Patrick regularly in hospital and the relationship with him was enhanced by getting to know him 'on his own turf' after discharge. The efforts made to find out how he survived, given his considerable adversity, offered him the knowledge that the nurse was concerned for him.

Patrick's survival skills are impressive, though essentially he remains vulnerable. On a few occasions he has been bashed and robbed by local youths, but generally most people leave him alone. He will give a cigarette if asked for one in the street. He uses a local cafe as his bank and for sustenance, as he carries only small amounts of money. The cafe proprietors seem genuinely interested in his welfare and appreciate him as a good customer. They have learnt over the years how to approach him when he is loud or irritable around other customers. For his part, Patrick respects their support and usually cooperates with their requests. In addition, Patrick attends the inner-city mission for a change of clothes, a shower and the occasional meal. He also frequently attends the TAB to place dollar bets, as he follows the horses.

*continued ...*

The community mental health nurse explored with Patrick his dislike of medication. Patrick explained that side effects prevented him from rolling cigarettes properly as he became too restless. He refuses medication to ease the side effects, and so a vicious circle sets in. Similarly, Patrick refuses offers of plastic sheeting to protect him from rain where he sleeps, for fear that others will rob him.

After each hospitalisation, Patrick's functioning is relatively stable. However, this does not last and eventually he becomes disruptive and difficult to communicate with. This usually coincides with his being hard to find, thwarting outreach interventions. Because of his lack of insight into his mental illness, crisis intervention usually includes involuntary hospital admission. Over the years a nurse–patient relationship has developed between Patrick and his case manager nurse along unobtrusive but supportive lines. The community team maintains the perspective that a longer-term vision is required for Patrick, and the mental health nurse perseveres with him without feeling too disappointed that improvement will not be immediate.

## Questions

1. What strengths and capacities assisted Patrick to survive his homelessness?
2. What assessment tools could be utilised in undertaking Patrick's functional assessment?
3. What strategies could be used to bolster the social support available to Patrick?
4. Why was mutual goal setting with Patrick difficult?
5. In the light of the nurse's role in Patrick's involuntary hospitalisation, what difficulties could there be in maintaining a therapeutic relationship with him?
6. Should Patrick be cared for in a long-stay hospital environment? If so, why? If not, why not?

## Exercises

1. List Patrick's strengths, deficits and needs and use them to draw up a tentative treatment plan and set of goals to discuss with him.
2. Describe the case management activities that could be utilised to address Patrick's homelessness.
3. Examine the clinical and social factors relevant to initiating interventions on Patrick's behalf.
4. Compare the advantages and disadvantages of collaborative goal setting with those of involuntary treatment.
5. Consider how the mental health team's interventions could both support and undermine Patrick's trust in team members.

# CASE STUDY 17.2: *Graham*

Graham is a 30-year-old single, unemployed man with a history of non-compliance with treatment for schizophrenia against a background of criminal activities related to past substance abuse. He was diagnosed with schizophrenia in jail eight years ago, and stopped treatment two years ago. Inner-city shelter staff became concerned with his strange account of a recent assault in a nearby country town, and asked the community mental health team for an outreach assessment.

At initial interview, Graham presented as calm and courteous, but his grooming was poor. He was obsessed with the alleged recent assault. Graham claimed he had been assaulted by a group of men he did not know, who held him down while they injected him with an unknown substance. He could give no reason for the incident and reported it to the local police the following day. He stated that the police had told him there was nothing they could do. He then went to the hospital to seek an 'antidote'. Now he says he feels too scared to sleep.

Graham was preoccupied with finding an antidote for the injection, but appeared to show no adverse effects from the event. Though he remained intractable in this belief, and was considerably agitated and worried, there were no unusual thought processes or disturbed behaviour to suggest psychotic illness. After consultation with the psychiatric registrar, Graham agreed to take a small dose of thioridazine (Melleril) to help him sleep.

With Graham's permission the police were contacted and they confirmed that he had reported the assault. They stated they did not consider him to be mentally unstable, only a little 'weird'. The team, again with Graham's permission, contacted his mother in an effort to obtain more information. She reported past relapses involving aggression, somatic delusions, and sexual delusions about his sister. He had believed he had 'holes in his head' and that his sister had sexually abused him as a child, and he had expressed verbal threats to 'get the family'.

Graham deteriorated quickly during the first two weeks of assessment. He started to phone the family home several times a week and this usually ended with him shouting at his mother. He attacked her verbally about their 'pretend' family. His father had died some years ago and had been convicted of child abuse years before. Graham blamed his mother for both events, and became even more preoccupied with both the assault and the antidote. He thought his veins had changed shape and that his proportions had been transformed, and insisted he could taste vanilla essence. He explained that this was all due to 'that injection'. He also became increasingly agitated and incoherent, and was at times verbally threatening to shelter staff.

Although he did not accept that he was mentally ill, Graham agreed that he needed medication to 'bring him down'. In this acute phase of illness, biological treatment took priority over other interventions, with several adjustments made to his medication. Involuntary admission was considered because of his quick

*continued ...*

deterioration and potential to be a danger to others. He was against being admitted to hospital, which he linked to a past experience of being raped in jail. As he was still able to maintain self-care functions, though he showed some difficulty with impulse control, he was seen at least daily by his nurse case manager and the crisis team.

Effective community care for Graham was enhanced by increased community team support, and education for shelter staff, his mother and local residents. Approaching Graham with clarity and a non-judgmental, supportive attitude developed his trust in the community team. By the third week his illness subsided and his ability to process information, maintain attention and develop rapport returned. He could now make use of more complex psychological interventions. The need to continue with pharmacotherapy and maintain some therapeutic contact was reinforced on many occasions and persisted over time. The nurse tested Graham's sense of reality, judgment and insight by encouraging him to verbalise his perceptions and feelings. Alternative coping strategies were explored and practised to assist Graham to deal with his anger.

With the acute aspects of his illness stabilised, interventions with Graham focused on rehabilitation, and a position in the shelter's kitchen was secured with the help of the shelter staff. Graham included finding work as a goal. He was encouraged to modify his expectations by concentrating on his strengths and remaining tactful but realistic about his deficits after his period of acute illness.

Continuing support was provided for the family, as well as teaching them to understand and identify possible warning signs of relapse. Graham's goals and desires were listened to and respected, and became part of his treatment plan. His dislike of medication was acknowledged and overcome through consultation and education. His wish to remain in the community was respected, with support for him and his carers compensating for his decline into psychosis.

These collaborative efforts contributed to overall treatment planning, and corresponded to Graham's needs, capacities, and desire to 'feel more settled'. The nurse as case manager complemented and coordinated other important interventions by a variety of people. Distinct advantages were achieved by decreasing the potential severity of Graham's relapse, by limiting stress for all concerned, by maintaining continuity of care and by enhancing Graham's community adaptation.

## Questions

1. What stressors and personal vulnerabilities contributed to Graham's relapse?
2. What long-term and short-term goals could the mental health team establish with Graham's cooperation?
3. What strategies helped the community mental health team to maintain continuity of care?

4. What actions specifically developed the nurse–patient relationship?

5. What interventions could have been made to reinforce Graham's links with his mother?

6. In what circumstances may hospitalisation have become necessary?

## Exercises

1. List Graham's strengths, deficits and needs and describe how they influenced the mental health team's interventions.

2. Outline the case management processes used in the overall treatment plan.

3. Explain how the mental health nurse prioritised interventions.

4. Evaluate how Graham's personal disabilities were made worse by his social environment.

5. Describe possible methods of intervention to assist with the problem of Graham's phone calls home.

6. Identify possible difficulties with goal setting when Graham was acutely ill.

# SUMMARY

- The biopsychosocial model of care provides for the variety and choice of interventions required for a comprehensive mental health service. Less complex biological needs take priority over more complex social and psychological needs in the treatment of mental illness.

- The effect of medication is enhanced by the addition of psychosocial interventions.

- Case management actively coordinates the services of different agencies and ensures continuity of care.

- The use of intersectoral links can assist people with mental illness to gain access to important social and welfare services.

- Wherever possible, therapeutic nurse–patient relationships are dependable and endure over time.

# DISCUSSION QUESTIONS

1. Explain how mental health nurses determine and prioritise their interventions.

2. Describe the process of goal setting with someone with a mental illness, paying particular attention to the person's motivation, enthusiasm and insight.

# EXERCISES

1. Identify the types of personal disabilities that may contribute to a person's social handicaps, and describe how they may interrelate.
2. Taking one of the case studies in this chapter, review the intersectoral services involved in the care of the client (see Chapter 8).
3. Identify the accommodation and income support services available to homeless people with a mental illness living in your community.

# FURTHER READING

- The following two papers are concerned with homelessness, co-morbidity, impairments, disabilities and handicaps:
  - Hawks, D. (1992) 'Commentary to addiction and the American debate about homelessness: can we assume that the community cares?' *British Journal of Addiction* 87, pp.11–12; and
  - Selzer, J.A. & Lieberman, J.A. (1993) 'Schizophrenia and substance abuse', *Schizophrenia* 16(2), pp.401–12.

- McFarlane, A.C. (1988) 'The International Classification of Impairments, Disabilities, and Handicaps: its usefulness in classifying and understanding biopsychosocial phenomena', *Australian and New Zealand Journal of Psychiatry* 22, pp.31–42. This paper explains the concepts of impairments, disabilities and handicaps referred to in the text.

# REFERENCES

American Psychiatric Association (1994) *Diagnostic and Statistical Manual of Mental Disorders* (4th edn) (DSM-IV), Washington: APA.

Anthony, W.A., & Liberman, R.P. (1986) 'The practice of psychiatric rehabilitation: historical, conceptual and research', *Schizophrenia Bulletin* 12(4), pp.542–58.

Anthony, W.A., Cohen, M., Farkas, M. & Cohen, B.F. (1988) 'Clinical care management: the chronically mentally ill Case Management—More than a Response to a Dysfunctional System', *Community Mental Health Journal* 24(3), pp.219–28.

Bachrach, L.L. (1989) 'Case management: toward a shared definition', *Hospital and Community Psychiatry* 40(9), pp.883–4.

Bachrach, L.L. (1992a) 'Case management revisited', *Hospital and Community Psychiatry* 43(9), pp.867–8.

Bachrach, L.L. (1992b) 'What we know about homelessness among mentally ill persons: an analytic review and commentary', *Hospital and Community Psychiatry* 43(5), pp.453–64.

Baumohl, J. (1992) Editorial: 'Addiction and the American debate about homelessness', *British Journal of Addiction* 87, pp.7–10.

Bellack, A.S. (1992) 'Cognitive rehabilitation for schizophrenia: Is it possible? Is it necessary?' *Schizophrenia Bulletin* 18, pp.43–50.

Bellack, A.S. & Mueser, K.T. (1986) 'A comprehensive treatment program for schizophrenia and chronic mental illness', *Community Mental Health Journal* 22(3), pp.175–89.

Borland, S., McRae, J. & Lycan, C. (1989) 'Outcomes of five years of continuous intensive case management', *Hospital and Community Psychiatry* 40(4), pp.369–76.

Cournos, F. (1992) 'Factors in homelessness among psychiatric patients', *American Journal of Psychiatry* 149(2), p.279.

Dixon, L., Haas, G., Weiden, P.J., Sweeney, J. & Frances, A.J. (1990) 'Acute effects of drug abuse in schizophrenic patients: clinical observations and patients' self-reports', *Schizophrenia Bulletin* 16, pp.69–79.

Dixon, L., Haas, G., Weiden, P.J., Sweeney, J. & Frances, A.J. (1991) 'Drug abuse in schizophrenic patients: clinical correlates and reasons for use', *American Journal of Psychiatry* 148, pp.224–30.

Drake, R.E., Osher, F.C. & Wallach, M.A. (1989) 'Alcohol use and abuse in schizophrenia: a prospective community study', *Journal of Nervous and Mental Disease* 177(7), pp.408–14.

Drake, R.E., Osher, F.C. & Wallach, M.A. (1991) 'Homelessness and dual diagnosis', *American Psychologist* 46(11), pp.1149–58.

Goffman, E. (1961) *Asylums*, New York: Doubleday.

Harris, M. & Bergman, H.C. (1988) 'Clinical case management for the chronically mentally ill: a conceptual analysis', *New Directions for Mental Health Services* 40, pp.5–13.

Holloway, F., McLean, E.K. & Robertson, J.A. (1991) 'Case management', *British Journal of Psychiatry* 159, pp.142–8.

Hooley, J. (1985) 'Expressed emotion: a review of the critical literature', *Clinical Psychology Review* 5, pp.119–40.

Kanter, J. (1989) 'Clinical case management: definition, principles, components', *Hospital and Community Psychiatry* 40(4), pp.361–7.

Khantzian, E.J. (1985) 'The self-medication hypothesis of addictive disorders: focus on heroin and cocaine dependence', *American Journal of Psychiatry* 142(11), pp.1259–64.

Lamb, H.R. (1988) 'Deinstitutionalisation at the crossroads', *Hospital and Community Psychiatry* 39(9), pp.941–5.

Leff, J., Kuipers, L., Berkowitz, R., Eberlein-Vries, R. & Sturgeon, D. (1982) 'A controlled trial of social interventions in the families of schizophrenic patients', *British Journal of Psychiatry* 141, pp.121–34.

Lehman, A.F. (1989) 'Strategies for improving services for the chronic mentally ill', *Hospital and Community Psychiatry* 40(9), pp.916–20.

Minkoff, K. (1987) 'Beyond deinstitutionalisation: a new ideology for the postinstitutional era', *Hospital and Community Psychiatry* 38(9), pp.945–50.

Mueser, K.T., Bellack, A.S. & Blanchard, J.J. (1992) 'Comorbidity of schizophrenia and substance abuse: implications for treatment', *Journal of Consulting and Clinical Psychology* 60(6), pp.845–56.

National Health Strategy Paper no. 12 (1993) *Healthy Participation: Achieving Greater Public Participation and Accountability in the Australian Health System*, Melbourne: Treble Press.

Overall, J.E. & Gorham, D.R. (1962) 'The brief psychiatric rating scale', *Psychological Reports* 10, pp.799–812.

Rosen, A., Hadzi-Pavlovic, D. & Parker, G. (1989) 'Life skills profile: a measure assessing function and disability in schizophrenia', *Schizophrenia Bulletin* 15(2), pp.325–7.

Sabelli, H.C. & Carlson-Sabelli, L. (1989) 'Biological priority and psychological supremacy: a new integrative paradigm derived from process theory', *American Journal of Psychiatry* 146(12), pp.1541–51.

Tarrier, N. (1991) 'Some aspects of family interventions in schizophrenia. 1: Adherence to intervention programmes', *British Journal of Psychiatry* 159, pp.475–80.

Taube, C.A., Morlock, L., Burns, B.J. & Santos, A.B. (1990) 'New directions in assertive community treatment', *Hospital and Community Psychiatry* 41(6), pp.642–6.

Torrey, E.F. (1986) 'Continuous treatment teams in the care of the chronic mentally ill', *Hospital and Community Psychiatry* 37(12), pp.1243–7.

Zisook, S., Heaton, R., Moranville, J., Kuck, J., Jernigan, T. & Braff, D. (1992) 'Past substance abuse and clinical course of schizophrenia', *American Journal of Psychiatry* 149(4), pp.552–3.

# PART VII

# PROFESSIONALISATION

P ART VII FOCUSES UPON professional and ethical issues in mental health nursing practice. Chapter 18 provides the context by discussing some of the contemporary influences on mental health nursing. Prominent among these influences are the changes to practice required by mental health legislation reform; the preparation of mental health nurses in the higher education sector; the greater emphasis now placed on standards and codes of professional practice; and the requirement for more accountability on the part of members of the mental health professions. Chapter 19 takes up the important issue of mental health nursing ethics by examining precepts and dilemmas relevant to practice. Readers are invited to use the ethical frameworks discussed as a basis for considering the ethical issues embedded in this book as a whole. These frameworks inform the everyday practice of mental health nurses and extend the analysis of nursing interventions presented in Part VI. The chapter on mental health nursing ethics has been presented as the final chapter in the book to leave readers with the thought that to practise ethically is the most important principle in mental health nursing.

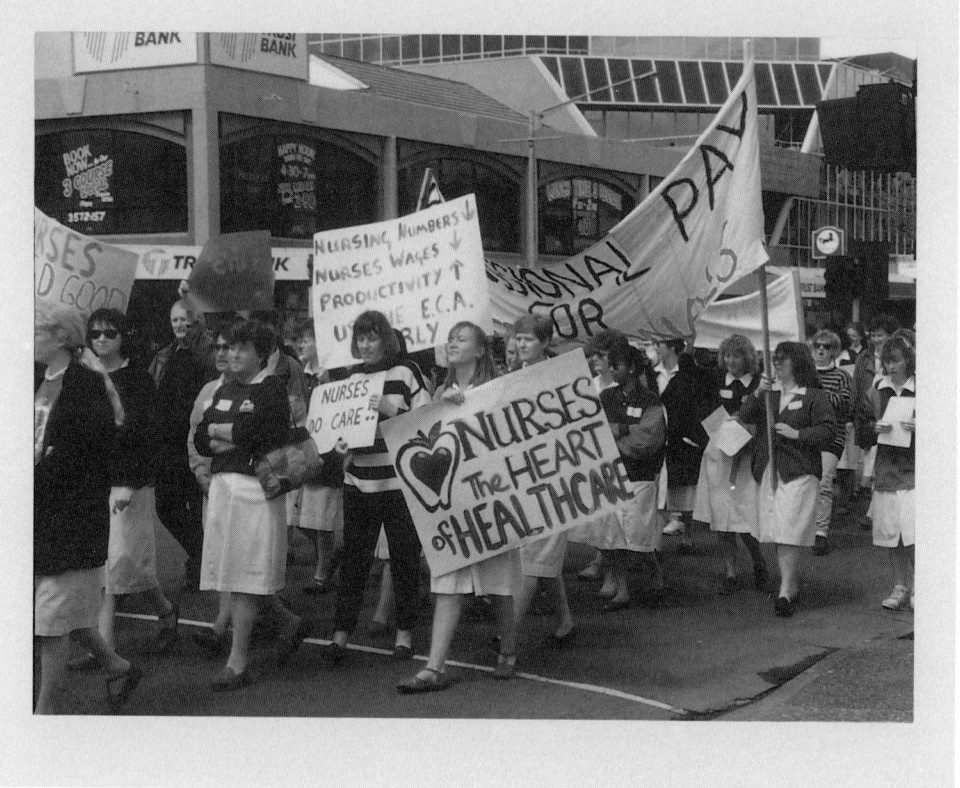

NURSING NEW ZEALAND – WELLINGTON, NZ

Progress is won not given. Only through their professional organisations and unions can nurses have an effective voice in the health care system.

## CHAPTER 18

# PROFESSIONAL ISSUES

Michael Clinton and Sioban Nelson

## CONTENTS

# LEARNING OBJECTIVES

This chapter will assist the reader to:

- discuss changes in the preparation, registration and practice of mental health nurses in Australia and New Zealand;
- explain the relationship between changes in mental health services and the preparation of mental health nurses;
- identify the characteristics of the settings in which the mental health nurses of the future will practise;
- discuss changes in mental health legislation;
- analyse the factors that influence the quality of mental health nursing practice;
- outline some of the activities of trade unions and professional organisations.

# INTRODUCTION

Mental health nursing occurs throughout all fields of nursing practice; it is an integral part of nursing practice. Nonetheless, mental health nursing is also a specialty. The care of people with serious mental illness is a branch of nursing with its own skill base and its own history. The separation of psychiatric nursing from 'general' nursing is a product of the history of mental illness, the development of the asylums and the emergence of the medical field of psychiatry. Although the term 'psychiatric nurse' is still used, increasingly nurses working with the mentally ill have adopted the term 'mental health nurse'. For example, the Australian and New Zealand College of Mental Health Nurses has used this term since its inception in 1974 at the Congress of Mental Health Nurses.

Over the past 10 to 15 years the profession of mental health nursing in Australia and New Zealand has been dominated by three events: the closure of many freestanding psychiatric hospitals, the transfer of nursing education to the higher education sector, and the preparation of generalist nurses. This chapter explores changes in the preparation, registration and practice of mental health nurses; the shifts in practice setting; the development of standards of practice; legal issues surrounding practice; the role of trade unions and professional associations; and the challenges ahead for nurses working with people with mental illness.

# PREPARATION, REGISTRATION AND PRACTICE

The preparation of mental health nurses has witnessed enormous changes over the past decade. In 1980 all psychiatric nurses were prepared by certificate courses conducted at psychiatric institutions. Training involved a rotation through the wards of large institutions and the study of a psychiatric nursing curriculum. Once studies were completed, these nurses were registered to work in psychiatric settings. Post-basic certificate courses were also available for nurses who had completed a course of training in general nursing—these were generally of 18 months duration.

This model is no longer used in any State or Territory of Australia, nor in New Zealand. The education of mental health nurses through direct entry courses has either been abandoned, or is proceeding through a sunset period. Although the registration requirement for specialised psychiatric training remains in the Australian Capital Territory, the Northern Territory and South Australia, psychiatric training is available only as a post-basic qualification. In the other States, university graduates (and New Zealand polytechnic graduates) are registered as 'generic' or 'comprehensive' nurses, although in some States nursing councils may endorse nurses to practise as psychiatric nurses. This registration allows the graduate to apply for employment as a beginning practitioner in any area of nursing, other than midwifery. Although the nurse registration bodies still control the registration of nurses and the regulation of nursing, it is the responsibility of the employer, not the State licensing body, to ensure the competence of nursing staff to practise in their area of employment.

Different requirements exist for registration and practice in all the States of Australia, and the imperative of mutual recognition among States has led to a review of the legal requirements for nursing practice. Queensland, New South Wales, Victoria, Western Australia, South Australia and Tasmania have reviewed existing nursing acts, or have implemented new acts in the 1990s. Mental health nursing is thus in a period of transition where the changes to education, registration and the scope of practice are being redefined and reforms implemented.

Yet, despite changes in the preparation and registration of mental health nurses, the category of psychiatric nurse is far from extinct. Within the field of mental health nursing most practitioners in the early 1990s remain psychiatric nurses (O'Brien 1994). The 1991 Australian census figures reveal that, out of a total number of 178 879 nurses, 5427 were classified by self-report as psychiatric nurses. Of these, 3215 practised in psychiatric hospitals (AIHW 1994).

The transfer of nurse education out of large institutions, and the development of comprehensive nurse registration in New Zealand and in most States of Australia, has not been accomplished without controversy. There have been serious concerns on the part of psychiatric nurses that their specialised area of practice is losing legitimacy (Curry 1993). The custodial model of care has been challenged and nurses have been under pressure to demonstrate their clinical skill base and to follow the patients out into the community (Bennett 1992; Curry 1993; Speedy 1993). The introspection and self-evaluation that has attended transformations in the field of mental health nursing have been absorbing tasks for psychiatric nurses as they have attempted to seize control of the direction of their profession and participate in the policy changes affecting mental health care (Curry 1993).

There have been three challenges for mental health nurses to negotiate over the past decade: deinstitutionalisation (see Chapter 8), the move to higher education, and the implementation of generalist nursing preparation. The challenge of deinstitutionalisation has had profound effects on mental health nursing, as it has eroded the organisational base from which psychiatric/mental health nurses used to function. This has necessitated a resiting of the professional development and practice of mental health nursing out of the large institutions to within the multidisciplinary teams of community mental health services and acute psychiatric facilities within acute general hospitals. These changes are most marked where deinstitutionalisation has proceeded rapidly, such as in New South Wales and Victoria. The challenge of higher education training courses has led to the need for psychiatric nurses to improve the preparation of new practitioners and to upgrade the educational base of skilled practitioners. There has also been a sense of urgency, fuelled by the fear that mental health is being left behind by advances in generalist nursing education (Speedy 1993). The challenge to mental health nursing posed by the dissemination of mental health nursing practice as part of comprehensive nursing has necessitated a re-examination of the specialty.

In fact, the entire move within the health system to **mainstream** services, provide comprehensive care and abandon the divided approach to care that has so often led psychiatric services to be the 'poor relation', has left mental health nurses concerned that the entire specialty was about to be absorbed, without trace, by either comprehensive (general) nursing, or generic mental health workers (Curry 1993). It is certainly the case that one could read documents concerning the direction of mental health care in Australia, such as the National Mental Health Policy and Plan (1992) or the *First National Mental Health Report* 1993 (DHS&H 1994), and have to look closely to find the word 'nurse'—a point of grave concern to the Australian and New Zealand College of Mental Health Nurses (ANZCMHN 1994).

In New South Wales the rapid downsizing of psychiatric institutions following the Richmond Report (1983), the preparation of comprehensive nurses (1985), and the adoption of the single register (1987) occurred in succession. Community psychiatric nurses adopted the name of community mental health workers, prizing their multidisciplinary case management approach, and mental health nursing—the specialty that was psychiatric nursing—looked set to fade from the map. A similar scenario occurred in New Zealand. Polytechnic graduates have been registered as comprehensive nurses since the 1980s and, although the psychiatric register remains, no New Zealand nurse has been added to the list since 1987. The institutions continue to downsize and the community sector grows. However, the new graduates who work in this field generally receive only on-the-job training. New graduate programs are available in some Australian States—in Western Australia and New South Wales, for example—to replace the student workforce, and provide some specialist psychiatric experience. However, this appears to be an interim measure. As the number of freestanding institutions declines, the available positions will follow suit.

# SERVICE SETTINGS

The National Mental Health Policy and Plan was launched in Australia in 1992 as a response to international trends in the further deinstitutionalisation of the mentally ill, the introduction of innovative methods of service delivery overseas, concern in Australia about the human rights of people with mental illness, and dissatisfaction with inadequate, underfunded and sometimes non-existent services. The implementation of the National Mental Health Policy and Plan and the introduction of similar reforms in New Zealand have had far-reaching effects on the practice of mental health nurses.

As a result of continued emphasis on providing cost-effective services through an ever more complex range of community services, hospitals are emerging as highly specialised facilities. Large psychiatric hospitals are being replaced by a mix of general hospital-based acute services, newly established residential facilities, scaled-down mental hospitals, and expanded community treatment and support services. Meanwhile, mental health nurses are being retrained and redeployed to take their place at the forefront of providing better and higher-quality services for the mentally ill. The largest proportion of mental health nurses in the future will be providing treatment and support services in the community.

However, a time lag exists between policy shifts and service modifications, and changes in funding arrangements. Large institutions still consume up to 80% of expenditure on mental health services (DHS&H 1994, p.31). Targets have been set across the States to achieve 50:50 spending in the community and institutional sectors (DHS&H 1994, pp.28,56) as financing and organisational arrangements move to 'reflect mainstreaming and integration principles' in the development of new services (see Chapter 8). Acute services are increasingly provided within mainstreamed facilities. This process is quite advanced in some States, with 84% of acute beds in Queensland, and 87% in Tasmania located within acute facilities in 1993 (DHS&H 1994, p.49).

The framework developed for services in Victoria has elements typical of those being developed in other States and Territories. As resources shift to the community, services are being delivered on a local basis to allow improved access to care, and to ensure continuity of clinical services between hospital and community treatment settings. Networks of community-based services have become the nucleus of mental health care, with hospital-based services functioning in a supportive role. The purpose of the adult mental health service to be developed under this framework is to assess and treat people with mental illness, to coordinate care, to deliver a range of community and residential treatment programs, and to undertake prevention activities and community education (*Victorian Government Department of Health and Community Services* 1994 p.26). Such frameworks acknowledge that, in community settings, nursing and other allied health staff will play a leading role in the provision of case management.

# MENTAL HEALTH LEGISLATION

To underline this climate of transition and uncertainty, the legal framework within which nurses practise and deliver mental health care to clients is itself under review in many States, or has recently been changed. Queensland, Tasmania, the Northern Territory and Western Australia are all reviewing their mental health acts or have implemented new acts. New Zealand proclaimed its new *Mental Health Act* in 1993. Students are advised to examine the reforms to mental health legislation that have occurred or are occurring in their area. (See also Chapter 19.)

The National Mental Health Policy (1992) emphasises the need to develop nationally consistent mental health legislation. The United Nations resolution on the Principles for the Protection of Persons with Mental Illness and the Improvement of Mental Health Care, and the Australian Health Ministers' Statement of Rights and Responsibilities provide the principles which State and Territory legislation must embrace (DHS&H 1994, p.116). Furthermore, the *Human Rights and Mental Illness Report* by the Human Rights and Equal Opportunities Commission (1993), better known as the Burdekin Report, emphasised the need to review procedures, to protect the rights of people suffering from mental illness and to demand minimum standards of practice and accountability of the health professions.

## Community treatment orders

Many governments, cognisant that human rights for people with mental illness have been poorly protected under legislation, are working within the framework of the directives of the National Mental Health Policy and Plan to mainstream services, increase care provision in the community and downsize psychiatric hospitals. Mental health acts have been adopted or developed to provide the framework for a new type of care, a new type of practice. One innovation has been the implementation of community treatment orders (CTOs). New Zealand, Victoria, New South Wales and South Australia have all implemented CTOs; Tasmania and Queensland are likely to do so in their new acts. The implications of this development for community practice of mental health nursing are profound.

CTOs represent an important innovation in the management of severe mental illness, allowing for flexibility to suit the special needs of clients. The provision of such care is negotiated among the client, doctor, carers and the nurse. (See Chapter 17 for a discussion of the role of the nurse in the management of clients under CTOs.) In rural or remote communities, the use of CTOs can overcome the need to transfer the client away from family and friends to the city or town where acute inpatient facilities are located. The use of CTOs in remote Australia, such as areas in the Northern Territory, and the development of schemes to run case management teams with Aboriginal health worker involvement (McCloud 1993) allows for the culturally sensitive management of acutely ill clients and avoids what may be the traumatic, and certainly costly, evacuation of clients to Darwin or Alice Springs.

However, the use of CTOs is not without its opponents. Concern has been raised as to whether community services have sufficient resources, in Australia and New Zealand, to manage compulsory patients (Mulvaney 1993; Street & Walsh 1994). The 'burden of care' experienced by families is similarly increased if extra resources are not available for support when the client becomes acutely ill. Nurses have expressed fears that their legal responsibilities vis-à-vis patients under legal treatment orders attenuate the therapeutic relationship (Street & Walsh 1994). Importantly, as nurses are increasingly caring for clients in the community who are very ill, without a concomitant increase in resources, the nurse's ability to provide preventive care is severely diminished.

## Guardianship and advocacy

A second area of innovation in mental health legislation is the adoption of new arrangements for guardianship and the development of **advocacy** codes. In both South Australia and Victoria, modifications to the mental health acts have occurred alongside changes to guardianship arrangements and advocacy laws so that, increasingly, the human rights of those with severe mental illness are safeguarded. The Queensland Human Rights Commissioner, Dr Ian Siggins, has argued that similar modifications should be adopted in Queensland (Siggins 1994). In fact, Dr Siggins argues that there is no need for mental health legislation at all if guardianship laws are comprehensive enough to cover issues of involuntary admission. According to Dr Siggins, the very existence of a mental health act is discriminatory, as it sets mental health apart from other health problems. This is despite the fact that mental illness is not the only condition that affects the ability of a person to consent to treatment (Siggins 1994).

## STANDARDS OF PRACTICE/STANDARDS OF CARE

In line with changes in mental health legislation, mental health nursing practice is itself undergoing voluntary regulation. However, standards for mental health nursing practice must be considered in the context of broader structural factors that influence the quality of mental health services, including:

- the settings in which nurses work;
- the characteristics of the mental health nursing workforce;
- funding arrangements for mental health services;
- the role of unions and professional organisations;
- relevant legislation; and
- changing social values.

Irrespective of whether mental health nurses practise in the hospital or community services of the future, or participate in both forms of care in integrated services, they will be part of services that will be held accountable for the quality and cost-effectiveness of care. Services as a whole will be accountable for their performance through systems of program evaluation and review. One aspect of this process will be the voluntary participation of services in the accreditation processes of organisations such as the Australian Council on Healthcare Standards (ACHS). Such accreditation is part of the quality movement that is sweeping service industries, including the health industry.

Mental health nurses participate in **quality assurance** procedures such as clinical audits, the monitoring of patient outcomes, and the use of clinical indicators to assess performance against service standards. These procedures are being used on a service- or organisation-wide basis to encourage systematic continuous improvement in service delivery. At the level of the individual nurse, such procedures extend to performance appraisal and training needs audits. All these management strategies are designed to stress the importance of the **consumer** perspective in the development and further improvement of services. Such measures are to the benefit of both consumers and service providers, hence the important role played by trade unions and professional organisations in ensuring the quality of services while protecting the interests of nurses as employees.

Standards for mental health services are '[a]greed and defined clinical procedures and practices for the optimal treatment and care of persons with mental illness' (National Mental Health Plan 1992). Such standards are part of a system of ensuring quality in health care that includes arrangements in States and Territories that play a vital role in monitoring the implementation of mental health legislation. Monitoring is carried out through mechanisms such as the operation of mental health tribunals, the appointment and reporting arrangements for official visitors to psychiatric facilities, and the arrangements for handling complaints about health services and health professionals through such bodies as the Queensland or New Zealand Health Rights Commissions. Some of the professional standards currently influencing the care of the mentally ill in Australia and New Zealand are shown below.

- The Royal Australian and New Zealand College of Psychiatrists (RANZCP) Code of Ethics and Clinical Memoranda.
- Australian Medical Association Code of Ethics.
- Australian Association of Occupational Therapy Code of Ethics.
- Australian Association of Social Workers Code of Ethics.
- Code of Ethics for Pharmacists (Pharmacy Board of Queensland).
- Australian Congress of Mental Health Nurses: Standards of Mental Health Nursing Practice.
- Australian Psychological Society Code of Professional Conduct.

(Queensland Health, *Mental Health Services in Queensland: Minimum Service Standards* 1993, pp 3–4.)

As well, the RANZCP Quality Assurance project has developed clinical practice guidelines as examples of best practice in assessment and clinical management for a number of mental disorders and mental health problems, including treatment outlines for schizophrenia, depression and agoraphobia.

The publications of professional organisations are an invaluable resource when developing service standards. For example, the Mental Health Branch of Queensland Health used the publications listed above to develop a set of minimum service standards. An example of a minimum standard for mental health workers developed by Queensland Health is shown in Figure 18.1. The standards proposed for mental health nursing practice by the Australian and New Zealand College of Mental Health Nurses are shown in Figure 18.2. The standard for advanced practice is met when the mental health nurse demonstrates the ability to integrate, at a level of excellence, the six standards listed in Figure 18.2, using skills in clinical practice, leadership, management, research and education.

## FIGURE 18.1: *Mental health standards in Queensland—minimum service standards*

### Standard 1: Privacy, Dignity and Confidentiality
**Each patient's right to privacy, dignity and confidentiality is recognised and respected.**

Minimum requirements to meet Standard 1

1.1  Each patient and his/her family or caregivers are treated with respect and consideration.

1.2  Mental health professionals provide care which respects gender, age, disability, cultural needs and religious beliefs.

1.3  The region/sector mental health service has a statement of patient and carer rights and responsibilities publicly available, consistent with the United Nations Resolution on the Protection of Persons with Mental Illness and the Improvement of Mental Health Care (1991) and the Mental Health Statement of Rights and Responsibilities (1991).

1.4  Each service has a clearly outlined and publicly available procedure for handling complaints and grievances. Allegations of violations of patient rights are reported immediately to the responsible authority.

1.5  All documentation on patients is relevant, clear and objectively stated.

1.6  Only those staff directly involved in the patient's care, formally monitoring the quality of care or with a statutory entitlement, have access to the clinical record or computerised information.

1.7  Research is approved and monitored by an Ethics Committee established according to National Health and Medical Research Council Guidelines.

1.8  The Quality Assurance program of the mental health service monitors these requirements with the aim of improving patient care.

# FIGURE 18.2: *Standards for mental health nursing practice*

The Australian and New Zealand College of Mental Health Nurses has published revised standards for mental health nursing. To meet the revised standards, mental health nurses must demonstrate that they:

1. ensure culturally appropriate personal practice through the sensitive and supportive identification of cultural issues;

2. establish partnerships as the working basis for therapeutic relationships;

3. provide systematic nursing care that reflects contemporary nursing practice and clients' health care/treatment plans;

4. promote the health and wellness of individuals, families and communities;

5. commit to ongoing education and professional growth, and develop the practice of mental health nursing through the use of appropriate research findings;

6. practise ethically, incorporating the concepts of professional identity, independence, interdependence, authority and partnership.

The development of standards is an important task for the professions, as standards form part of the process of defining the domain of practice and the body of skills encompassed by practitioners. More specific indicators need to be developed at unit level in order to translate these broad professional standards into applicable guidelines for practice, and to facilitate best practice. Minimum standards that have direct clinical applicability are in the process of being developed in practice settings, and broad guidelines for professional standards have provided the framework to set practice standards that will improve nursing care. The identification of such specific clinical indicators ensures that a minimum standard of documented practice is benchmarked (Rosen, Miller & Parker 1989).

A primary objective of the standards movement in mental health is to ensure that all services satisfy the requirements of the United Nations Principles for the Protection of Persons with Mental Illness and the Improvement of Mental Health Care (1991). In keeping with increasing concern about the cost-effectiveness of services, the National Mental Health Policy and Plan (1992) has placed renewed emphasis on ensuring that national outcome standards are developed and used as a basis for assessing the performance of services. Two broad options are available:

1. standards can be assessed by monitoring the inputs and processes of care; or

2. standards can be assessed in terms of whether services are effective in achieving positive client outcomes, by ensuring that consumers are satisfied with the care they receive (DHS&H 1994, p.101).

In practice, both approaches are used in mental health care, hence both are relevant to the practice of mental health nurses. However, the first approach has the most immediate implications for mental health nurses, because codes of practice are available for nurses in Australia and New Zealand. The availability of such codes raises the important question of the relationship between the quality of care and the role of unions and professional organisations.

# ROLE OF TRADE UNIONS AND PROFESSIONAL ORGANISATIONS

National organisations play a key role in influencing nursing practice. The Code of Ethics developed under the auspices of the Australian Nursing Federation, the Australian Nursing Council Incorporated and the Royal College of Nursing, Australia, is a good example of what can be achieved through cooperation between national organisations (ANCI 1994; Parkes 1994; Parkes 1993). The Code is intended to help nurses to reflect on the ethical dilemmas inherent in their work, rather than to assist them to resolve dilemmas they confront in their practice on a daily basis. The Code contains six broad statements of value that can aid in exploring and considering the ethical concerns that arise from nursing practice. It makes it clear that nurses have the moral right to refuse to participate in procedures that are at variance with their personal philosophies of care. For example, nurses may refuse to assist with the forceful administration of medication to patients. But in so doing they may leave themselves open to disciplinary procedures on the part of employers. Codes of ethics and the Code of Conduct currently under development in Australia by the registration authorities are important in shaping the quality of nursing practice. The preamble to the Code of Ethics is particularly important in reminding nurses of their role in 'supporting and enabling individuals, families and groups to maintain, restore or improve their health status, or to be cared for and comforted when deterioration of health has become irreversible' (ANCI 1993).

These and similar sentiments have underpinned statements on nursing practice that have been published by professional nursing organisations in Australia and New Zealand (ANCI 1994, New Zealand Nurses' Association 1990). Such standards have been part of a broader framework that seeks to improve the quality of health services. International trends in best practice, national policies, the influence of legal reforms, and increasing emphasis on the responsibilities of service providers and the rights of consumers have all played their role in focusing attention on the quality of services and patient outcomes.

The increasing focus on the quality of mental health services raises issues that are at the forefront of the roles of unions and professional organisations. The quality of mental health nursing practice is determined not just by the preferences of individual nurses and the policies and procedures of their employers, but also by the context in which nurses are employed. The changes to the practice of mental health nurses that have been outlined in this chapter have been presented in isolation from important factors that shape the possibilities for practice. The industrial context in which nurses are employed has a major influence on what can be achieved in any practice setting, whether it be the home of the patient, a new small-scale residential facility, a refurbished hospital, or a psychiatric unit in a local general hospital.

Among the factors that shape nursing practice are the conditions under which nurses are employed and the quality of the relationship between nurses and their employers. In recent years, in Australia and New Zealand, there has emerged:

> ... an implicit acceptance of the ability of competition to improve efficiency and of the general applicability of competitive market theories to the funding and provision of health services. (Beaumont 1992, p.7)

Uncritical acceptance of these principles on both sides of the Tasman has resulted in the advent of enterprise bargaining in Australia, and the introduction of employment contracts negotiated outside national award agreements in New Zealand and in a number of Australian States. The emphasis on more flexibility in employment contracts in both countries has raised major concerns in professional nursing organisations. The workplace approach to the negotiation of pay and conditions has the potential to be divisive as professional organisations struggle to maintain conditions of employment against a background of increasing fragmentation and complexity.

Changes in the New Zealand health care system, described in Chapter 8, have resulted in the need for the New Zealand Nurses' Organisation (formed by amalgamation of the New Zealand Nurses' Society and the New Zealand Nurses' Association) to pursue negotiations with individual employers rather than participate in negotiating one major national award every year. Further problems have arisen in New Zealand because nurses who have entered into individual agreements on pay and conditions with their employers have signed contracts that prevent them discussing the contents of their contracts with any third party because of alleged 'commercial sensitivity' (Beaumont 1992, p.7).

Such developments are important at any time, but particularly so during the present period of change in mental health services. However, it is important to stress that professional organisations and unions are not concerned solely with the pay and conditions of their members. These organisations have a strong commitment to safeguarding and improving the quality of health services. For example, the ANF (Victorian Branch) *Policy Statement on the Integration of Psychiatric Services* (1992) states explicitly that all nurses have an invaluable contribution to make to the overall advancement of the profession, as well as to the advancement of patient care.

The ANF has demonstrated concern over the interests of its members in such matters as psychiatric hospital closures. However, it stresses the inextricable relationship between conditions of employment and the quality of mental health services (*The Lamp* 1993). Mental health nurses and the organisations that represent them must be satisfied that any reforms introduced will improve access to better services for all who need them, and that the interests of staff will be protected. In negotiating issues such as the closure of hospitals, there is a need for strategic planning of the size, composition and characteristics of the mental health workforces in Australia and New Zealand. Questions about the portability of entitlements for staff in existing mental health services, funding arrangements, the ability of services to meet reasonable standards of care and to achieve better outcomes for the consumers of mental health services need to be addressed. These broader determinants of the quality of mental health services were raised by the 100 000-strong Australian Nursing Federation in its response to the discussion paper, *Mental Health Workforce Issues* (ANF 1993). In its response the ANF stressed the need for proper workforce planning for mental health services and emphasised the importance of preparing the existing mental health workforce for new roles. These issues were later taken up by the Australian Health Ministers' Council, and consultants were appointed to advise on the training needs of the mental health workforce. The consultants recommended that a strategy be implemented to initiate, coordinate and support a national training approach (KPMG Consulting 1994). At the time of writing, the recommendations of the consultants are under consideration by Commonwealth and State departments.

## FUTURE CHALLENGES

Mental health nurses face a period of challenge. The field of education and professional preparation of mental health nurses has undergone, and continues to undergo, major transformation. So too the practice domain has been dramatically affected by policy and service shifts

### Preparation

It is essential that a national training strategy is devised and implemented for the preparation of new practitioners in mental health nursing, and for the development of existing staff, in order to accommodate new service requirements. In each State and Territory of Australia, and in New Zealand, the matter is one of ongoing negotiation. In most States, post-basic courses have been only slowly phased out and thus the number of nurses with specialist psychiatric qualifications registered in the 1991 census remains substantial.

A national training strategy requires the implementation of an evaluation process. One such process is the measurement of competencies. *Competencies* are values, attitudes and behaviours that can be demonstrated to have been achieved by the end of an award course, a post-basic nursing course, or program of personal development. Formal competencies for registered and enrolled nurses have been developed by the ANCI and adopted by the registration boards throughout Australia. Moves to implement mutual recognition of qualifications throughout Australia are the subject of continuing negotiation between the

States, the Commonwealth, the Australian Nursing Council Incorporated, and the registration bodies. Once standards have been agreed, registration and/or enrolment will be based first on qualifications, later on standards of competence. In New Zealand, competency-based standards of practice in mental health nursing are considered to

> ... represent the standard of performance which can be expected from a registered nurse who has been working for a period of the equivalent of twelve months full-time in any mental health context (New Zealand Branch, ANZCMHN 1994).

As Australia and New Zealand continue to reform mental health services, pressure will increase for mental health nurses to clarify their contribution to caring for people with mental illness. Mental health nurses must demonstrate a distinctive body of knowledge that enables them to assist people with mental illnesses and their carers to access services, to cope with symptoms and functional disability, and to enjoy a reasonable **quality of life** free from prejudice and discrimination. Therefore, if the expense of preparing them is to be justified, mental health nurses must be able to articulate their knowledge, show how it is applied in practice, and demonstrate that what they do makes a difference to health care outcomes (Bennett 1992, p.66).

For mental health nurses to articulate their knowledge it will be necessary for them to identity, clarify and systematise the knowledge they draw on in practice. It will be necessary, too, for the universities involved in nursing education in Australia and New Zealand to expand the knowledge base of mental health nursing through research and scholarship. Finally, the research capacity of mental health nurses in the universities will need to be directed to collaborative research with practitioners, to identify what mental health nursing practice achieves for the consumer.

Similarly, collaboration between universities and health agencies will be necessary to develop high-quality courses leading to graduate certificates, graduate diplomas and master's degrees in mental health nursing, with easy credit transfer between clinical settings and the universities. Recognition of prior learning and maximum credit transfer will enable the expertise of the health care industry and the higher education sector to be brought together to ensure the efficient use of scarce resources (Bennett 1992, p.67). Such arrangements will continue to be put in place as increasing pressure on budgets forces health agencies to discontinue post-basic nurse education.

## Practice

The manner in which mental health nurses negotiate opportunities to practise in the community and the hospital setting will be determined to a great extent by the strength of their professional identity. In the community it takes a confident and positive professional identity to adapt to practice in a multidisciplinary team. The community-based team setting demands that mental health nurses define their area of practice and expertise and defend its application as being in the best interests of the client. In the field of rehabilitation, the role of nursing assistants, enrolled nurses, residential workers and others raises serious concerns over the erosion of the role of the mental health nurse. In the hospital setting the same challenge exists. The decline of hospital-based specialty training, and the gradual replacement of psychiatric nurses with generic nurses, also challenges the field to define and justify its existence. The focus on competencies, quality assurance and outcome measures provides the imperative for nursing care to establish and conform to standards that guarantee consistent and valuable care. As Professor Sandra Speedy argues, 'we need to show that our nursing has a measurable and demonstrative impact upon our clients' (Speedy 1993, p.330).

One area for mental health nurses to come to terms with is that of independent nursing practice. Although independent practice for nurses, with rights to prescribe medication, refer patients to medical specialists, and charge a fee under health insurance schemes has been a fact of life for some years in the United States, Canada and, increasingly, in New Zealand, independent practice in Australia is at a very early stage. In New South Wales, there were positive moves in this direction early in 1992, with an assessment of the feasibility of extending the limits of nursing practice, particularly in specific fields such as remote area health and women's health. The introduction of independent nursing practitioners will have considerable impact for mental health nursing practice. In a survey of two independent nursing practices in Auckland, the main reasons for consultation of the nurse by men and women were **stress**, insomnia and **depression** (McDonald 1989, pp.20–37). Speedy predicts that declining numbers of nurses in institutional roles could lead to expanded opportunities for independent practice in the community as: 'community mental health nurses, women's health nurses, and nurse therapists' (Speedy 1993, p.332). Furthermore, early discharge programs and other cost-containment measures in hospitals are among the health care trends that are creating opportunities for independent nursing practice. The outcome of the New South Wales pilot scheme will have significance for the development of independent nursing practitioners elsewhere. Thus, in the future, mental health nurses could play a key role in the field of **prevention**, particularly in rural and remote communities.

## SUMMARY

- The preparation and practice of mental health nurses is undergoing profound change.
- Further changes in mental health nursing are needed to support the implementation of the National Mental Health Policy and Plan (1992).
- The mental health nurses of the future will work in more flexible integrated and mainstreamed mental health services.

- Changes in mental health legislation will continue to influence mental health nursing practice.
- The consumer movement and the need for mental health professionals to be accountable will result in continuing pressure for the quality of mental health services to be improved.
- Trade unions and professional organisations will continue to play a key role in the development of mental health practice.

## DISCUSSION QUESTIONS

1. Of all the changes taking place in mental health nursing, which do you regard as the most significant and why?
2. Why have the mental health services in Australia and New Zealand become such important areas for reform?
3. What is the purpose of mental health legislation?
4. What factors do you believe have most impact on the quality of mental health nursing practice?
5. Select a standard for nursing practice from any published source and critique its application to mental health nursing.
6. Arrange with your lecturer to have an independent nursing practitioner talk to your group. Discuss with the practitioner the mental health aspect of his or her role.

## EXERCISES

1. Analyse any chapter in *Human Rights and Mental Illness: Report of the National Inquiry into the Human Rights of People with Mental Illness* and identify the implications for improving mental health nursing practice.
2. Next time you undertake clinical experience in a mental health setting, compile a profile of the strengths and weaknesses of direct entry courses into psychiatric nursing by interviewing two registered nurses, one prepared in a direct entry course, the other prepared in a tertiary education institution.
3. Arrange with your lecturer for a representative of a local consumer organisation to brief your class on the role played by the organisation in reforming mental health legislation in your State.
4. Identify the factors that influence the quality of nursing practice. Pay particular attention to the application of explicit standards for practice and processes of quality assurance.

# FURTHER READING

- Speedy, S. (1993) 'Claiming the future: mental health nursing—2000 and beyond', *Australian Journal of Mental Health Nursing* 2(7), pp.329–37. This paper examines the current state of mental health nursing and its future direction. Professional issues from preparation and practice to higher education and research are addressed.

- Rosen, A., Miller, V. & Parker, G. (1989) 'Standards of care for area mental health services', *Australian and New Zealand Journal of Psychiatry* 23, pp.379–95. In this paper the authors outline the function of standards, the challenge to develop and implement such standards, and their role in achieving a high-quality integrated community and hospital mental health service.

- Street, A.F. & Walsh, C. (1994) 'The legislation of the therapeutic role: implications for the practice of community mental health nurses using the New Zealand *Mental Health (Compulsory Assessment and Treatment) Act* of 1992', *Australian and New Zealand Journal of Mental Health Nursing* 3(2), pp.39–44. This paper examines the implications of the introduction of community treatment orders in New Zealand. Issues of practice, resources and ethics are discussed in this report on preliminary research in the area.

# REFERENCES

Australian and New Zealand College of Mental Health Nurses (1994) *Preliminary Position Paper on the Australian National Mental Health Policy and Plan*. Greenacres, SA: ANZCMHN.

Australian and New Zealand College of Mental Health Nurses (1995) *Standards for Mental Health Nursing Practice (revised)*. Greenacres, SA: ANZCMHN.

Australian Nursing Incorporated Council (1993) *Code of Ethics for Nurses in Australia*. Canberra.

Australian Nursing Incorporated Council (1994) *Draft Code of Conduct for Nurses 1994*. Canberra.

Australian Institute of Health and Welfare (1994) 'Number of persons employed by occupation by establishment type'. Data compiled for Centre for Mental Health Nursing Research, Queensland University of Technology, extracts from 1991 Census.

Australian Nursing Federation (1990) *Submission to National Inquiry concerning the Human Rights of People with Mental Illness*. Unpublished document.

Australian Nursing Federation (1993) Response to discussion paper, *Mental Health Workforce Issues*. Unpublished paper, March 1993.

Australian Nursing Federation, Victorian Branch (1992) *Policy Statement on the Integration of Psychiatric Services*. Unpublished paper, 11 February 1992.

Beaumont, M. (1992) 'Health reforms—lessons', *Australian Nurses Journal* 22(4), October, pp.6–7.

Bennett, M.J. (1992) 'Psychiatric nursing education in Victoria: future directions', *Australian Journal of Mental Health Nursing* 2(2), pp.65–70.

Curry, G. (1993) 'Self-actualisation or self-destruction: an historical perspective on psychiatric nursing', *Australian Journal of Mental Health Nursing* 2(5), pp.234–42.

Department of Health, Housing and Local Government (1992) *Mental Health Policy and Plan*, Canberra: AGPS.

Department of Human Services and Health (1994) *First National Mental Health Report, 1993*, Canberra: AGPS.

Human Rights and Equal Opportunities Commission (1993) *Human Rights and Mental Illness: Report of the National Inquiry into the Human Rights of People with Mental Illness*, Canberra: AGPS.

KPMG Management Consultancy (1994) National mental health workforce education and training consultancy, Melbourne.

*The Lamp* (1993) New South Wales Nurses Association concerns about the future of the Gladesville Hospital, August, p.4.

McDonald, J. (1989) Two independent nursing practices: an evaluation of a primary health care initiative, Ministry of Health, Discussion papers, Wellington.

Mental Health Branch Queensland Health (1993) *Minimum Standards for Mental Health Services in Queensland. The Standards Implementation Kit.* Internal document, Queensland Health.

Mulvaney, J. (1993) 'Compulsory community treatment: implications for community health workers', *Australian Journal of Mental Health Nursing* 2(4), pp.183–9.

New Zealand Nurses' Association (1990) *Standards for nursing practice.* Wellington: New Zealand Nurses' Association.

O'Brien, A. (1994) 'A review of the problems and prospects in mental health nursing educationa qualitative review', *Australian and New Zealand Journal of Mental Health Nursing* 3(3), pp.95–106.

Parkes, R. (1993) Code of ethics for nurses in Australia. *Australian Nursing Journal*, September 28–30.

Parkes, R. (1994) Update on national practice standards. *Australian Nursing Journal*, April 24–38.

Rosen, A., Miller, V. & Parker, G. (1989) 'Standards of care for area mental health services'. *Australia and New Zealand Journal of Psychiatry* 23, pp.379–95.

Richmond, D. (1983) *Inquiry into health services for the psychiatrically ill and developmentally disabled.* Sydney: New South Wales Depart Health.

Siggins, I. (1994) 'Should we have a mental health act?' A paper presented to the Northern Queensland Mental Health Conference, Hamilton Island, North Queensland, 19 March.

Speedy, S. (1993) 'Claiming the future: mental health nursing—2000 and beyond', *Australian Journal of Mental Health Nursing* 2(7), pp.329–37.

Street, A.F. & Walsh, C. (1994) 'The legislation of the therapeutic role: implications for the practice of community mental health nurses using the New Zealand *Mental Health (Compulsory Assessment and Treatment) Act* of 1992', *Australian and New Zealand Journal of Mental Health Nursing* 3(2), pp.39–44.

United Nations General Assembly Resolution (1992) The Protection of Persons with Mental Illness and the Improvement of Mental Health Care: Resolution 98B. Adopted Dec. 1991, Geneva: UN.

Victorian Government Department of Health and Community Services (1994) *Victoria's Mental Health Service: The Framework for Service Delivery.* Melbourne: Department of Health and Community Services.

# Hygieia

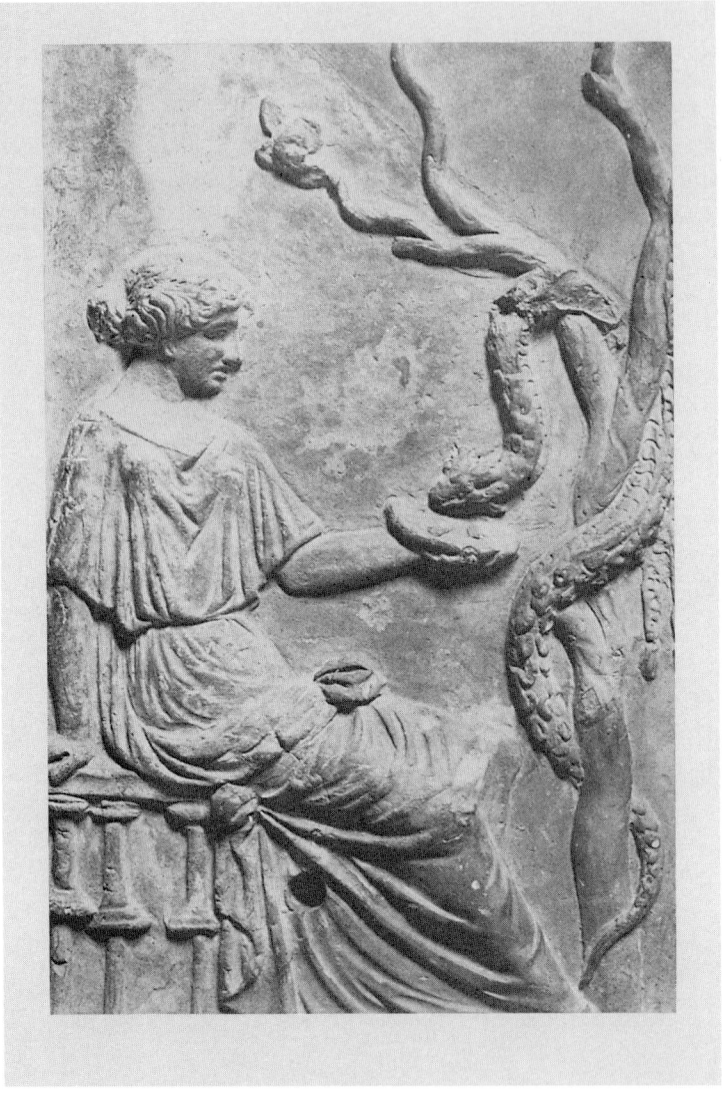

Hygieia: Goddess of health and wisdom in Ancient Greece, compassionate
friend of humanity. Hygieia symbolises the essence of virtue
in ethical nursing practice.

## CHAPTER 19

# ETHICAL ISSUES

Gail Tulloch and Gail Hart

## CONTENTS

## LEARNING OBJECTIVES

This chapter will assist the reader to:

- argue the relevance of ethical principles to mental health nursing;
- identify ethical issues in mental health nursing practice;
- assess mental health nursing practice within the framework of United Nations human rights conventions;
- apply ethical principles in clinical decision making and nursing practice;
- outline the contribution of the feminist critique of traditional ethics to the understanding of key issues concerning women and mental health;
- formulate an approach to ethical issues in mental health nursing that incorporates both a personal and professional perspective.

## INTRODUCTION

Ethical issues abound in mental health nursing. Consider discovering poor standards of patient care involving a nursing colleague or a doctor; or being asked to force a patient to take medication; or to tell a 'white lie' to patients or relatives. All too frequently, there is conflict between the imperative to act immediately and the need to provide a considered response to a complex situation. All these situations can pose acute ethical dilemmas for the nurse working in a mental health setting.

## ETHICS

What then is ethics? *Ethics* is a branch of philosophy which centres on the study of good and bad, right and wrong, and attempts to formulate principles that guide us in deciding what to do and how to act morally. The Golden Rule, 'Do unto others as you would have them do to you', is one well-known example of such a principle. Ethics is to do with morals, not mores (i.e. customs, such as driving on the right or left of the road). Importantly, ethics involves giving reasons why it is right or good to act in a given way in a particular situation, and these reasons are universal and are concerned with human welfare and human interests. Ethics thus involves our deepest notions of human nature, and what it is to be a person.

There have been two main traditional approaches to ethics: *deontological* and *consequentialist*. Consider your own experience: sometimes you apologise to someone by saying, 'I'm sorry, I didn't mean that to happen', and sometimes you might say, 'I'm sorry, I didn't know that would happen'. Sometimes, that is, you appeal to your intention, or state of mind, to excuse yourself, and sometimes you appeal to your inability to predict the consequences. *Deontologists* hold that what makes an action right is your state of mind, that ethics is a matter of determining which actions are required or prohibited as a matter of duty. *Consequentialists* hold that the moral worth of an action is measured by its consequences. In practice, consequentialists tend to be associated with **quality of life** arguments (Singer 1993), recognising that circumstances alter cases, and deontologists with **sanctity of life** arguments, based on respect for people and individual rights that are not to be traded off as means to ends. In practice, too, both tend to emphasise rationality and autonomy as the basis of respect for people—an emphasis that is still frequently appealed to in ethical contexts.

Immanuel Kant (1724–1804) is the most influential deontologist. He argued that the only thing intrinsically good in the world—that is, good for its own sake—is a good will, and that a good will acts out of duty, out of obedience to the moral law. Kant grounded the basis of moral justification on what he called the Categorical Imperative, and gave two important formulations of it:

1.  Act always so as to treat humanity, whether in your own person or in that of another, never merely as a means, but always at the same time as an end.
2.  Act only according to a maxim which you can at the same time will to become a universal law.

Self-interest and individual feelings were no basis for morality; instead, human dignity was grounded in rationality.

Consequentialists, on the other hand, hold that an action is right if it maximises what is desirable in its outcome. *Utilitarianism* is the most familiar form of consequentialism, where consequences are evaluated in terms of the effects of an action on the welfare and happiness of people (or, more broadly, sentient beings), and the greatest good for the greatest number is aimed at. Jeremy Bentham (1748–1832) was the founder of utilitarianism and formulated the Principle of Utility, according to which:

> Actions are right in proportion as they tend to promote happiness, wrong as they tend to produce the reverse of happiness. By happiness is intended pleasure and the absence of pain; by unhappiness, pain and the privation of pleasure.

For Bentham, there would have been no difference between a computer game such as Nintendo and poetry, as far as pleasure goes.

John Stuart Mill (1806–73) modified Bentham's utilitarianism by referring to 'utility in the largest sense grounded on the permanent interests of man as a progressive being', and by distinguishing between higher and lower pleasures. The higher pleasures are those that develop perception, discriminative feelings, mental activity and moral choice, and the pleasures derived from the highest faculties are preferable in kind, and yield greater happiness. Mill also stresses 'the sense of dignity which all human beings possess' (Mill vol.10, p.212).

If Mill's richer, more complex utilitarianism is applied, the best course of action is always the way that promotes respect for autonomy and individual self-determination. **Paternalism,** or doing something for another's good as *you* see it, is taboo, as is force in dealing with an individual, except in the case of protecting some third party from harm. 'White lies', or force-feeding someone with medication would run counter to the liberal emphasis on voluntary actions, and free, undeceived consent. In the nursing context, this clearly applies in situations involving euthanasia, not for resuscitation (NFR) orders and informed consent, to name a few obvious examples from medical ethics.

In the early days of medical ethics (the 1970s), bioethical dilemmas were fitted into the framework of standard moral theories, particularly utilitarianism and Kantian deontology. Case studies became a common strategy, generally handled using the standard moral principles—justice, autonomy, beneficence ('do good'), non-maleficence ('do no harm') and utility—as a way of contextualising and applying moral principles (Beauchamp & Walters 1989; Mappes & Zembaty 1991).

## FEMINIST CRITIQUE OF TRADITIONAL ETHICS

Standard moral themes later became identified with a male-dominated ethics model that came to be seen as overwhelmingly physician-dominated, and sexist in that gender was likely to be deemed irrelevant. Frustration with the level of abstraction and generality of much of traditional ethics, and a concern for a more contextually based moral theory produced a feminist critique. Feminists wished to take account of specific relationships, and give added weight to particular qualities like care and responsibility. Gilligan's (1982) work in defending a 'different voice' in moral reasoning, and an ethic of care to complement (not displace) the Piagetian–Kohlbergian ethic of justice and abstract reasoning is a well-known and influential example. Further examples are the work of Ruddick (1989) and Noddings (1984), with their emphasis on caring and mothering. These three theorists may be called 'feminine ethicists'.

Feminine ethics arose out of a recognition that the ideals of western rationality, including scientific thought, devalue contextual modes of thought and emotional components of reason. Sherwin (1992), among others (Jaggar 1993; Card 1993), has pointed to an 'antiwoman' bias that pervades much of existing theoretical work in ethics, in that the audience is seen as exclusively male, and a different set of virtues applies for women, with only male virtues being treated as of philosophical interest or moral worth. This 'blatantly misogynistic vision' (Sherwin 1992, p.43) applies to Aristotle, Kant, Aquinas, Rousseau, Hegel, Nietzsche and Sartre—with Plato and Mill being honourable exceptions. The tendency persists today, and even the presumption that philosophy can be done in a gender-neutral way can perpetuate male privilege. While women are assumed to fall under the general notion of 'the agent', the moral concerns that are examined are frequently those that arise from a male perspective.

The presumed norm of the moral subject is therefore male-biased, premised on male norms, interests and lifestyle, while attention to context and consideration of the emotions are associated with the feminine. A luminous example of male=norm can be found in the Broverman et al. study into sex role stereotypes. The Broverman study of 'Sex role stereotypes and clinical judgements of mental health' in the United States is now a generation old (published in 1970), yet unfortunately remains relevant. In this study, clinicians were asked to describe a healthy man, a healthy woman, and a healthy adult. The healthy man and the healthy adult were all but identical. A healthy woman, however, was described as more submissive, more emotional, less objective, less independent, less adventurous and less aggressive than a healthy man—hardly a description of a mature, healthy individual. Moreover, this stereotype represents pressure to 'adjust' to such a model or have one's 'femininity' and 'normality' questioned. The report by the Human Rights and Equal Opportunities Commission, *Human Rights and Mental Illness* (1993), better known as the Burdekin Report, affirms that some women believed they had been labelled as 'dysfunctional' because they did not conform to such a stereotype, and quoted the National Health and Medical Research Council Report of 1991 on Women and Mental Health which highlighted discriminatory and often negative consequences of **labelling**, such as identifying non-acceptable behaviour in women as madness.

Similar views about women and moral agency abound. As Sherwin (1992, p.45) points out, Freud regarded women as incapable of justice because of their commitment to the personal, while Kolberg found women deficient in moral development relative to men on the basis of tests developed from male norms for moral development. This was the basis of the critique by Gilligan (1982).

The question of whether women's nature is different from men's, and the related question of whether women pursue morality differently from men are therefore central issues in feminist philosophy today. Feminist ethics derives from the explicitly political perspective of feminism, which sees the oppression of women as morally and politically unacceptable (Jaggar 1993; Card 1993; Sherwin 1992; Holmes 1992; Holmes & Purdy 1992). Hence, it goes further than the call of feminine ethics for recognition of women's actual experiences and moral practices, to a critique of the specific practices that constitute women's oppression, stressing the significance of the social situation of people to their moral perspectives.

Feminist ethicists therefore stress the importance of reflecting the political dimension, and charge that discussion in medical ethics has been myopic, in that the institution of medicine has been accepted as given, and legitimated, its patriarchal practices and authoritarian nature not critiqued (Sherwin 1992; Rowland 1992; Holmes 1992; Holmes & Purdy 1992). They emphasise that the relation between the physician and the patient is far from equal, and problematise inequalities and sexist occupational roles. These issues pose basic questions in nursing ethics.

In particular, feminist ethics offers a fruitful perspective for understanding the experience of women with mental health problems, by critiquing the patriarchal practice and institutions of society, the equation of 'male' with 'human' (already noted), the constraints imposed by notions of 'femininity' and what is 'natural' and 'normal' in labelling women, and the adverse effects on women who lack economic independence, particularly those women who have suffered abusive relationships (see Chapter 3).

Mental health nursing brings many of these issues into sharp relief: paternalism, autonomy, informed consent, respect for persons, confidentiality, rights and duties. However, to date, mental health has rarely been the focus of a feminist perspective in its own right. Rather, feminist ethics and bioethics have focused on the importance of agency and/or caring—either as complementary or as an alternative to an ethic of justice. The clinical area of interest has been the new reproductive technologies: IVF, surrogacy, and similar issues. This is not surprising, given that one of the original planks in the women's movement platform since the 1970s has been reproductive autonomy (contraception, the option to choose abortion), as reproductive autonomy was an obvious and necessary precondition if women were to avail themselves of increased educational and employment opportunities, and move fully into the public arena.

Table 19.1 summarises some key terms which have emerged so far. Box 19.1 lists the three key ethical principles which will form the basis of our discussion of ethics and mental health nursing.

## TABLE 19.1: *Ethical principles*

| | |
|---|---|
| • autonomy | • avoidance of paternalism (informed consent) |
| • beneficence (do good) | • non-maleficence (avoid harm) |
| • justice/fairness | • rights |
| • equity | • respect for persons |
| • equality | • dignity |
| • sanctity of life | • quality of life |

## BOX 19.1: *Formulae: Key ethical principles*

The Golden Rule

The Categorical Imperative

The Principle of Utility

Three of the key principles stated in Table 19.1—beneficence, paternalism and autonomy—will now be examined to see how they might apply in mental health nursing.

# BENEFICENCE

The ethical ideal of beneficence requires the nurse to practise in a way that benefits rather than harms the client. It may be difficult, however, to determine what constitutes 'benefit' and what constitutes 'harm'. Underpinning beneficence is the assumption that the expertise of the nurse is important in determining what constitutes benefit and harm. For example, a nurse may judge that adherence to a medication schedule will benefit the client by controlling hallucinations and delusions. The same client may view the medication as harmful because it is associated with feelings of lethargy, a loss of libido, weight gain or tremor.

The report of the Royal Commission into Ward 10B, the psychiatric unit of Townsville General Hospital, criticised the heavy use of psychotropic drugs as a form of chemical restraint (Alavi & Frow 1991). Staff relied on medication as a means of controlling behaviour and maintaining order on the unit. The use of medication was justified by staff on the grounds that it ensured quick relief from symptoms, which then allowed the clients to participate in group therapy. The clients, on the other hand, expressed frustration and concern about lack of information regarding the side effects of medication and the intrusive nature of group therapy. The Royal Commission found evidence of an almost complete loss of individual civil rights. Is the nurse ever justified in urging, or even forcing, clients to accept medication, believing that compliance is in the best interest of the clients, their carers and the wider community?

## CASE STUDY 19.1:  Lucy: The right to choose

Lucy was diagnosed with paranoid schizophrenia when she was 21 years old. She was admitted to a psychiatric facility but was quickly discharged. Her attractiveness and intelligence belied the seriousness of her illness. She was homeless and transient. She found shelter in Salvation Army crisis centres, lived and worked on a Hare Krishna farm, moved to a hostel and then outstayed her welcome with a circle of friends and family. Although she was often unable to assess her own level of wellness, she was not a danger to herself or others. Three years after her initial diagnosis, Lucy decided to stop taking medication and her health began to deteriorate. At the same time she became pregnant. She was advised that any medication might affect the foetus. Her mother urged her to have an abortion. One of her doctors, who had a personal commitment to the 'Right to Life' movement, urged her to have the baby.

Nurses working in the area of mental health are frequently confronted with situations that create ethical conflicts on a personal level, within their professional practice and in their relationships with colleagues. Both Lucy's mother and her doctor may assert they are acting on the principle of beneficence with their conflicting advice. From their personal perspectives, medication and abortion are both benefits and harms. Neither has taken time to determine Lucy's perspective. The very nature of mental illness means that family members, friends and health professionals often override a client's right to self-determination. Is Lucy's refusal to take medication a thoughtful and informed personal decision, or is it a symptom of her paranoid thinking?

## AUTONOMY AND ADVOCACY

The ethical ideal of **autonomy** or self-determination (Charlesworth 1993) requires the nurse to respect an individual's freedom as far as possible. In order to demonstrate respect for patient autonomy and to avoid paternalism, a nurse could leave decision making to the client and assume a passive, non-interventionist approach. However, carried to its extreme, this position could be life-threatening to a client who was suicidal. In a study of the ethical conflicts experienced by mental health nurses (Forchuk 1991), most of the situations described involved an attempt by the nurses to balance beneficence with autonomy. Gadow (1980) argues that nurses are unable to practise without making a choice between beneficence, which implies a professional responsibility to identify benefit and harm, and client autonomy. She describes advocacy nursing as an alternative to either beneficence or autonomy. She describes advocacy as 'assisting patients in their own actions and decisions rather than substituting professional actions and decisions for those of patients' (Gadow 1980, p.53).

In applying an **advocacy** model to the case history outlined above, the nurse could actively assist Lucy to make an informed decision of her own determination. This can be achieved by providing Lucy with information that the nurse considers relevant (e.g. the potential consequences of refusing medication, or the option of modifying the dosage to reduce undesirable side effects). The advocacy model also requires attention to the client's concerns and questions. The nurse must ensure that Lucy has the opportunity to determine and ask for the information she requires to make an informed decision. For example, Lucy may want information about abortion or support services for single mothers.

It is important that the nurse and other relevant health professionals disclose their personal viewpoints. If Lucy understood the doctor's commitment to the 'Right to Life' movement, it would give her a perspective for judging the relevance of the advice for her own decision making. By discussing personal values and the values of relevant others, the nurse has the opportunity to ascertain the client's values. It would be important to know the significance and meaning of pregnancy, childbirth and parenting from Lucy's perspective. It would also be important to understand her values related to health, independence and medication. Therefore, in assisting Lucy to make a decision, it is important to consider Lucy's values, her individuality, and her unique understanding of herself and the situation.

Before a nurse is able to self disclose personal values with a client as a means of assisting self-determination, the nurse must have achieved an appropriate level of self-awareness and confidence. This requires a commitment to reflective practice and peer consultation. Street (1990) argues that 'it is imperative that nurses closely examine their role, their nursing actions, the clinical setting in which they practise the process of reflection itself in order to reject mythical thinking and easy solutions'. Schon (1983) notes that professionals often engage in 'reflection-in-action' or a 'reflective conversation with the situation'. He suggests that the value of this practice-based reflection can be extended by encouraging colleagues to join in the reflection as a collaborative process. This happens in an informal way when nurses consult with one another about a client's response to a visit by a family member or a reduction in medication. It happens more formally when nurses are encouraged to share a case study or incident from their professional practice. Nurses have a professional and ethical responsibility to examine their own practice, to contribute to the professional development of their peers, and to ensure that the insights and knowledge they gain find expression in the care they provide to clients.

*C*ASE STUDY 19.1: *Continued ...*

## Lucy's decision and what followed

Lucy decided to continue with the pregnancy and found accommodation in a caravan park. Despite her wish to give birth in the caravan, the community midwife persuaded her to go into hospital when labour began. Although two psychiatrists agreed that she was psychotic after the birth of her baby, she was deemed by the magistrate to be fit and discharged with a five-day-old daughter. Distressed by Lucy's agitated behaviour and the incessant crying of the baby, the caravan park manager called the doctor. Police and medical staff arrived at midnight to find Lucy showering in the public ablutions block while feeding her baby. In a violent and traumatic scene the baby was removed from Lucy and placed in foster care. The father of the child was subsequently awarded custody and, most hurtfully of all, Lucy's mother described her as unfit to care for the child. The support that could have been provided for Lucy to assist her in her role as a mother does not seem to have been considered.

Lucy's story is a series of ethical dilemmas, involving a balance of beneficence and autonomy. Her wish for a home birth was discouraged by the community midwife; her choice to live alone and care for her child was overridden by the caravan park manager, her doctor, child welfare authorities, her mother and the father of the baby. All acted on the principle of beneficence—a subjective determination of what was 'best' for Lucy and her baby. The magistrate, in contrast, chose to disregard the psychiatrists' opinions and support Lucy's decision to leave hospital.

While beneficence and autonomy have been described as 'moral duties' of the nurse, it is also appropriate to consider mental health care in terms of the rights of clients. The approaches and actions of professionals, family and community members are both supported and contraindicated by human rights legislation. There is *the right to freedom of movement and choice of residence*. Those 'caring' for Lucy recognised a conflict between her right to freedom and her own well-being and that of her baby. The NSW *Mental Health Act* indicates, however, that if the magistrate is not satisfied on the balance of probabilities that the individual is mentally ill, the person must be discharged (HREOC vol.1, p.65). This principle (the right to freedom of movement and choice of residence) supported the magistrate's decision to discharge Lucy. The hearing before the magistrate placed an onus on the physician to justify a decision to limit the freedom of the client. At the same time, the hearing ensures the patient has an advocate. In this way, the ethical responsibility to respect the client's rights and ensure beneficent action is assured.

# THE UNITED NATIONS HUMAN RIGHTS FRAMEWORK

One of the conundrums that arises in the case of people with psychiatric illness is the feeling that consent, as it is enshrined in the law, is perhaps out of place in dealing with mental illness. (Dr Ian Siggins, then Victorian Health Commissioner, now Queensland Health Commissioner, HREOC, 1993, p.71)

Clearly, it is an extremely serious matter to deprive a person of civil liberty or legal capacity, yet these are routine matters inherent in the area of mental health. The framework adopted by the Human Rights and Equal Opportunities Commission in its report, *Human Rights and Mental Illness* (1993), is grounded firmly in the United Nations rights approach, developed since the 1945 Charter and encompassing the international instruments which Australia has ratified. These include the 1948 UN Declaration of Human Rights, the 1966 International Covenant on Civil and Political Rights, the 1958 Discrimination (Employment and Occupation) Convention, and the 1975 Declaration on the Rights of Disabled Persons. The Convention on the Elimination of all Forms of Racial Discrimination (ratified by Australia in 1975) and the Convention on the Elimination of all Forms of Discrimination against Women (ratified by Australia in 1983) are also applicable.

Principles for the Protection of Persons with Mental Illness and For the Improvement of Mental Health Care were adopted by the UN General Assembly in 1991 and, although they have not been formally incorporated in Australian legislation, they have been endorsed in the National Mental Health Policy of 1992, which sets 1998 as the target date for ensuring full compliance by Australian mental health legislation. Principles and other UN instruments serve, therefore, as basic international benchmarks.

Essentially, these UN human rights instruments offer basic rights to which everyone should be entitled, without discrimination. This does not require that everyone be treated alike. Special measures to cater for special needs are not precluded; rather, it is recognised that special measures of assistance or protection may be needed to ensure the equal enjoyment of human rights by groups of people who are particularly vulnerable or disadvantaged—such as the mentally ill. The Declaration on the Rights of Disabled Persons defines 'disabled person' as:

> ... any person unable to ensure by himself or herself, wholly or partly, the necessities of a normal individual and/or social life, as a result of deficiency, whether congenital or not, in his or her physical or mental capacities.

This definition includes people with a mental illness, and recognises (among other rights) their entitlement to the right to protection from exploitation or discriminatory, abusive or degrading treatment, and the inherent right to respect for their human dignity.

The Principles also affirm that discrimination on the basis of mental illness is not permitted, and that people with mental illness should not be stigmatised or disadvantaged in the care available. Therefore, it is not permissible to have lower standards for mental health care than for general health care. The Principles are not restricted to a remedial approach; they emphasise the 'least restrictive alternative' for treatment, and the right to be treated and cared for as far as possible in the community, as well as treatment suitable to each person's cultural background. Treatment is to be aimed at 'enhancing personal autonomy'; hence, privacy and freedom of communication (post, telephone) are rights, and informed consent is required, except where the patient is held as an involuntary patient, or when an independent authority is satisfied that the patient lacks the capacity to give or withhold informed consent, or is unreasonably withholding consent, and the independent authority is satisfied that the proposed plan of treatment is in the best interests of the patient's health needs.

In considering Lucy's story, other human rights, apart from beneficence and autonomy, are relevant and suggest a different course of ethical action. For example, there is *the right of children to special protection* and *the right to marry and found a family* (HREOC vol.1, p.22). Where there is a conflict between the rights of the child and the rights of the parent, most would agree that the child's rights should be given preference. In custody disputes, Family Law Court rulings are determined in the best interests of the child. In this respect, it could be argued that the caravan park manager, doctor, child welfare authorities and family members were acting in the best interests of Lucy's baby. The Declaration of the Rights of the Child indicates that a child has the right to 'grow and develop in health and for this purpose is entitled to special care and protection' and 'where possible, grow up in the care and protection of his or her family' (HREOC vol.1, p.26).

Despite the involvement of a range of professionals, the experience of Lucy and her immediate family was emotionally painful, socially isolating and guilt-provoking. Sadly, Lucy did not have the benefit of a case manager to act as an advocate on her behalf. The case manager might have provided continuity of services between hospital and home, and organised supportive services to help Lucy to care adequately for her child. Similarly, the case manager may have been able to assist the family through a referral to a non-government agency such as the Schizophrenia Fellowship or the Association of Relatives and Friends of the Mentally Ill (ARAFMI). Both organisations provide mutual support, information sharing and advocacy services. With such assistance Lucy and her family may have been able to create an environment that was safe for Lucy and her baby and conducive to ethical decision making.

## A MILLIAN FRAMEWORK: PATERNALISM AND HARM

The UN rights agenda is clearly applicable to the consideration of ethical issues in mental health nursing. Equally relevant is the framework articulated in John Stuart Mill's classic essay 'On Liberty', where he investigated 'the nature and limits of the power which can be legitimately exercised by society over the individual'. He argued the principle that:

> The sole end for which mankind are warranted, individually or collectively, in interfering with the liberty of action of any of their number, is self-protection. The only purpose for which power can be rightfully exercised over any member of a civilised community, against his will, is to prevent harm to others. His own good, either physical or moral, is not a sufficient warrant. (Mill vol.10, p.233)

This is the anti-paternalism principle, which proscribes acting on someone else's behalf, in their best interest as you see it. Harm to others is a clear ground for restraint; harm to self is more equivocal. The passage continues:

> The only part of the conduct of anyone, for which he is amenable to society, is that which concerns others. In the part which merely concerns himself, his independence is, of right, absolute. Over himself, over his own body and mind, the individual is sovereign. (Mill vol.10, p.233)

This standpoint applies to 'human beings in the maturity of their faculties', and so it might be thought to be easily waived in the case of a person suffering mental illness, who by definition is no longer sovereign over his or her own mind. Yet its influence remains as an ideal standard, a benchmark of treating someone's rights as autonomous, only to be infringed as a last resort, for a clearly specified good reason, which meets the necessary onus of justification. This is clearly evident in the area of mental health.

The NSW *Mental Health Act* of 1990, for example, requires not only that a person suffers from mental illness, but also that there are, as a result, 'reasonable grounds for believing care, treatment or control of the person is necessary', for the person's own protection from serious physical harm, or for the protection of others from serious physical harm. Alternatively, the 'reasonable grounds' may be for 'the person's own protection from serious financial harm or serious damage to the person's reputation, including damage to important personal relationships'.

The report, *Human Rights and Mental Illness* (HREOC 1993, Appendix 5, pp.989–1005), outlines twenty-five principles 'for the protection of persons with mental illness and for the improvement of mental health care'. Given the aim of protecting dignity, self-respect, privacy and self-determination, 'even—and especially—when they seem not to have the wit to function' (HREOC, p.229), the decision that someone lacks legal capacity is a weighty one, and must be made by an independent tribunal (Principle 1). Involuntary admission is similarly problematic, and every effort should be made to avoid it (Principle 15). The grounds given in Principle 16 are very similar to those in the NSW *Mental Health Act*, in the preceding paragraph:

(i) That, because of that mental illness, there is a serious likelihood of immediate or imminent harm to that person or to other persons; or

(ii) That, in the case of a person whose mental illness is severe and whose judgement is impaired, failure to admit or retain that person is likely to lead to a serious deterioration in his or her condition or will prevent the giving of appropriate treatment which can only be given by admission to a mental health facility in accordance with the principle of the least restrictive alternative.

# UNETHICAL ISSUES IN MENTAL HEALTH

Involuntary admission does not, however, justify the forcible administration of medication. This was clearly brought out by the Carter Report on Ward 10B in Townsville, which found the care and treatment that occurred there between 1975 and 1988 negligent, unsafe, unethical and unlawful. In discussing unlawful situations, involving force, it was noted that:

> Some staff members believed that force could be lawfully used to medicate a patient if the patient was regulated but not so if he/she was a voluntary admission … This view misconceives the true position.

Commissioner Carter quoted Section 260 of the Criminal Code, preventing a breach of the peace, which lawfully protects from criminal liability a person who, in the process of preventing a breach of the peace, commits an assault, but found this 'inappropriate for the purpose of containing violence and overcoming resistance in a psychiatric unit'. The Carter Report gave the following definitions of 'negligent' and 'unsafe' care and treatment:

> '*Negligent*' *care and treatment*: that which is characterised by a lack of necessary or ordinary care, that which is careless and that which demonstrates a want of attention to what ought to be done.
>
> '*Unsafe*' *care and treatment*: that which exposed patients to danger or risk; that which involved or was not free from danger or risk. (p.377)

It is generally recognised that it is for one's peers to determine whether conduct is unethical—that is, self-regulation—in normal circumstances. In these extraordinary circumstances, Commissioner Carter found that much more than 'a departure from the proper standards of clinical practice was involved and that the conduct had been unethical'. He further found that those courageous enough to speak out were identified as troublemakers, 'the usual fate of whistleblowers'.

The Inquiry provided a legal perspective on the 'moral duty' of staff towards clients by defining ethical practice and negligent or unsafe care. It didn't explain how the unethical practice in Ward 10B was tolerated by health professionals or the wider community for over 12 years. Neither does it give much insight into the clients' experience of such practice. In contrast, the account in Voice Box 19.1, written by a former Ward 10B patient, highlights the powerlessness and terror engendered by such unethical practice.

# $V$OICE BOX 19.1:   The case of Ward 10B

> The woman's nakedness was exposed to male patients passing in the corridor. Heavily drugged, she had been dragged into the showers, stripped and held under the running water.
>
> Just days before, the woman had presented for admission with her baby daughter. She was perhaps 35, well groomed, mature, co-operative. She was apparently suffering from depression following the death of her father. On the decision of a nurse, she was immediately administered 1200 mg of chlorpromazine, a major tranquilliser, which severely impaired her ability to maintain consciousness. The woman's condition was not diagnosed, and she was denied consultation with a psychiatrist, doctor or allied health professional. During the following days, she was physically forced to attend group therapy, spending much of this time semi-comatose on the floor. Junior nurses monitored the condition of the baby.
>
> After several days, the Director of Psychiatry ordered that no assistance whatsoever was to be given to the woman by staff in the care of the baby.
>
> *continued …*

Independently of this decision, a senior nurse ordered that her 'medication', the major tranquilliser, be increased by one-third.

The woman's maternal instincts saw her cling to consciousness part of the time, attempting to care for her baby. She attempted on two occasions to give the baby boiling water direct from the bottle, attempts prevented only by the chance appearance of another patient.

Patients and junior nurses became extremely concerned for the baby. A secret meeting was held, after professional and most senior nursing staff had gone home for the day. It was decided that the patients, many themselves suffering from acute illness and drug overdose, would care for the child. Late that night, a middle-aged male patient was wakened in the ward by a young nurse and handed the baby. The nurse then left the room. The man had been transferred to the ward from a maximum security prison for the criminally insane …

*Kim Jewell*

The story in Voice Box 19.1 is related by a client who survived the experience of Ward 10B. The woman and her baby also survived, although the woman was left with permanent ocular damage as a consequence of the extremely high doses of chlorpromazine administered during her admission. Kim Jewell, the narrator of the story, was the client transferred from the maximum security prison and entrusted with the care of the child. He gave evidence at the Carter Inquiry and continues to be an active lobbyist for the rights of consumers of mental health services (see Chapter 1).

This story, and Kim Jewell's commentary, signals how important it is for nurses to be reflective about their clinical practice. Through reflection nurses have a responsibility to identify ethical issues. They should seek opportunities to share their experiences and reflections with peers and colleagues to ensure that they are not unwittingly seduced by a charismatic individual, or a persuasive theory, to practise in a manner that could be described as unethical. Possibly the most powerful safeguard against unethical practice is a strong focus on client care. If the staff working in Ward 10B had conveyed an empathic understanding of the clients they cared for, if they had demonstrated a commitment to individualised, client-centred care, the events described would be inconceivable. However, this is not to blame nursing staff for what happened, nor to suggest that a different approach from the nurses would have prevented the tragedy of Ward 10B. For nurses to have been more effective in limiting the excesses of Ward 10B, a fundamental shift in the power relationship between the psychiatrists and the nurses would have been necessary.

Ethical dimensions are involved in doctor–nurse relations, nurse–patient relations, confidentiality, communicating the truth (to patients and relatives), and experimentation. The key issues of informed voluntary consent and paternalism, as well as involuntary hospitalisation and behaviour control, are particularly problematic in the field of mental health nursing. In some States it is, after all, up to the nurse's judgment whether a patient meets the criteria for involuntary admission (see the Victorian *Mental Health Act*). Nurses are likely to be the first to recognise adverse side effects of medication, and community health nurses become involved as virtual enforcers of medication under community treatment orders (CTOs). What is the advisable course of action in these situations?

Nurses have a duty of care to take action whenever they judge the behaviour of a colleague to be unethical. Likewise, they have a responsibility to report negative outcomes for clients resulting from a particular policy or procedure. In most instances this can be dealt with without creating an ethical issue for the nurse. It is appropriate to speak to the colleague directly at the time that unethical or inappropriate behaviour is observed. This allows both parties to clarify the issue and minimise misunderstanding. When an issue cannot be resolved at an individual level, it may be necessary to discuss the concern with a supervisor and/or document the incident. If the safety or well-being of a client is likely to be compromised, further action is always warranted.

It is important to be aware of the appropriate processes and procedures that apply within a particular health care agency for dealing with these and similar concerns about the quality of client care. By using these processes and procedures, many such issues may be resolved. It is only when an issue is not resolved, and when the organisation threatens the well-being of a client, staff member or member of the wider community that a nurse may decide to take further action. This step can contribute to an ethical dilemma for the nurse, unless there is strong peer support for such action. Peer support can be fostered through regular formal and informal opportunities to talk with colleagues about clinical practice (Hart et al. 1994). By sharing issues of concern and listening empathically to the perspectives of others, nurses are more likely to have a consensual view of ethical practice. When confronted by a serious issue they are also more likely to be united in their approach.

## W HISTLEBLOWING AND CONFIDENTIALITY

Mental health nurses may experience an ethical dilemma in the area of confidentiality. They have a professional obligation to hold all information relevant to clients in confidence, yet they may also be required by law to disclose information. For example, nurses are required to report incidents of child sexual abuse (Smith 1990). Similarly, nurses may experience a moral obligation to divulge confidential information in order to protect others. Recently, in New Zealand, the media highlighted the experience of a charge nurse, Neil Pugmire (O'Connor 1994). Pugmire wrote to the Minister for Health and the police to express his moral and professional concerns about recent changes to mental health legislation. Pugmire believed that psychiatric patients who were considered dangerous to the public might be released through a new loophole in the law. When this occurred a few months later, an Opposition spokesman released the contents of Pugmire's letter to the media. Pugmire was suspended from his position—the reason given: 'issues of confidentiality'.

Although Pugmire was reinstated after a hearing in the Auckland Employment Court, he paid a high personal cost for his actions. He chose to take paid leave because of the ongoing stress associated with the incident. Pugmire's experience is not unique. Whistleblowers frequently suffer social, emotional and financial hardship. Witt (1983) lost her job, her home and her health when she complained of inhumane, abusive and life-threatening treatment of patients in a private psychiatric facility. At the same time, nurses who fail to blow the whistle may also suffer. Nurses employed at Townsville General Hospital on Ward 10B were implicated and held responsible for their failure to intervene when faced with inadequate and inappropriate care. Consider the telling summation of the Judge during the New Zealand inquiry into cervical cancer screening experiment in 1987:

> I know you say that nurses feel very vulnerable but would you forgive me for thinking that they have been rather less than brave in bringing matters before this Inquiry?

Nurses are in an excellent position to monitor the impact of mental health services and treatments on patients. Without the right, and indeed the obligation, to speak out when faced with threats to patient safety and care, mental health nurses will be unable to undertake an advocacy role.

Feliu (1983) describes **whistleblowing** as 'speaking out on your own initiative about activity within your organisation that otherwise would not come to public attention' (p.1387). He suggests that whistleblowing is an extraordinary step with serious consequences. He cautions nurses to be thoughtful about their motives for whistleblowing and the methods they choose.

He advises the following four steps before taking action.

1. Verify facts and document claims to ensure that you have a defensible story.

2. Begin by making your concerns known within the organisation in order to try to solve the matter informally.

3. Exhaust all internal remedies by pursuing all avenues to resolve the issue within the organisation, allowing time for remedies to be implemented.

4. Secure legal advice and support.

# SUMMARY

- A concern with duty and a concern for consequences characterise the two main approaches to ethics—deontological and consequentialist.

- Feminist ethics developed from a recognition of male bias in traditional ethics.

- Beneficence is an ethical principle that emphasises the importance of doing good.
- Personal autonomy means self-determination and is a central ethical principle within mental health care.
- Ethical principles underpin the nurse's duty of care while the United Nations provides legal protection for the client's rights.
- Paternalism is acting on another's behalf for their good as you see it.
- Unethical behaviour has been highlighted by the Carter Report on Ward 10B, Townsville General Hospital.
- Women are particularly disadvantaged in relation to mental health because of stereotypes of femininity on one hand and the burden of care on the other.

# DISCUSSION QUESTIONS

1. What is the basis of the feminist critique of traditional approaches to ethics?
2. How can mental health professionals adhere to the principle of beneficence and, at the same time, avoid being paternalistic?
3. How might you facilitate personal autonomy for a client whose mental judgment is compromised by a serious mental illness?
4. How is the United Nations human rights framework relevant to mental health nursing practice?
5. What course of action is appropriate for a nurse who observes unethical practice?

# EXERCISES

1. Select an ethical dilemma in mental health nursing, and compare and contrast the application of a deontological and consequentialist approach to its analysis.
2. Review the case study of Lucy and demonstrate the relevance of the concept of beneficience.
3. Analyse the Ward 10B experience and identify any evidence of paternalism.
4. Consider the mental health services in your area; identify those offering support for women who are primary caregivers and also experiencing mental health problems.
5. Consider a mental health nursing dilemma of your choice and compare the application of the feminist critique with at least two other approaches to ethics.

6. You are a nurse working in an acute psychiatric unit. You become concerned that a number of quite common nursing practices contravene patients' legal rights (such as the use of seclusion on voluntary patients). What do you do? What would you do if you were (a) a relief staff member, (b) a permanent staff member, or (c) a student nurse on clinical placement?

# FURTHER READING

- For an understanding of the human rights issues and the extent of the problem, the student is referred to either one of these texts:

    Carter Report (1991) *Commission of Inquiry into the Care and Treatment of Patients in the Psychiatric Unit of Townsville General Hospital*;
    and
    Human Rights and Equal Opportunities Commission (1993) *Human Rights and Mental Illness*, Canberra: AGPS.

- For a further discussion of ethics in nursing, refer to:

    Forchuk, C. (1991) 'Ethical problems encountered by mental health nurses', *Issues in Mental Health Nursing* 12(4), pp.375–83;
    Gadow, S. (1980) 'A model for ethical decision making', *Oncology Nursing Forum* 7(4), pp.44–7.

# REFERENCES

Alavi, C. & Frow, J. (1991) 'From judgements on uncertain issues', *Australian Society* August.

Beauchamp, T.L. & Walters, L. (1989) *Contemporary Issues in Bioethics*, Belmont, California: Wadsworth.

Broverman, I.K., Broverman, D., Clauson, S., Rosencrantz, P. & Vogel, S. (1970) 'Sex role stereotypes and clinical judgements of mental health', *Journal of Consulting and Clinical Psychology* 34(1).

Card, C. (1993) *Feminist Ethics*, University Press of Kansas.

Carter Report (1991) *Commission of Inquiry into the Care and Treatment of Patients in the Psychiatric Unit of Townsville General Hospital*.

Charlesworth, M. (1993) *Bioethics and the Liberal Society*, Cambridge: Cambridge University Press.

Feliu, A.G. (1983) 'Thinking of blowing the whistle?' *American Journal of Nursing* 83, pp.1387–8.

Forchuk, C. (1991) 'Ethical problems encountered by mental health nurses', *Issues in Mental Health Nursing* 12(4), pp.375–83.

Gadow, S. (1980) 'A model for ethical decision making', *Oncology Nursing Forum* 7(4), pp.44–7.

Gilligan, C. (1982) *In a Different Voice*, Cambridge: Harvard University Press.

Hart, G., Bull, R., Mungomery, L., & Albrecht, M. (1994) 'Peer consultation: options and opportunities in Queensland hospitals', *Australian and New Zealand Journal of Mental Health Nursing* 3(4).

Holmes, H.B. (1992) *Issues in Reproductive Technology*, New York: Garland Publishing Inc.

Holmes, H.B. & Purdy, L.M. (1992) *Feminist Perspective in Medical Ethics*, Bloomington: Indiana University Press.

Human Rights and Equal Opportunities Commission (1993) *Human Rights and Mental Illness*, Canberra: AGPS.

Jaggar, A. (1993) *Living With Contradictions*, Boulder: Westview Press.

Mappes, T.A. & Zembaty, J.S. (1991) *Biomedical Ethics*, New York: McGraw-Hill.

Mill, J.S. 'On Liberty', in *Collected Works*, Toronto: Toronto University Press.

Noddings, N. (1984) *Caring*, Berkeley: University of California Press.

O'Connor, T. (1994) 'Whistling up a storm', *Nursing New Zealand* 2(2), p.2.

Rowland, R. (1992) *Living Laboratories*, Sydney: Sun Books.

Ruddick, S. (1989) *Maternal Thinking*, Boston: Beacon Press.

Schon, D. (1983) *The Reflective Practitioner*, London: Temple Smith.

Sherwin, S. (1992) *No Longer Patient*, Philadelphia: Temple University Press.

Singer, P. (1993) *Practical Ethics*, Cambridge: Cambridge University Press.

Smith, J. (1990) 'Privileged communication: psychiatric/mental health nurses and the law', *Perspective in Psychiatric Care* 26(4), pp.26–9.

Street, A. (1990) *Nursing Practice: High Hard Ground, Messy Swamps and the Pathways in Between*, Geelong: Deakin University Press.

Witt, P. (1983) 'Notes of a whistleblower', *American Journal of Nursing* 83, pp.1649–51.

# GLOSSARY

**abuse,** *see* **domestic violence**

**adaptation**   The process by which a migrant adjusts to the host society.

**advocacy**   Speaking on behalf of a person or group, often used in nursing to refer to the role of the nurse in speaking up for clients who are unable to speak for themselves.

**affect**   Emotional responsiveness, specifically the external expression of emotions.

**agoraphobia**   Intense fear in and of open spaces.

**agranulocytosis**   A sudden drop in white blood cells that leaves the body defenceless against bacterial infection, a notable side effect of drugs and chemicals that affect the bone marrow and depress the formation of granulocytes.

**alogia**   The inability to speak due to a lesion in the brain.

**Alzheimer's disease**   A brain disease of unknown cause with characteristic features of **dementia**. The disease has an insidious onset and progresses slowly. It affects older people, especially those over 70 years of age.

**anxiety**   Unpleasant sense of unease associated with a perceived threat or general sense of concern.

**anxiolytic**   A therapeutic substance effective in controlling anxiety.

**Australian Council on Health Care Standards**   An independent organisation established to promote, in cooperation with health care professionals, continuing improvement in the quality of care delivered by Australian health care organisations.

**autonomy**   The degree of freedom one has to make choices according to one's will.

**avolition**   The lack of interest and sense of purpose found in some serious mental illnesses.

**bipolar disorder**   Disorder characterised by one or more manic or hypomanic episodes, usually with a history of depressive illness.

**body image**   `The subjective appreciation a person has of his or her body.

**cognitive**   Elements and processes involved in thinking, memory and recall.

397

**coming out**    The empowering process of declaring oneself in public to be a person with a mental health problem or disorder, thereby breaking down the secrecy and shame that results from the stigma of mental illness.

**consumers—(a) primary consumer**    A person who has, or has had, a mental illness; may also be referred to as a **survivor** (of the psychiatric system); (b) **secondary consumer**    Someone who cares for such a person.

**crisis intervention**    Short-term actions initiated by the nurse with people in crisis, to ensure their safety, decrease the impact of the crisis, and help them to mobilise personal resources, regain equilibrium and, if possible, move to a higher level of functioning.

**delirium**    A mental disturbance of usually short duration brought on by a toxic state and marked by illusions, hallucianations, delusions, excitement, restlessness and incoherence.

**delusions**    Recurring false beliefs.

**dementia**    A syndrome due to changes in the brain which results in reduced intellectual functioning (e.g. thinking, memory). Deterioration in emotional and social control is also common. The term 'dementia' refers to all stages of the dementing process.

**demography**    The vital statistics of communities and human populations.

**depersonalisation**    A sense of strangeness about the self and/or the environment.

**depression**    A mood disorder characterised by exaggerated feelings of sadness, melancholy and hopelessness; involving disturbed thought patterns, and physical symptoms such as loss of appetite and sleep disturbances. The term refers to all forms of depression.

**derealisation**    A sense of strangeness or unreality about one's surroundings.

**disabilities**    Physical or mental restrictions on the ability to undertake ordinary activities within the normal range for a human being. **Impairments** associated with serious mental illness include poor self-care and personal grooming, and other social and employment incapacities.

**domestic violence**    Violence that occurs in the home usually perpetrated by men against women and children.

**empathy**    The process of fully understanding the thoughts and emotions of another person from that person's perspective.

**epidemiology**    The study of the distribution of health risks and diseases in communities and populations.

**ethnicity**    A policy term identifying some migrants as sharing a culture that is markedly different from that of Anglo-Australians. In practice, used to refer to migrants of non-English speaking background (NESB).

**family therapy**    Treatment of the entire family for problems in relationships.

**handicaps**    Social disadvantages—that may be due to stigmatisation, discrimination, or lack of supportive or compensatory environments—which limit the person's social role within the normal range for a human being. Handicaps include substandard housing, or no accommodation, and lack of vocational, social and recreational opportunities. Such social handicaps can arise from personal **disabilities**.

**insight**  The understanding that clients have about their mental health problem and how it affects their thoughts, feelings and behaviours.

**intersectoral**  Involving government sectors other than the health sector, and by extension non-government sectors, in the development of policy and service delivery.

**labelling**  The social process of stripping away the identity of a person by conferring a label, often a psychiatric diagnosis, that governs thereafter the way the person is perceived by and responded to by others.

**learned helplessness**  The process of progressively withdrawing from taking responsibility for control over one's life due to structural factors in the social environment, notably inequalities in power relations and institutionalised practices, prejudices or assumptions.

**mainstreaming**  A policy term used to describe the process of incorporating the treatment and care of the mentally ill into general health services.

**mania**  A disorder characterised by elevation of mood, hyperactivity, agitation, and accelerated thinking and speaking.

**mental disorder**  Persistent, repetitive, recognisable and exaggerated expressions of disordered thought, disturbed feeling and disruptive behaviour.

**mental health**  The capacity of individuals and groups to interact with one another in ways that promote individual and collective well-being, while achieving personal and collective goals consistent with social justice.

**milieu therapy**  The purposeful use of the social environment for therapeutic purposes. Every interaction with the client is seen as having potentially beneficial outcomes in promoting optimal functioning.

**mood**  Internal emotional state.

**negative symptoms**  Include restricted range and intensity of emotional expression (flat affect), limitations in initiation of goal-directed behaviour, and restricted clarity in thought and speech.

**NESB**  Non-English speaking background.

**NGO**  Non-government organisation.

**normalisation**  The process of helping people with a mental illness or mental disability to meet their needs by living as much as possible like other members of the community with access to appropriate housing, a home-like atmosphere in which to live, and with access to the same facilities and services as everyone else.

**paranoia**  Systematised delusions of persecution sometimes accompanied by delusions of grandeur.

**paternalism**  A form of behaviour in which people in authority assume without consultation the responsibility for making decisions on behalf of others, especially people in their care.

**pharmacokinetics**  The study of the movement of drugs in the body, especially the processes of absorption, distribution, transformation and excretion.

**positive symptoms**  Demonstrated features of mental illness, including **delusions, hallucinations,** disorganised speech, and grossly disorganised behaviour.

**prevention:** **(a) primary prevention** sets out to alter forces in the community that are thought to influence mental health adversely; **(b) secondary prevention** involves activities that reduce the prevalence of mental illness in the community; **(c) tertiary prevention** involves effective rehabilitation.

**psychoeducation** A generic term used to refer to education and training programs designed to help people live with mental illness.

**psychosis** An extreme response to stress, causing the possible development of **delusions** and **hallucinations,** and affective, psychomotor and physical disturbances.

**puerperal psychosis** A serious episode of psychosis that occurs in the period or state of confinement and requires urgent treatment to safeguard the health of the mother and baby.

**quality assurance** Any structured program developed to continuously improve quality in a service or organisation.

**quality of life** A subjective judgment about the degree to which life holds meaning, purpose and the potential for happiness from the perspective of the individual.

**sanctity of life** A term used to emphasise the distinctiveness, value and dignity of human life, and the duty of protecting people from harm.

**self-advocacy** Speaking up for oneself and representing oneself to people in authority, especially to members of the mental health professions.

**self-efficacy** A person's conviction that he or she can successfully execute the behaviour required to produce a desired outcome.

**self-help groups** Groups founded on the principles of informality and mutual aid.

**serial reciprocity** The process whereby people in a relationship take turns in supporting one another through difficult periods such as bereavement, unemployment and illness.

**serious mental illness** A group of specific disorders which, although varying in cause, course and treatment, share common characteristics and produce long-term adverse effects or significant levels of impairment.

**somatisation** The expression of mental illness through physical symptoms.

**stigma** A mark of disgrace; people who have been labelled as mentally ill are marked out as different and discriminated against because of their health status. Stigmatisation results in shame and social isolation.

**stress** The reaction to a broad class of events, distinguished by the fact that they result in demands that tax the ability of the individual to cope.

**suicide** The act of voluntarily and intentionally taking one's life. The term 'suicide' may refer to parasuicide (attempts at suicide or suicidal gestures), suicidal ideation (ideas about taking one's life), or threatened suicide (expressions of suicidal intent).

**survivor,** *see* **consumers.**

**time out** A nursing intervention that involves short periods of segregation in a quiet room or bedroom to provide time for the patient to reflect on his or her actions. Generally used to decrease patient alienation from peers as a result of unacceptable (often violent) behaviour. An effective strategy for protecting patients from personal harm or potentially dangerous behaviour towards others.

**transference**   A psychoanalytical term that refers to the tendency of clients to attribute to their therapists feelings and emotions that relate to other people in their lives, for example when a client projects feelings about his or her father onto the therapist. Countertransference occurs when the therapist projects such feelings onto the client, or when the therapist has an otherwise irrational response to the client. Transference is positive when it facilitates therapy, negative when the client resists understanding its significance. Countertransference is positive or negative to the degree the therapist is able to control his or her irrationality.

**whistleblowing**   Taking action to expose unethical activities within an organisation that would not normally come to the attention of the relevant authorities, or which the relevant authorities have ignored or failed to act upon.

# INDEX